A Vision of

SEMIR ZEKI

UNIVERSITY COLLEGE LONDON

the Brain

OXFORD

BLACKWELL SCIENTIFIC PUBLICATIONS

LONDON EDINBURGH BOSTON
MELBOURNE PARIS BERLIN VIENNA

© 1993 by
Blackwell Scientific Publications
Editorial Offices:
Osney Mead, Oxford OX2 0EL
25 John Street, London WC1N 2BL
23 Ainslie Place, Edinburgh EH3 6AJ
238 Main Street, Cambridge
  Massachusetts 02142, USA
54 University Street, Carlton
  Victoria 3053, Australia

Other Editorial Offices:
Librairie Arnette SA
2, rue Casimir-Delavigne
75006 Paris
France

Blackwell Wissenschafts-Verlag GmbH
Meinekestrasse 4
D-1000 Berlin 15
Germany

Blackwell MZV
Feldgasse 13
A-1238 Wien
Austria

First published 1993

Set by Setrite Typesetters, Hong Kong
Printed and bound in Spain by
Printek SA, Bilbao

DISTRIBUTORS

  Marston Book Services Ltd
  PO Box 87
  Oxford OX2 0DT
  (Orders: Tel: 0865 791155
          Fax: 0865 791927
          Telex: 837515)

USA
  Blackwell Scientific Publications, Inc.
  238 Main Street
  Cambridge, MA 02142
  (Orders: Tel: 800 759−6102
          617 876−7000)

Canada
  Oxford University Press
  70 Wynford Drive
  Don Mills
  Ontario M3C 1J9
  (Orders: Tel: 416 441−2941)

Australia
  Blackwell Scientific Publications Pty Ltd
  54 University Street
  Carlton, Victoria 3053
  (Orders: Tel: 03 347−5552)

A catalogue record for this title
is available from the British Library

ISBN 0−632−03054−2

Library of Congress
Cataloging-in-Publication Data

Zeki, Semir.
    A Vision of the Brain/Semir Zeki.
        p.   cm.
    Includes bibliographical references
    and index.
    ISBN 0- 632−03054−2
    1. Visual cortex. 2. Visual pathways.
    3. Vision. 1. Title.
    [DNLM: 1. Visual Cortex − physiology.
    2. Visual Perception − physiology.
    WL 307 Z48v]
    QP382.022Z45   1993
    612.8'255 − dc20

There is, it seems to us,
At best, only a limited value
In the knowledge derived from experience.
The knowledge imposes a pattern, and falsifies,
For the pattern is new in every moment
And every moment is a new and shocking
Valuation of all we have been.

T.S. Eliot, from *The Four Quartets* (East Coker)

For Anne-Marie

Contents

Preface

In this book I give a personal view of the brain, based largely on my own work and on other work which seemed to me to be particularly relevant and interesting. I wrote it partly to satisfy my curiosity and partly for the enjoyment of my friends and colleagues and others interested in the subject. If, after reading it, you find that you have learned something about the brain and about vision which you did not know before, then I shall have been rewarded. If reading the book provides you with new insights about brain function, then I shall have been amply rewarded. But my greatest reward will be if the book inspires you to develop new ideas about the brain and design new experiments to test one aspect or another of brain function. The study of the brain is still in its infancy and many exciting ideas about it remain to be generated and to be tested. I hope that no one will be deterred from asking new questions and suggesting new experiments simply because they are not specialists in brain studies. Leaving it to the specialist is about the greatest disservice that one can render to brain science in its present state. The question that the most humble person can ask about the brain is often surprisingly sophisticated and one to which the most accomplished specialist has no answer. Moreover, with the rapid development of new techniques, experiments which would have seemed outrageous even five years ago have moved into the realms of the practical. Perhaps what is needed most in brain studies is the courage to ask questions that may even seem trivial and may therefore inhibit their being asked. I once learned a good lesson from my then five-year-old son who, having seen the selective responses to colour of a single cell in the anaesthetized brain, asked somewhat hesitantly, 'But how does this reach the mind?' It was a child's question but a deeply profound one nevertheless and one to which we still have no answer; no one will understand the workings of the visual cortex or of the brain until they can answer his question. No one should therefore fear that they are making a fool of themselves by asking such questions. You may find that you are making a fool of the specialist, not because he does not have an answer to your question, but because he may not have even realized that there is a question to answer. On the other hand, no one should be disappointed or surprised if an answer turns out to be wrong in the end. The cerebral cortex is a great and complex organ about which we know very little. It has been the graveyard of great and brilliant men and of exciting and new ideas. In studying the cerebral cortex, what is required above all is humility. Even <u>Santiago Ramon y Cajal</u>, one of the most brilliant and dogmatic neuroscientists, was subdued with humility when he approached the cerebral cortex. What he wrote in his book *Histologie du Systéme Nerveux* almost sixty years ago remains true today:

> A dire vrai, il n'est pas possible, dans l'etat actuel de nos connaissances, de formuler une théorie definitive du plan...fonctionnel du cerveau....Il est inutile de dire que nous ne prétendons pas donner à notre hypothése un caractére dogmatique; nous savons trop bien que des faits imprévus modifient ou renversent, du jour au lendemain, nos conjectures scientifiques. Tout ce que nous pouvons souhaiter, c'est qu'il reste de notre conception quelquesuns des principes sur lesquelles nous l'avons basée....*

The reader must not seek to find in this book a detailed coverage of all that is known about the visual cortex. There are many areas, such as the pharmacology of the visual cortex or its development, which have been given scant coverage or none at all. This can be explained partly by the fact that I have written about what has interested me, and partly by the fact that I have tried to write for the more general reader who may want to have an idea of how the visual cortex, and the brain, works without getting lost in too many details. Some details are nevertheless necessary and these are described in a few brief chapters. The more general reader can skip these without losing the main thrust of the argument while the contents of the chapters may be too well known to the specialist, who may therefore also want to skip them. The more serious readers will have to endure them in order to better understand the more exciting part of the story. I hope that they find themselves adequately rewarded for the minimum of patience necessary to read these brief chapters.

Above all, I hope that all who read the book will begin to understand what great fun the study of the brain can be.

S. Zeki
London

---

* In truth, it is not possible, in our present state of knowledge, to formulate a definitive theory of the functional plan of the brain.... It is obvious that we do not wish to give our hypothesis a dogmatic character; we know only too well that unforseen facts modify and even reverse, from one day to the next, our scientific conjectures. All that we could hope for is that there should remain of our concept something of the principles on which it is based.

Acknowledgements

I acknowledge with gratitude the help that I have received from many colleagues in preparing this book. I am grateful in particular for the detailed comments made on earlier versions of the manuscript by Bernard Katz, Richard Morris and Eric Kandel. Bernard Katz also translated many of the critical papers in the German literature for me. Without that help, it would not have been possible to write an account of the historical developments which have dominated our views of how the visual cortex functions. It was a collaboration which I much enjoyed. I am also indebted to Stewart Shipp for the many discussions on the relative merits of various arguments and for his comments on some of the chapters, and to Richard Frackowiak and his laboratory for the experiments on the human brain and for the comments he has made on the relevant chapters here.

There is a huge gulf that separates the desire to write a book and the realization of that desire. I was fortunate in finding in Harvey Shoolman an outstanding editor, whose great enthusiasm for the book was instrumental in helping me to complete it.

Prologue

Books about the brain, even small parts of the brain, are not easy to write. If asked what they want to know about the brain, most laymen would probably say that they would wish to know what brain states correspond to consciousness and to learning and memory, what characterizes the brain of a Newton or a Leonardo and what it is that moves the mind of man. These are all legitimate questions. But the answers to them lie in a millenial future so distant that most neurobiologists would today recoil with horror at the thought of being asked them at all. If pressed, the answers that they might give would be so imprecise as to be useless; indeed, they would be far less precise than the answers that one may find in the poetry of Shakespeare or the music of Wagner, both of whom might be considered, perhaps somewhat unconventionally, to have been among the greatest of neurologists. For they, at least, did know how to probe the mind of man with the techniques of language and of music and understood perhaps better than most what it is that moves the mind of man. The neurobiologist, by contrast, has only a very sketchy knowledge of what the brain does and how it does it. He has hardly begun to understand the elementary functions of the brain and is still incapable of accounting in anything more than a vague outline for even the simple operations of the brain, for example of how it sees forms and colours and how it interprets sounds. He therefore fears to stray into the subjective world of thoughts and feelings and into the problems of consciousness and of the mind, preferring to leave the former to the psychoanalyst and the latter to the philosophers. Yet, however grand these problems may seem, it is a mistake to suppose that one will acquire anything more than a superficial understanding of the brain unless one addresses them, even when studying an elementary function of the brain such as seeing.

The brain's knowledge of the external world

In this book I have tried to explore something of what the brain, and more particularly the cerebral cortex, does. I have used the visual cortex as the terrain for this enquiry because vision is the most developed sense in man and much of our knowledge of the external world comes through it. Correspondingly, the visual cortex constitutes a relatively large part of the cerebral cortex. Any general rules about the functioning of the visual cortex are therefore likely to apply to other parts of the cerebral cortex as well. This is not an idle hope. The architecture of much of the visual cortex is very similar to the architecture of other cortical areas, the pattern of cortical connections in it resembles that found elsewhere and many general features of its functional organization are reflected in other cortical areas, though the details will of course vary from one area to another. I have used colour vision as a major, though by no means the only, tool in this exploration. In spite of its apparent complexity and the detailed mathematical treatment that it often receives, colour vision is perhaps the simplest visual attribute to understand. It well illustrates how the brain, living in a continually changing environment, is able to acquire a knowledge about certain constant, unchanging, physical characteristics of objects from the ever-changing information reaching it from these objects, and thus make itself as independent as possible from the vicissitudes of constant change. This is a common theme in vision and, indeed, in sensation generally, for objects and surfaces are rarely seen (or sensed) in one condition only. Instead, they are viewed from different angles and distances, in different surroundings and in continually changing conditions of illumination, and yet they maintain their identity. This property, often called constancy, is therefore not unique to colour vision but is perhaps easiest to understand in terms of it. It implies that to acquire a knowledge about the external world, the cerebral cortex cannot passively analyze it. It must instead undertake some operation to discard the ever-changing information reaching it and approximate its own constructs as nearly as possible to the true physical constants of objects, and thus be able to categorize objects according to colour, to form, or to motion and so on.

This book is therefore an enquiry into the brain's knowledge of the external world through the sense of vision, though it is not a philosophical enquiry but rather a physiological and neurological one. In discussing problems of knowledge and of the mind, many philosophers have used vision as an example to a greater or lesser extent, since vision constitutes such an important medium for acquiring knowledge about the external world. It seems therefore a little incongruous, and something of a disappointment, that those practitioners of the neurobiology of vision have rarely seen it fit to address, in return, the problems of knowledge and of consciousness. There are at least three reasons for this. First, neurobiologists in general, or at least the more respectable ones amongst them, tend to be wary of problems such as knowledge, understanding, experience and consciousness, problems that not only seem to them insoluble at present but also ones that belong in the private and unobservable world of subjective mental states. They prefer instead to concentrate on the observable and the measurable — the connections of cells, their responses to particular stimuli, their metabolic rates and their membrane properties — studies in which they have had a high degree of success and which have contributed so much to our understanding of the elementary physiology of the brain. Next, until the last two decades and possibly even today, most visual neurobiology was concerned with relatively low levels of vision and in particular with the retina. Most would agree that it would seem a little silly to discuss the mind in retinal terms. Finally, there has been a tendency, dictated partly by philosophical speculation and partly by neurological speculation, to separate the problem of sensing from that of understanding. Most neurobiologists would regard it as necessary to unravel the first process before they can start to unravel the second.

Seeing and understanding

The genesis and lineage of this idea of a separation between the two causally linked faculties of seeing and understanding, the former a passive and the latter an active process, are not easy to trace. Whatever the origins, the idea is unmistakably there in the speculations of the German physiologist Hermann Munk and his compatriot, the neurologist Heinrich Lissauer,[1] although one might find at least a superficial resemblance between such a view and Kant's belief in the two faculties of Sensing and Understanding, the former being passive and the latter active. In accepting this doctrine neurologists had come, by the turn of the century, to develop a deeply philosophical attitude about the brain, usually without realizing it. As well, they had succeeded in tying the two separate processes to separate cortical areas, or so they imagined. Their evidence for this was partly anatomical and partly pathological. The anatomical evidence was derived from a study of how the eye connects to the brain and of how the architecture of the cortical area receiving the visual projections differs from that of the surrounding areas. This evidence seemed compelling until the last few years. The pathological evidence was controversial from the very start. It relied mainly on the demonstration that, whereas lesions in one part of the visual cortex led to blindness, lesions in another part led to a condition in which patients could see but could not understand what was seen, a condition which Munk called 'mind-blindness' (*Seelenblindheit*) and which is now commonly referred to as 'agnosia', following the term introduced by Sigmund Freud. Not everyone accepted this idea and from the very beginning it has had its critics.[2] But such criticisms did little to lessen the profound impact on the neurobiology of vision that this belief generated. It gradually became, and continues to be, such a central dogma in visual neurobiology that, in its service, important evidence which spoke otherwise came to be dismissed. Indeed, it would be no exaggeration to say that adherence to this doctrine retarded our present notion of the organiz-ation of the visual cortex and of brain function by well over a century[3] which, given that the discipline of neurology is not much older, is a very long time.

The impact of history and inherited opinion

This is one reason why I have traced the history of the subject to the present time and tried to demonstrate the weakness of the evidence on which the premise is based. This book is perhaps a little unusual in devoting a relatively large amount of space to the history of the subject and the reader might well enquire whether this is at all necessary. The answer is yes. It is almost impossible to comprehend the thinking in many papers, written as recently as a decade ago and even today, without a knowledge of that history. Why is one area of the cortex alone called the visual cortex while the areas surrounding it are known as 'association' cortex, when all the evidence points to the fact that there are perfectly respectable visual areas in association cortex? Why was the evidence from early clinical papers, suggesting that the visual cortex is more extensive than the one usually described as 'visual', so easily dismissed? Why was there such a powerful resist-ance to the idea of a functional specialization in the visual cortex? And why does the doctrine of a separation between seeing and under-standing continue to play a powerful role in the interpretation of many neurological syndromes and even physiological results? *It is impossible to understand these issues and impossible to understand, too, the new directions that research and thinking about the visual cortex and the brain in general are taking without at least a superficial knowledge of that all-important history.*

Colour vision as a guide to cerebral mechanisms

Because colour vision has played so central a role in interpreting the organization of the visual cortex, I have naturally devoted relatively more space to it. But there is another, and more profound, reason why I have dwelt on the subject. I happen to hold the view that the problem of vision is the problem of knowledge, knowledge about the external world acquired through the sense of vision. For why do we need to see at all, except to acquire that knowledge? It is my view that one cannot unravel the first process, that of seeing, in any profound sense unless one unravels the second process, that of under-standing what is seen, because there is no real division between the two. In other words, seeing is understanding, and colour vision happens to be a perfectly good example of this. Indeed, it is very likely that had the early neurologists really understood the nature of vision in general and of colour vision in particular, progress in the field of visual neurobiology would have taken a different course, as it has during the past few years. The study of colour vision has thus been instrumental in modifying our views on the cerebral processes involved in vision. Indeed, it has provided us with powerful insights into brain function. Understanding the role of the cortex in colour vision has therefore philosophical and epistemological implications which go far beyond understanding the detailed physiological mechanisms underlying the perception of colours. In short, the study of colour gives us a vision of how the visual cortex works. The study of the visual cortex in turns gives us a vision of how the brain works.

The new insights into the role of the cerebral cortex in vision have not been obtained by studying colour in isolation, but rather in relation to how the cerebral cortex handles other attributes of vision, such as form, motion and depth. To grasp this requires a fairly detailed, though not exhaustive, description of the anatomy and physiology of the visual pathways. Central to this description is the theory of functional specialization.[4] This theory supposes that different attributes of the visual scene are processed simultaneously, in parallel, but in anatomically separate parts of the visual cortex. The study of colour vision and of motion vision have provided the cornerstones on which the theory of functional specialization in the visual cortex is based and have thus given us some insights into how the brain is organized to acquire its knowledge of the visual world.

The problem of knowledge and consciousness

The problem of understanding and of knowledge cannot be tackled unless one tackles the problem of consciousness, for how can one acquire knowledge or understanding without consciousness? Indeed, one will find that there are pathological conditions affecting the visual cortex in which the problem of consciousness cannot be avoided at all.[5] Nor should one be deterred by the fact that consciousness belongs in the private and unobservable world of subjective mental states. After all, evolution has produced brains in which a critical and cardinal feature is the presence of subjective mental states and therefore no theory of the brain is complete if it cannot give a scientific account of the subjectivity of mental states. I have therefore addressed these problems, though not exhaustively. No one should imagine that I have a ready answer to them or indeed that there is one in the present state of knowledge. But little is served by not addressing the problem and much is gained by doing so. There are of course dangers too, in particular the danger of trying to explain too much on the basis of too little and the danger of relying too much on the facts with which one is well acquainted and ignoring those of which one has only a sketchy knowledge or none at all. It is of course inevitable that, of the good many facts known about the brain in general and about the visual cortex in particular, I should have chosen those which seem to be particularly relevant to my theme. I hope that those who find themselves unjustly not referred to will look at these omissions in this context and in a forgiving way. They must realize that my vision of the brain is obviously filtered through the prism of my own researches and thinking, and therefore necessarily includes a great deal of my own work. This is not to imply that my views have been reached without my being lifted onto the shoulders of giants in the field. However, any view is obviously a subjective one to an extent, and that very subjectivity must be conditioned by the work that I have done.

The poverty of our neural language

Anyone interested in learning about how the brain works, and particularly about the higher functions of the brain, must accept that we are ignorant of much in this area. Our language tends therefore to be imprecise, tentative and vague — a reflection of our ignorance. As the reader will soon discover, this imprecision of language, the wrestle with words and meanings, is also encountered in the study of vision in general and of colour vision in particular. We use words such as 'translation' or 'operation' to signify that something is happening, that the process is more complex than we had previously imagined, but we are not able to be more precise about what it is that is happening. Even terms such as 'information' are commonly vaguely used, or at least used in ways which philosophers, trained to think about the precise meaning of words, would strongly disapprove of. Yet, however much philosophers might disapprove of the imprecise way in which we use terms, the terms themselves often serve a very useful purpose in indicating important facts about the brain. A term such as the 'unconscious inference', used by Helmholtz to describe the fact that the brain must somehow 'discount the illuminant' in assigning a constant colour to a surface viewed under different conditions of illumination, would, I imagine, be one that philosophers feel uncomfortable with. Yet Helmholtz made a real contribution when, using this term, he implied that colour vision must entail much more than the passive reception of sensory impressions from the retina, as many had then supposed and still do. Today, we might use the term 'operation' to emphasize the same point, without being able to specify any more precisely the details of the operations that the brain must undertake to achieve this. However vague both terms may be, they are nevertheless important in underlining a certain fact about what the brain does, in introducing new concepts of brain function. It is therefore fortunate that neurobiologists are not philosophers, for they might otherwise find themselves immersed, like the philosophers, in an endless and ultimately fruitless discussion on the meaning of words such as 'unconscious' or 'inference' or 'knowledge' and 'information' instead of trying to unravel important facts about the brain. They would, in brief, end up contributing as meagrely to an understanding of the brain and of the mind as philosophers have. This last point is not a trivial one for ultimately the problems that cortical neurobiologists will be concerned with are the very ones that have preoccupied the philosophers throughout the ages — problems of knowledge, experience, consciousness and the mind — all of them a consequence of the activities of the brain and ultimately only understandable when the brain itself is properly understood. The path towards that millenial future lies more with neurobiologists and some philosophers acknowledge this. 'Neuroscience', writes one of them, 'must change the philosophy of mind, and to a great extent has already done so'.[6] It is only through a knowledge of neurobiology that philosophers of the future can hope to make any substantial contribution to understanding the mind. And it is only by gaining sufficient confidence to address problems such as knowledge, consciousness and the mind that visual neurobiologists will begin to understand vision and the brain in any profound sense.

References

1 Lissauer, H. (1890). Ein Fall von Seelenblindheit nebst einem Beitrage zur Theorie derselben. *Arch. Psychiatr. Nervenkr.* **21**, 221–270.
2 Stauffenberg, F. von (1914). Uber Seelenblindheit. *Arb. Hirnanat. Inst. Zurich* **8**, 1–212; Critchley, M. (1964). The problem of visual agnosia. *J. Neurol. Sci.* **1**, 274–290; Bender, M.B. & Feldman, M. (1972). The so-called 'visual agnosias'. *Brain* **95**, 173–186.
3 Zeki, S. (1990). A century of cerebral achromatopsia. *Brain* **113**, 1721–1777.
4 Zeki, S.M. (1974). The mosaic organization of the visual cortex in the monkey. In *Essays on the Nervous System: A Festschrift for Professor J.Z. Young*, edited by R. Bellairs & E.G. Gray, pp. 327–343. Clarendon Press, Oxford; Zeki, S.M. (1978). Functional specialization in the visual cortex of the rhesus monkey. *Nature* **274**, 423–428.
5 Weiskrantz, L. (1986). *Blindsight*. Clarendon Press, Oxford.
6 Hondrich, T. (1987). Mind, brain and self-conscious mind. In *Mindwaves*, edited by C. Blakemore & S. Greenfield, pp. 445–460. Basil Blackwell, Oxford.

Chapter 1: The retina and the visual image

A great deal has been written about colour vision. Most of this relates to the role of the retina. This is not surprising. All the input into our visual brain must pass through it. Moreover, until relatively recently there was a misconception, popular among scientists and laymen alike, that an image of the visual world in all its forms and colours is impressed on the retina and then transmitted to be analyzed and interpreted by the cerebral cortex. This idea was no doubt reinforced by superficial notions of the eye acting as a camera, which nevertheless became ingrained enough in the popular mind to become part of our scientific, and indeed linguistic, culture.

There is no doubt that the study of the retinal mechanisms involved in colour vision has enhanced immeasurably our knowledge of the subject and has provided the key to our understanding of the inherited retinal colour blindnesses. Perhaps one of the greatest advances in this area was made by Thomas Young (Figure 1.1). In his Bakerian

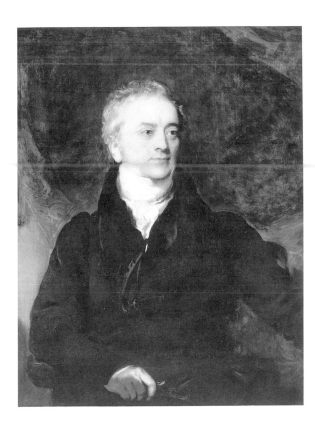

Fig. 1.1 Thomas Young (1773–1829), the great polyhistor of nineteenth century British science. He proposed a brilliant theory of the receptors for colour vision, which became inappropriately called a theory of colour vision. (Reproduced by permission of the President and Council of the Royal Society.)

Lecture to the Royal Society in 1802,[1] he wrote, 'As it is almost impossible to conceive each sensitive point of the retina to contain an infinite number of particles, each capable of vibrating in perfect unison with every possible undulation, it becomes necessary to suppose the number limited, for instance to the three principal colours, red, yellow and blue'.[1] By undulation, Young meant wavelength. We should note here that Young was equating wavelength directly with colour, for he speaks of undulations in the first part of his sentence and of colour in the second. Because colour is a sensation, he was also implicitly equating the response of particular 'particles' in the retina with particular sensations, a view which came to dominate thinking about colour vision for a long time. Young's statement was in the nature of an aside, in a lecture whose subject was the wave properties of light. But what an aside! It was a revolutionary idea, not only in colour vision, but also in sensory physiology. For what Young was saying was that it would be difficult to imagine that a sensory surface would necessarily provide its possessor with a receptor for every possible sensation or experience. Instead, a sensory surface may possess only a limited number of receptor types, and endow them with such potential that an individual may experience a wide variety of sensations. This is the approach the brain uses for colour vision. It is not necessarily the same for all sensations. Where an experience is specified by some unique feature, as for example when an odour is uniquely specified by a unique molecular structure, there may in fact be a very large number of receptors,[2] each one corresponding to a unique molecular structure, in the manner of a lock and key mechanism.

Young's idea was soon forgotten, or so historians of science claim. It was to be resurrected many years later by Herman von Helmholtz, the great German physicist and the father of the discipline of psychophysics. Helmholtz drew curves for how he would expect the three 'retinal fibres', as he called them, to respond to different wavelengths of light (Figure 1.2).[3] He imagined that each would respond to lights of different wavelengths but that each would be maximally sensitive to a different part of the visible spectrum. This notion gained considerably when scientists began to measure in detail how the cones of the primate retina absorb light.[4-6] They found that there are indeed three and only three classes of cone. Each class absorbs light of many different wavelengths, but has a maximal sensitivity to light at a particular part of the spectrum, precisely as Helmholtz and Young had anticipated (Figure 1.2). But Helmholtz, like Young before him, had tried to account for the sensation of colour directly in terms of the absorption characteristics of the cones. He wrote, 'Red light stimulates the red sensitive fibres strongly and the other two weakly, giving the *sensation* red; green light stimulates the green sensitive fibres strongly and the other two weakly, giving the *sensation* green;

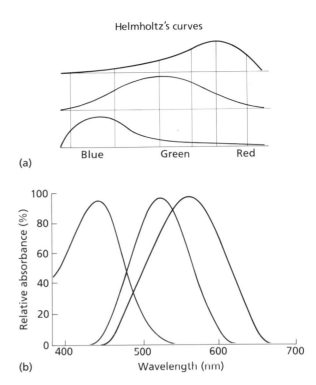

Fig. 1.2 (a) Helmholtz imagined that the three retinal colour receptors would respond to lights of different wavelengths, with each responding to a considerable portion of the visible spectrum but having a maximal sensitivity at a certain part only. (b) The actual sensitivities of the three cones in the primate retina, revealed by more sophisticated techniques.

blue light stimulates the blue sensitive fibres strongly and the other two weakly, giving the *sensation* blue', adding that, 'when all three fibres are stimulated about equally, the *sensation* is that of white or of pale hues'[3] [my emphasis]. Notice that, here again, Helmholtz is equating sensation directly with retinal activity, explicitly stating that stimulation of the red-sensitive fibres, for example, leads to the sensation of red. This view of how the brain codes for colour is now commonly called the Young−Helmholtz Trichromatic Theory of colour vision. The theory is the basis of the so-called colour matching studies. In its simplest form, it states that any given coloured light can be matched precisely by adjusting the intensity of three other lights of different colour and that colour vision is therefore trivariant. It has proven to be an indispensable tool for determining the nature of the inherited retinal colour blindnesses, since the matches made by people with inherited retinal abnormalities differ from those of normals. But to account for the complexities of colour vision in retinal terms alone or in terms of the trichromatic theory alone was impossible then, and is impossible today. In no sense therefore is the Young−Helmholtz theory a theory of colour vision. It is instead a theory of the receptors for colour vision.

In fact, of course, Helmholtz was well aware of the limitations of trying to account for colour vision in these terms. In particular, it was difficult to account for the phenomenon of colour constancy, which refs to the fact that colours change little when viewed in different illuminants, conditions under which the wavelength composition of the light reflected from them would be different. A green leaf, for example, looks green when viewed at dawn, dusk or at noon on a sunny or cloudy day. There will naturally be changes in the shade of green. But the leaf will nevertheless remain green. This in spite of the fact that if one were to measure the amount of lights of different wave-lengths reflected from the leaf under these different conditions, one would find considerable variations. Indeed, if it were not for colour constancy, colour vision would lose its significance as a biological signalling mechanism. For if an object were to appear green in one set of conditions, yellow in another and orange in a third, then the object could no longer be recognizable by its colour but only by some other attribute. Helmholtz, like others, invoked vague cerebral factors to account for this process, which to him entailed 'discounting the illuminant' through a process which he called the 'unconscious inference'.[3]

Why did colour constancy play such a subsidiary role in enquiries on colour vision? Almost certainly because, until only very recently, it has been treated as a departure from a general rule, although it is in fact the central problem of colour vision. That general rule supposes that there is a precise and simple relationship between the wavelength composition of the light reaching the eye from every point on a surface and the colour of that point. Most deemed it necessary to understand what they thought to be the sensory process first and defer the second process, which involves the problem of knowing how and when to discount the illuminant, until the first stage was understood. Most also deemed it more important to account for what they imagined to be the normal condition, one in which there is a precise relationship between wavelength composition and perceived colour.

That idea too has a great tradition. It takes its origin from an experiment of Newton's, one of the greatest ever performed in colour vision. This is the celebrated experiment in which Newton passed sunlight through a prism and broke it up into its components, the different wavelengths, observing in the process that long-wave light looked red, middle-wave light looked green and short-wave light looked blue. To Newton, the conclusion was obvious. He wrote, 'Every Body reflects the rays of its own Colour more copiously than the rest, and from their excess and predominance in the reflected Light has its Colour'.[7] In other words, a green object looks green because it reflects more green (or middle-wave) light, a red objects looks red because it reflects more long-wave light, and so on. Some two centuries later, physiologists discovered wavelength-selective cells in the visual pathways. These cells respond selectively to lights of specific wavelengths, in ways which we shall consider in more detail later. A cell might, for example, respond to long-wave (red) light only, and not to light of other wavelengths or to white light. On the other hand, it might give opposite responses to lights of different colour. For example, it might increase its on-going electrical discharge when stimulated with long-wave light (ON response) and decrease its response when stimulated by middle-wave light, the cell increasing its response when middle-wave light is switched off (OFF response). Having found such cells, neurophysiologists naturally imagined that the way that the nervous system codes for the colour of an object is through cells which will respond to the predominant wavelength of the light reflected from every point in that object, and hence 'determine' its colour.

Neurologists adopt a simplistic view of colour vision

It all seemed to fit very nicely into the general conception of neurologists, especially since there is a topographic, 'point-to-point' projection from retina to the primary visual receptive centre in the cortex. Clues to concepts that are popular, or to the thinking of men, are often provided by the language that they use to describe their scientific discoveries, even if they themselves are not very explicit about the concepts. To neurologists, an 'image' of the visual world, together with all its forms and colours and movements, was 'impressed' upon the retina and these 'visual impressions' were subsequently 'received' to be 'analyzed' by the primary visual cortex, referred to by Henschen, the Swedish neurologist, as the 'cortical retina'.[8] Thus, the colour of every point in the field of view, determined by the wavelength composition of the light reaching the retina from that point, would be transmitted to the corresponding point in the 'cortical retina', there to be 'analyzed'. There might, to be sure, be other cortical influences at work, such as memory or experience. These would modify somewhat the 'received colour impression'. But the colour itself was determined at the retina. If anyone doubted this, one could show that among the cells of the retina are ones which respond selectively to long-wave light, that is to say to light which, when seen in isolation by the human observer, looks red. Such cells would respond to red objects, or so one supposed, precisely because red objects reflect more red, or long-wave, light. Indeed, many authors described such cells as 'red' or 'green' cells, implying that they could themselves signal the presence of a red or green object. Or one could point to the presence of 'feature detectors' in the retina of the frog[9] or motion detectors in the retina of the rabbit.[10]

Many physiologists would today protest loudly that they did not mean that the responses of a long-wave selective cell led directly to the sensation which we call red. Nor did they mean that the responses of a long-wave (red) ON and middle-wave (green) OFF cell, which they commonly referred to as a red-on, green-off cell, led directly to the common visual experience of seeing a green after-image when one looks at a red patch and then at a neutral, grey, screen. Yet, by commonly referring to these cells as red cells or blue cells, they had at the very least imbibed the culture of the times and supposed, perhaps even without thinking much about it, that a red surface looks red because it reflects more long-wave light and because there are cells in the visual system that respond selectively to the predominant wavelength of the light reflected from it, that is, to long-wave or red light. Supposing them to have been aware of the complexities of colour vision, they have been singularly ineffective in conveying to the general scientific public the notion that colour is a far more complex phenomenon. Psychologists and psychophysicists were in general a good deal more cautious. More conversant with the complexities of colour vision, which they study in minute detail, they have been more careful to distinguish between wavelength and colour for the very good reason that, as we shall see later, the relationship between the wavelength composition of the light reflected from a surface and its perceived colour is not quite as obvious or straightforward as one might think. But they too have been singularly ineffective in communicating their thoughts to the neurologists who were charting the way in which vision is represented in the cerebral cortex. But it is likely that, even if they had tried to explain, neurologists of that epoch would not have taken the slightest notice of their explanation.

The prevailing concept, then, among neurologists at least, was of a visual image with all its various attributes, in which the colour of every point had already been determined by the wavelength composition of the light reflected from it, being transmitted from the retina to be 'received' and 'analyzed' by the cortex; so powerful was this concept that for a good century almost all explanations of colour vision were given in retinal terms and much of the work on colour was undertaken on the retina. This is surprising because eminent authorities on colour vision, in England and Germany, had emphasized, at least implicitly, the importance of higher cortical activities in colour vision and had even come close to suggesting that the problem of colour vision is a problem of knowledge. Helmholtz (Figure 1.3) had spoken of colour as being 'due to an act of judgement, not an act of sensation',[3] Hering[11] (Figure 1.3) had emphasized the importance of memory and Clerk Maxwell[12] had written of colour vision as a 'mental science'. That these eminent authorities on colour vision should have had not the slightest influence on the thinking of neurologists debating the question of a colour centre in the cerebral cortex, and dismissing it, is perhaps testimony to the power of the prevailing neurological doctrines in those times. The determination of the colour

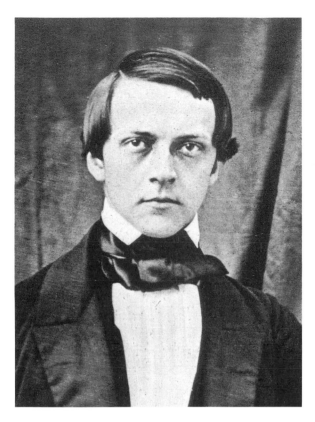
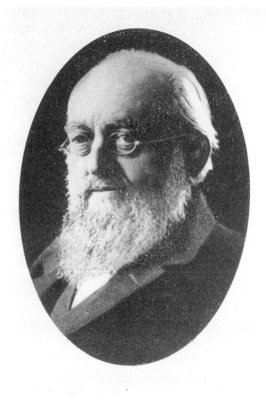

Fig. 1.3 Hermann von Helmholtz (1821–1894) (left), one of the most brilliant of nineteenth century scientists and founder of the discipline of psychophysics. (Reproduced by permission of the President and Council of the Royal Society.) His preeminence in the world of learning and in colour vision in particular was much resented by his compatriot, Ewald Hering (1834–1918) (right), whose opponents theory of colour vision was considered for a long time to be in opposition to the trichromatic theory. (Reproduced by permission from Polyak, S. (1957). *The Vertebrate Visual System*. University of Chicago Press, Chicago.)

of every point in the field of view by the retina, the transmission of that 'colour impression' to the 'cortical retina' in the well-documented point-by-point system connecting the two structures, and the fact that a small lesion anywhere along this pathway led to a total blindness for a small part of the field of view (a scotoma), were all strong arguments in favour of this simple analytic doctrine of vision, including colour vision, or so it seemed at the time. It led to the concept of a cortex passively receiving and 'analyzing' the visual image, a doctrine which is only now beginning to be modified, due in large measure to a much more sophisticated technology for studying the brain. At any rate, the adherence of neurologists to the concept of a visual image formed on the retina and received by the cortex was to retard the study of colour vision and of cortical function by at least a century. It was obvious to the hard-nosed men of neurology that the area of the cerebral cortex that received the visual 'impressions' must be the very one that also received the colour 'impressions', since this was part of the visual scene, and thus must be 'analyzed' in the same cortical area as the rest of the visual scene. There could not be a separate cortical area dealing with colour, or so they believed. But events elsewhere in cortical studies were taking a different turn.

References

1 Young, T. (1802). The Bakerian Lecture: On the theory of lights and colours. *Philos. Trans. R. Soc. Lond.* **92**, 12–48.
2 Axel, R. & Buck, L. (1991). A novel multigene family may encode odorant receptors: a molecular basis for odor recognition. *Cell* **65**, 175–187.
3 Helmholtz, H. von (1911). *Handbuch der Physiologischen Optik*, 2. Voss, Hamburg.
4 Stiles, W.S. (1978). *Mechanisms of Colour Vision*. Academic Press, London.
5 Rushton, W.H. (1956). Chemical basis of colour vision and colour blindness. *Nature* **206**, 1087–1091.
6 Marks, W.B., Dobelle, W.H. & MacNichol, E.F. (1964). Visual pigments of single primate cones. *Science* **143**, 1181–1183.
7 Newton, I. (1704). *Opticks: Or, A Treatise of the Reflexions, Refractions, Inflexions and Colours of Light*. S. Smith and B. Walford, London.
8 Henschen, S.E. (1910). Zentrale Sehstörungen. In *Handbuch der Neurologie*, 2, edited by M. Lewandowsky, pp. 891–918. Springer-Verlag, Berlin.
9 Lettvin, J.Y., Maturana, H.R., McCulloch, W.S. & Pitts, W.H. (1959). What the frog's eye tells the frog's brain. *Proc. Inst. Rad. Eng.* **47**, 1940–1951.
10 Barlow, H.B., Hill, R.M. & Levick, W.R. (1965). Retinal ganglion cells responding selectively to direction and speed of image motion in the rabbit. *J. Physiol. (Lond.)* **173**, 377–407.
11 Hering, E. (1964). *Outlines of a Theory of the Light Sense*, translated by L.M. Hurvich & D. Jameson. Harvard University Press, Cambridge.
12 Maxwell, J.C. (1872). On colour vision. *Proc. R. Instn. GB* **6**, 260–271.

Chapter 2: Functional specialization in human cerebral cortex

The idea of functional localization in the human cerebral cortex was born in Paris in 1861, though it was not an easy delivery. It was then that the first definitive conclusions about it, derived from a study of the human brain, as opposed to the endless empty speculations of the phrenologists, were put forward. This was done by Pierre Paul Broca (Figure 2.1) at a meeting of the Société d'Anthropologie, of which he was secretary at the time, on 18 April 1861.[1] Broca had been studying a patient who had lost the ability to speak twenty-one years previously. The brief description given by him is testament to the extraordinary insight of a neurologist possibly tainted with adventurism, for the same material would almost certainly have escaped the attention of a lesser person, as the attack on Broca at that same and subsequent sessions shows.

When Broca's patient had been admitted to hospital, he had lost the ability to speak and was only able to utter a single syllable, *tan*.

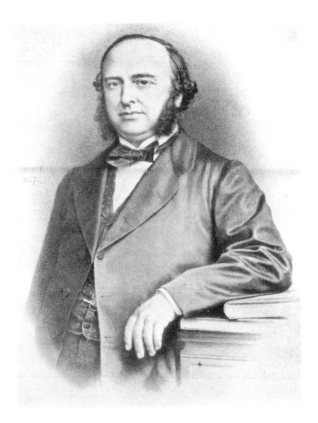

Fig. 2.1 Pierre Paul Broca (1824–1880), one of the greatest French neurologists. His ability to identify the precise location of the lesion causing aphasia and locate it in the left frontal lobe, when the lesion itself had been more extensive and of very long duration, is regarded by some as a sign of an outstanding insight and by others as a sign of profound adventurism. (Reproduced by permission from Polyak, S. (1957). *The Vertebrate Visual System.* University of Chicago Press, Chicago.)

He therefore became known as *Tan* to all in the hospital. Ten years after admission he became paralyzed on the right side. Subsequently his vision began to fail and there was a general diminution in his intelligence as well. Broca began studying him on 12 April 1861. The patient died on 17 April 1861. At autopsy the damage to the brain was found to be quite extensive. There was a softening of the left frontal lobe in its entirety. The destruction had resulted in a cavity sufficiently large 'to accommodate an egg'. The softening had extended posteriorly to the parietal lobe and to the base of the temporal lobe (Figure 2.2). It had also invaded subcortical structures such as the basal ganglia and the insula. 'But it is sufficient to glance at the brain to recognize that the primitive seat of the softening is the middle part of the left frontal lobe; this is where one finds the most extensive, the most advanced and the oldest lesions...one can consider it as certain that there had been a long period when the disease occupied only the convolutions

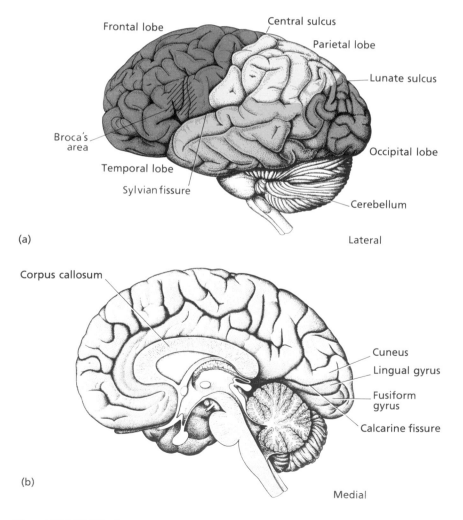

(a)

(b)

Fig. 2.2 The human brain seen from (a) the outside (laterally) and (b) when one half is cut away (medially). Broca's area is located in the left frontal cortex.

of the frontal lobe. This period probably corresponds to the eleven years which preceded the paralysis of the right arm and during which the patient, having retained his intelligence, had only lost the ability to speak'. Perhaps a more careful, but less insightful, intelligent and speculative neurologist than Broca would have demurred. He would have wanted to learn more about the lesions in other parts of the brain or about the involvement of subcortical structures. He may even have decided, as some neurologists were to later with cases of cerebral colour blindness, to conduct a detailed microscopic study, perhaps based on many brains. Today, he would almost certainly be applying for a large grant to pursue his studies. Broca was different. His conclusion was firm. It was delivered to the Société d'Anthropologie on the afternoon of the autopsy. He simply said, 'Everything allows us then to believe that, in the present case, the lesion in the frontal lobe had been the cause of the loss of speech'. Was Broca so insightful or merely an adventurer? Young[2] writes, 'Neither the conception of a faculty of articulate language nor its localization in the frontal lobes was novel. It might be argued that Broca was the first to confirm this localization...but the fact is that the quality of the evidence of his original case was very dubious indeed. What Broca seems to have contributed was a demonstration of this localization at a time when the scientific community was prepared to take the issue seriously'.

However that may be, Broca's conclusion, brief but incisive, was not to the liking of all. Immediately after Broca's presentation, Gratiolet stood up to deliver an attack.[3] Gratiolet was no mean neuroanatomist; indeed he is almost a household name in neurological circles for we attach his name to the optic radiations, the great nervous pathway that carries visual signals from the subcortical visual centre (the lateral geniculate nucleus) to the primary visual cortex. This pathway is also known as the bundle of Gratiolet. At any rate, in a long speech, much of it devoted to the relationship between brain weight and intelligence, Gratiolet denounced those findings, using arguments that appear surprisingly tenuous today. He cited evidence which purported to show that people can retain the faculty of language after damage to the frontal lobe. He quoted from Wepfer's *Historiae Apoplecticorum* about a husband who, in a fit of rage, had delivered a blow to his shrew of a wife. The blow had been sufficiently nasty to damage her frontal lobes and lead to death within less than twenty-four hours. And yet, even though the blow had been mortal, his wife had been able to hurl one last verbal insult at him, threatening to wring his neck, before dying. This showed, Gratiolet believed, that she had retained the faculty of speech which, in turn, proved that Broca must be wrong. Moreover, '...monkeys too have anterior lobes, and these lobes are subdivided as in man. One finds the same sulci and the same gyri... But do monkeys speak? Do they present the smallest vestige of human language?' He of course did not wish to belittle the efforts of Broca and of others. 'These are without doubt great, Titanic, efforts! But when we want to seize the celestial truth from the heights of Babel, the edifice crumbles'.

Broca was later to study the relationship between aphasia and brain damage in greater detail and to present a better argument. But, however convinced Broca may have been of his case, and however ready the scientific community may have been to accept it, the fact nevertheless remained that, to demonstrate functional localization convincingly, reliance on a single function was not enough. It was important to show that another, different, cerebral function is localized in another, distinct, part of the cerebral cortex. The case for localization would become more convincing if it could be shown that architecturally distinct parts of the cerebral cortex are involved in distinct functions. That evidence was not long in coming. It was provided by Gustav Fritsch and Eduard Hitzig in Germany in 1870.[4] They undertook systematic studies of the motor cortex in the dog and they summarized their results equally succinctly, 'One part of the convexity of the brain is motor in function, another part is not. In general, the motor part is situated anteriorly and the non-motor part posteriorly. By stimulating electrically the motor part, one obtains combined muscular contractions of the opposite half of the body'. The subsequent detailed study of the architecture of the cerebral cortex and the demonstration that the excitable motor cortex has a distinct architecture, different from that of the frontal cortex, laid down the foundations of cerebral localization in the cerebral cortex. It also made architecture an important feature in defining an area. In general, neurologists began to think of an area as one which has a distinct function, such as vision or audition, or a distinct architecture, and preferably both. Since then, neurologists and neurobiologists have defined many cortical areas associated with different functions, and many more subdivisions continue to be added. By the 1930s Lashley could write that, 'in the field of neurophysiology no fact is more firmly established than the functional differentiation of various parts of the cerebral cortex... No one can today seriously believe that the different parts of the cerebral cortex all have the same functions, or can entertain for a moment the proposition of Hermann that because the mind is a unit, the brain must also act as a unit'.[5] Here was an admission, by one who was more hostile to the idea of cerebral localization of function than most, that functional specialization may be a characteristic feature of the cortex at large, at least for different sensations, and that the integration evident in thought and behaviour does not preclude the existence of specialized subdivisions in the cerebral cortex.

Yet it was the very integrated and unitary nature of the visual image in the brain, one in which all the attributes of vision — form, colour, motion, distance — are seen in precise spatio-temporal registration, that was to mislead neurologists into thinking that all these attributes must be 'analyzed' in one and the same cortical area, and to dismiss any evidence which even hinted at a specialization for colour or, indeed, for other attributes of vision. No matter what Lashley said in 1930, neurologists before and after found it difficult to believe that the unitary visual image did not imply a unitary visual process, or indeed a single visual area, a manner of thinking to which Lashley himself, as we shall see, contributed in no small measure.

References

1 Broca, P.P. (1861). Perte de la parole, ramollisement chronique et destruction partielle du lobe antérieure gauche du cerveau. *Bull. Soc. Anthropol.* **2**, 235−238.
2 Young, R.M. (1990). *Mind, Brain, and Adaptation in the Nineteenth Century.* Oxford University Press, Oxford.
3 Gratiolet, L.-P. (1861). Reprise de la discussion sur le volume et la forme du cerveau. *Bull. Soc. Anthropol.* **2**, 239−275.
4 Fritsch, G. & Hitzig, E. (1870). Uber die elektrische Erregbakeit des Grosshirns. *Arch. f. Anat. Physiol. u. wiss. Med.* **37**, 300−332.
5 Lashley, K.S. (1931). Mass action in cerebral function. *Science* **73**, 245−254.

Chapter 3: The representation of the retina in the primary visual cortex

Many of the earlier cases of colour blindness due to specific cerebral lesions (*cerebral achromatopsia*), as well as other visual syndromes resulting from brain damage, are still of interest today and indeed are of importance in establishing the principle of functional specialization in the visual cortex of man. After a period of about eighty years, when the syndrome was hardly referred to, cases of cerebral achromatopsia are being cited again. It is therefore interesting to enquire why this evidence, which gives us so important an insight into the organization of the visual cortex, was dismissed so successfully and for so long. I shall return to that topic. But first I want to give a brief account of the nature of the retinal representation in the primary visual cortex, *as we know it today*, and an account of the terminology used to describe various levels of the visual pathways from the retina to the cortex. This will help in understanding not only the arguments which were used to dismiss the syndrome of cerebral achromatopsia, but also many of the descriptions given later in the book. It might also help the reader to appreciate the difficulties which earlier neurologists, not privy to the facts at our disposal today, had to face in trying to account for these syndromes.

Subdivisions of the retina

To understand how the retina is mapped or represented on the cerebral cortex, we can divide each retina into four segments — nasal and temporal, and upper and lower (Figure 3.1). It is best to refer these subdivisions to the part of the field of view which each registers. Thus, the nasal retina looks at the temporal field of view and the temporal retina at the nasal field of view. Because of the curvature of the eye, the nasal retina of the left eye and the temporal retina of the right eye look at the left half of the field of view, the *left hemi-field*, while the nasal retina of the right eye and the temporal retina of the left eye look at the right half of the field of view, the *right hemi-field*. Again, because of the curvature, the lower part of the eye looks at the upper field of view and the upper part of the eye looks at the lower field of view. Thus each hemi-field can, in turn, be subdivided into *upper and lower quadrants*. These subdivisions are important to bear in mind when considering the arrangement of the retinal map over the surface of the primary visual cortex.

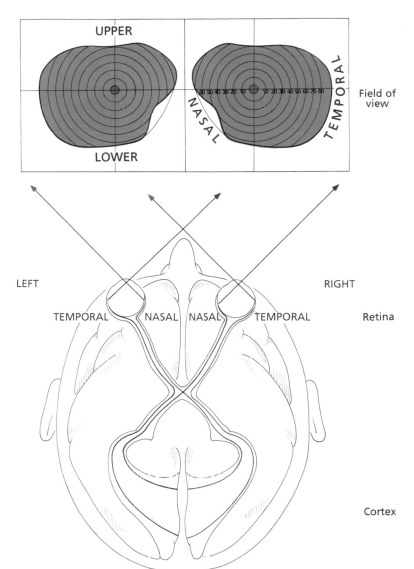

Fig. 3.1 The subdivisions of the retina and the manner of their connection to the cerebral cortex. The temporal retina of the right eye and the nasal retina of the left eye (shown in red) which, between them, look at the left half of the field of view, project to the right hemisphere (also shown in red) which consequently also 'looks' at the left half of the field of view. The left hemisphere, by contrast, 'looks' at the right half of the field of view.

The retina can also be subdivided into central and peripheral portions (Figure 3.2), though the terms have not been used consistently. The central retina is that part of it with which one fixates and sees detail. Structurally, it consists of a highly sensitive region, the *foveola*, which lies at the centre of the *foveal pit*. The foveola contains only the receptors for daylight vision, the *cones*, it is consequently known as the rod-free area of the retina, the rods being the receptors which are active at night or in low levels of illumination. It is usual to express retinal representation in terms of degrees subtended at the eye, a degree being a solid angle. This way one does not have to measure the distance of objects from the eye or determine their absolute size. The fovea represents the central 1° of vision; this is

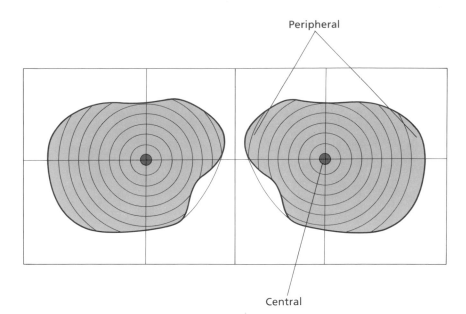

Fig. 3.2 The subdivisions of the retina into central (red) and peripheral parts. For details see text.

normally referred to as central vision. For many authors, however, central vision implies the central 5°. The macula lutea, a yellowish region of the retina, is concerned with the central 5° of vision. Thus, to many authors central vision and *macular vision* are used interchangeably. In general, the integrity of the central 5° of the retina and its cortical representation are necessary for fixation and detailed vision, as well as for colour vision, since the receptors for colour vision — the cones — are most numerous within the central retina and decline rapidly in more peripheral parts of the retina (Plate 1, part (a), facing p. 68).

Regions beyond the central 5° are referred to as peripheral parts of the retina, though it is of course best to be accurate and refer to the precise periphery in angular extent. The definition of the precise position on a retina is made by reference to the fixation point (i.e. the fovea). One can then speak of a point situated *peripherally* at an eccentricity of 15° from the fixation point in the upper left quadrant, and subtending 8° (Plate 1, part (b)). This will specify absolutely the position of the stimulus in the field of view, with respect to the observer. Or one can speak, with the same precision, of a stimulus viewed centrally, at an eccentricity of 3° and located in the lower right quadrant.

Projections from the retina to the brain

The terminology is slightly more complicated if one wants to describe retinal position in relation to the cerebral hemisphere. This is because of the manner in which the retina projects to each cerebral hemisphere (Figure 3.3). The fibres of the *optic nerve*, which carry the impulses

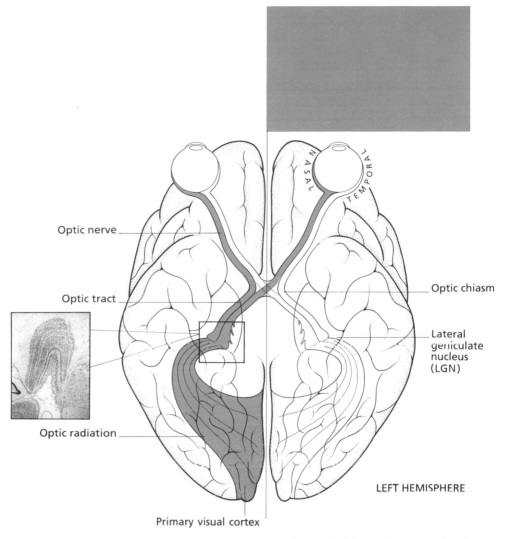

Fig. 3.3 The connections from the retina to the cerebral hemispheres. For details, see text. Inset to the left shows the multi-layered lateral geniculate nucleus (LGN).

from the retina, cross over at the *optic chiasm* in a very specific way. The fibres which have their origin in the nasal part of the retina cross over to the opposite hemisphere, while those which have their origin in the temporal retina do not, but continue to the same side of the brain. It follows that the fibres from the temporal retina of the left eye and from the nasal retina of the right eye pass to the left cerebral hemisphere, which therefore looks at the *contralateral* or right half of the field of view (the *right hemi-field*). By contrast, fibres from the nasal retina of the left eye and the temporal retina of the right eye pass over to the right hemisphere, which therefore looks at the *contralateral* or left half of the field of view (the *left hemi-field*). Thus, when looking at the field of view in relation to the cerebral hemispheres, one can speak of the *contralateral field of view* (the side opposite the hemisphere being considered) or the *ipsilateral field of view* (the same side as that of the cerebral hemisphere in question).

Beyond the optic chiasm the visual pathway becomes known as the optic tract. This relays visual signals to a subdivision of the cerebral hemispheres entitled the *lateral geniculate nucleus* (LGN) (Figure 3.4). This nucleus is a complex, six-layered structure. It has several noteworthy features, of which we need to emphasize two. The first is the remarkable specificity of connections between the eyes and the LGN. The inputs from the two eyes to the LGN are segregated, so that the optic nerve fibres coming from the *ipsilateral eye* (i.e. the eye on the same side of the LGN in question) terminate in layers 5, 3 and 2, whereas those fibres coming from the *contralateral eye* terminate in layers 6, 4 and 1. Superimposed on this strict segregation according to eye is a very detailed, point-to-point projection from the retina, so that adjacent points on the retina project to adjacent points in each layer of the LGN. Moreover, the layers are stacked upon one

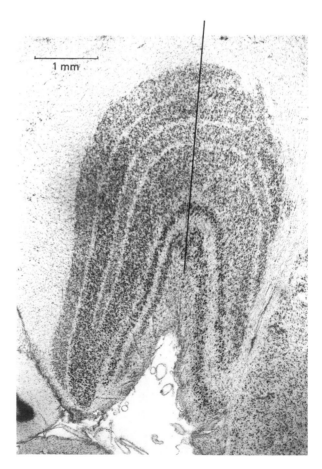

Fig. 3.4 The layers of the lateral geniculate nucleus (LGN). Each layer receives an input from one eye or the other only. But cells along the line shown here would be receiving inputs from homologous points in the two retinas and would therefore register identical points in visual space, though for different eyes. The upper four layers of the LGN have small cells and are known as the parvocellular (P) layers; the lower two have large cells and are known as the magnocellular (M) layers.

another in precise registration in terms of retinal representation. Hence, if the cells at a point A in layer 6 receive their input from a particular point in the left retina, the cells in point B in the layer below it will receive their input from the corresponding point in the right retina. The LGN thus shows to a high degree a feature which one encounters everywhere in the nervous system, namely the amazing specificity of connections. Since there are six layers in the LGN of each side, one might say that the retina is represented six times over in each LGN, three times for each eye. Thus, for each point in every layer representing a particular point in one retina, there is a corresponding point in the other layers representing the corresponding point in the other retina. We still have no real clue for this multifold representation, but it carries with it the implication of a functional segregation which is subsequently exploited in the visual cortex.

The second interesting point about the LGN concerns its subdivision into the upper four layers and the lower two layers (Figure 3.4). The upper four layers contain cells with small cell bodies and are therefore termed the *parvocellular* or *P layers*, whereas the lower two layers contain cells with large cell bodies and are termed the *magnocellular* or *M layers*. These subdivisions have assumed a great significance in recent years because the cells in the upper four layers are concerned with colour vision whereas those in the lower two are not. This is a theme developed more fully later on. Here, it is interesting to note that the first person to suggest such a functional dichotomy in the LGN was Henschen,[1] though his arguments were based on nothing more substantial than cell size, since he believed that small cells code for colour and large ones for light.

The projection to the primary visual cortex

The axons of the LGN cells on which the optic nerve fibres terminate then travel in the *optic radiation* to terminate in the cortex (Figure 3.3). The projection from each LGN is to the primary visual cortex of its own side, in an orderly, point-to-point manner. The consequence of this is twofold; first, that the cortex of each hemisphere receives signals from the contralateral half of the field of view and, second, that adjacent retinal points are mapped at adjacent points in this cortex, just as they are in the LGN. We speak of this map of the retina on the cortex as being a *topographical map*. Each part of the retina, including the fovea and the temporal crescent, is represented in a given part of the primary visual cortex[2] (Figure 3.5).

The optic radiation (*bundle of Gratiolet*) terminates in a part of the cortex situated in the occipital lobes, at the back of the brain. For a long time it used to be thought that this is the only part of the cortex that receives the output of the LGN in the primate, which is

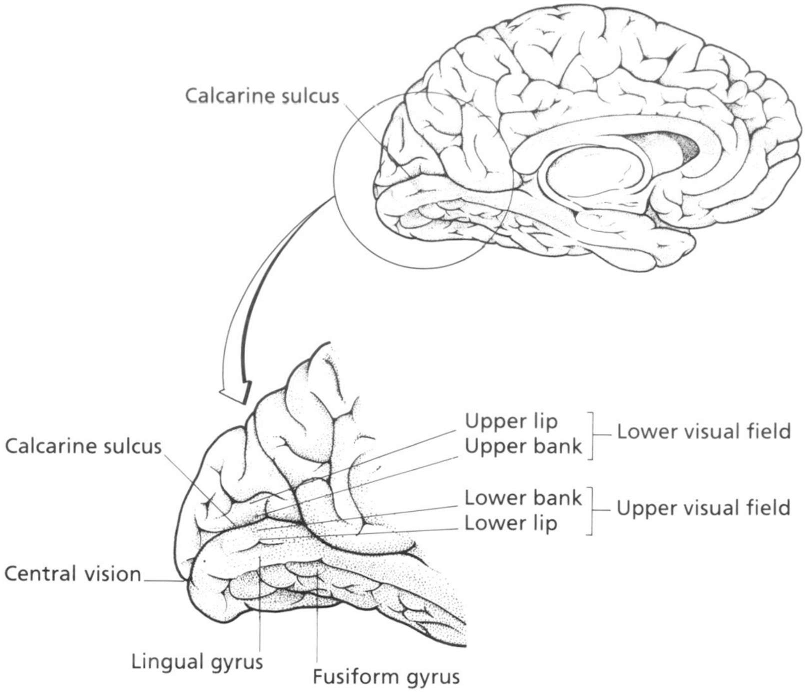

Fig. 3.5 The retina connects with the primary visual cortex (area V1) which lies mostly buried within the calcarine sulcus. The connections between retina and cortex are topographical, thus reproducing a map of the retina (and hence of the contralateral field of view) in each area V1. The left V1, shown here, 'looks' at the right half of the field of view. The lower part of the field of view is represented in the upper calcarine cortex and the upper part in the lower calcarine cortex, while central vision is represented at the occipital pole.

one reason why the area is commonly called the *primary visual cortex* or, more simply, *V1*. More recently, it has become apparent that there is a small projection from the LGN to the visual areas lying outside V1.[3] This latter knowledge is important in the interpretation of certain types of 'blindness', to be described later, in which the patient can 'see' in a rudimentary way but has no conscious awareness of having seen (blindsight). V1 has a very distinctive architectural appearance, making it visible at a glance. The characteristic feature of this architecture is a striation, and hence the term *striate cortex* (Figure 3.6). Much of the striate cortex is buried within a sulcus situated on the medial surface of the hemisphere and known as the *calcarine sulcus*. Only a small part, located posteriorly at the occipital pole, is visible from the external surface. Hence, another common term for V1, especially in the clinical literature, is the *calcarine cortex*. The German anatomist Korbinian Brodmann, who studied the architecture of the cerebral cortex in much detail, developed an esoteric and egocentric terminology to describe his areas — he numbered them according to the order in which he studied them — though no one has yet come up with a better terminology. The seventeenth area which he studied was the striate cortex, and hence the term *area 17* is also used to describe the primary visual receptive centre. From this it should become evident that the primary visual cortex parades under different names.

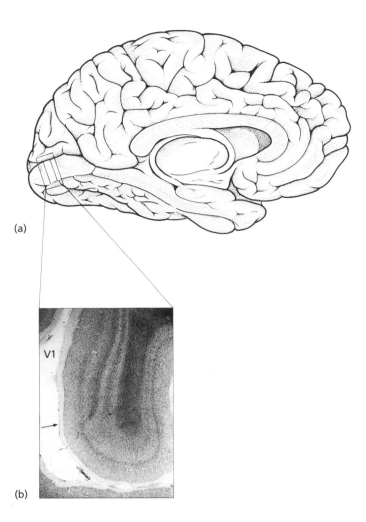

(a)

Fig. 3.6 (b) A section taken through the region of the occipital lobe of the brain shown in (a). It is stained to reveal the manner in which cells are stacked upon one another in layers in area V1. This constitutes the cytoarchitecture of V1. Note that it differs sharply from the cytoarchitecture of the neighbouring cortex, commonly called the visual 'association' cortex (transition point marked with an arrow).

(b)

Within the striate cortex the retina is mapped in the following manner. The right striate cortex receives projections (via the LGN) from the right (ipsilateral) temporal retina and the left (contralateral) nasal retina, with the consequence that it registers events in the left (contralateral) hemi-field of view. The left striate cortex registers events in the right hemi-field of view. In each striate cortex, the upper retina, registering events in the lower field of view, is represented in the upper lip of the calcarine cortex, while the lower retina, registering events in the upper field of view, is located in the lower lip of the calcarine cortex. Central vision, corresponding to roughly the central 5°, is represented at the pole of the occipital lobe (Figure 3.5). The connections between the retinas and the primary visual cortex, via the LGN, were worked out in great detail in the human brain towards the latter half of the last century by Salomon Henschen in Sweden, and later by Tatsuji Inouye in Japan and Gordon Holmes in England. The one great mistake that Henschen made was to suppose that macular or central vision was represented anteriorly in the striate cortex and peripheral vision posteriorly. As we shall see, this major blunder was one of the reasons why he denied, to the very end, the presence of a colour centre outside the striate cortex.

The consequences of damage to the optic pathways

We can see from this that damage to the retina in one eye, or to its optic nerve, leads to absolute blindness in that eye. The extent of the blindness is related strictly to the extent of the damage. Complete damage to the visual pathways beyond the optic chiasm, i.e. to the optic radiation of one side, or to the LGN or the striate cortex, also leads to blindness but this time the blindness is restricted to the contralateral field of view and is known as a *homonymous hemianopia* (same half of the field of view for each eye). Hence, the term *hemianopic field* refers to a blind field. There are many cases of hemianopia which spare the central 5° of vision, a phenomenon known as *macular sparing*. This phenomenon was the basis of a somewhat fantastic theory of visual representation in the cortex, postulated by Constantine von Monakow, and which we shall examine later. Macular sparing is now usually explained by the fact that the occipital pole receives a dual blood supply, from the posterior and middle cerebral arteries, and that it is consequently protected in cases of vascular accidents affecting one artery only, whereas the rest of the occipital cortex, which receives its blood supply from the posterior cerebral artery only, will be compromised with every vascular accident affecting it.

Damage to the upper lip of the calcarine sulcus will result in blindness in the *lower contralateral field of view*, a phenomenon known as *quadrantanopia*. Equally, damage to the lower lip of the calcarine cortex will lead to blindness in the upper field of view, hence an *upper contralateral quadrantanopia* (Figure 3.7).

When damage does not affect the entire striate cortex but is restricted to a small part of it, the blindness is correspondingly restricted. It is usual to refer to such a small area of blindness as a *scotoma*, thus distinguishing it from hemianopia (Figure 3.7). In general, any blindness which is not hemianopic or quadrantanopic is referred to as a scotoma. The position and extent of the scotoma is usually determined by *perimetry*. The patient faces a hemisphere and fixates a point at its centre. Small spots of light are flashed in different positions on this hemisphere and the patient is asked to report a sensation of light. The positions at which the patient is not able to report a sensation of light are marked and constitute the scotomatous region. Because of the very precise manner in which the retina connects with the primary visual cortex one can, by determining the extent and position of the scotoma, predict the precise region of the cortex affected with a great degree of accuracy. Of course, the scotoma or the hemianopia need not be due to a cortical lesion. A lesion anywhere from the LGN to V1 will yield much the same picture, although in every case the cortex, by being deprived of its input, will be affected. Commonly, blindness is total in the hemianopic or scotomatous field. But there are many interesting cases, discussed later, in which the scotoma is selective, i.e. one in which the patient is able to detect some visual attributes, e.g. motion, but not others, e.g. form.

The manner in which the retina connects with the visual cortex dictates, then, the topographical position of the blind field. In hemi-anopia the blindness is total. But there are other conditions, when there is blindness for only one attribute of vision. When restricted to colour vision such a condition is known as a *hemiachromatopsia*

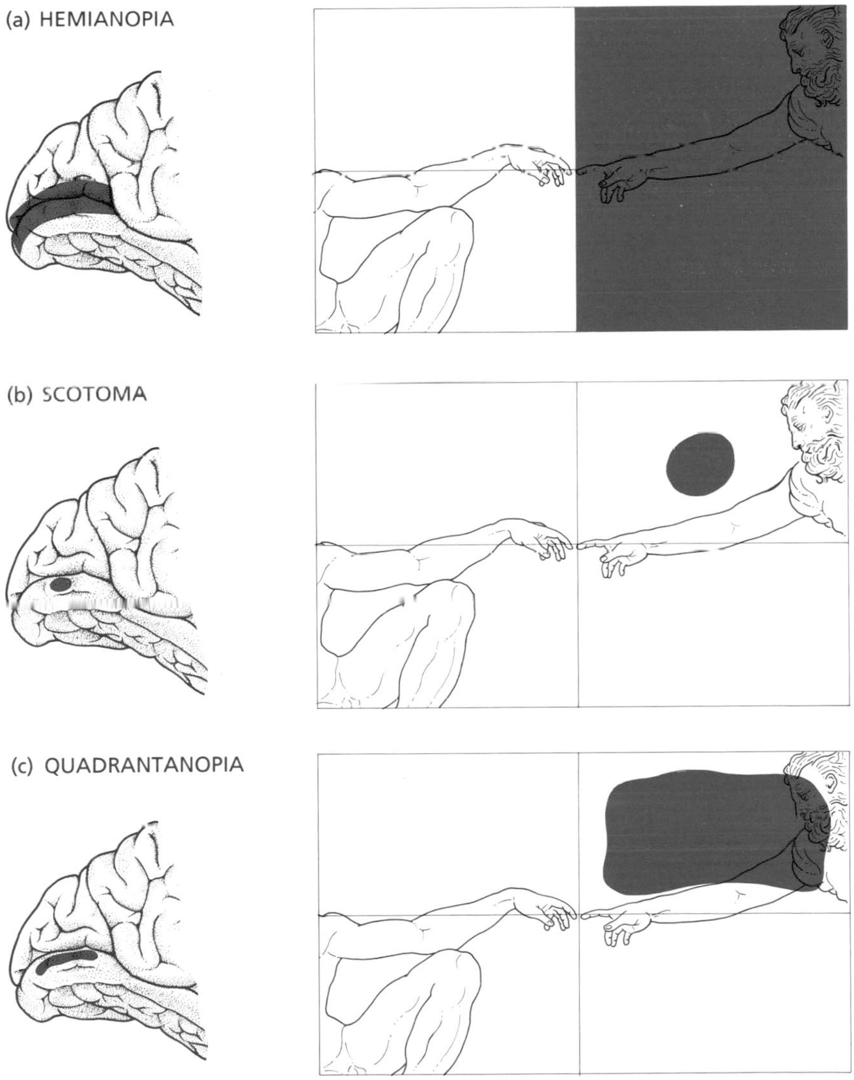

(a) HEMIANOPIA

(b) SCOTOMA

(c) QUADRANTANOPIA

Fig. 3.7 The consequences of lesions in the striate cortex (area V1). (a) The consequence of a total lesion affecting area V1 of the left hemisphere in its entirety; the result is a hemianopia affecting the right half-field of view. (b) A small lesion in the lower lip of the left area V1; the result is a scotoma in the upper quadrant of the right field of view. (c) A larger lesion affecting the lower lip of the left area V1; the consequence is a quadrantanopia restricted to the contralateral upper quadrant of the field of view. Because of the topographical retinal map in V1, one can predict with great accuracy the position of damage to the striate cortex, by noting the area of blindness in the field of view.

when it is confined to one hemi-field and *achromatopsia* when both hemi-fields are involved. In the former case, the cause is a specific lesion in one cerebral hemisphere only, while in the latter both cerebral hemispheres are involved. A rarer condition is one which we shall call *akinetopsia*, in which the subject is specifically unable to see motion in the field of view. So far, no case of *hemiakinetopsia* has been described.

We shall add here that the retina itself, in addition to connecting with the LGN, also connects with a subcortical, midbrain structure known as the superior colliculus and has a direct input to another thalamic nucleus, the pulvinar. We shall not be much concerned with these pathways, though they are important in understanding the symptomatology of certain blindnesses which will be discussed later.

References

1 Henschen, S.E. (1930). *Pathologie des Gehirns*, 8. I. *Lichtsinn—und Farbensinnzellen im Gehirn*. Verlag des Verfassers, Stockholm.
2 Talbot, S.A. & Marshall, W.H. (1941). Physiological studies of neural mechanisms of visual localization and discrimination. *Am. J. Ophthalmol.* **24**, 1255−1264; Daniel, P.M. & Whitteridge, D. (1961). The representation of the visual field on the cerebral cortex in monkeys. *J. Physiol. (Lond.)* **159**, 203−221.
3 Yukie, M. & Iwai, E. (1981). Direct projection from the dorsal lateral geniculate nucleus to the prestriate cortex in macaque monkeys. *J. Comp. Neurol.* **201**, 81−97; Fries, W. (1981). The projection from the lateral geniculate nucleus to the prestriate cortex of the macaque monkey. *Proc. R. Soc. Lond.* B **213**, 73−80.

Chapter 4: Colour in the cerebral cortex

The two cerebral functions, the production of articulate language and of willed movements, localized by Broca and by Fritsch and Hitzig to two geographically distinct parts of the cerebral cortex, nevertheless have a common denominator in that they both involved movement. Given this, is it plausible that two different attributes which share a common denominator in vision, say colour and motion vision, could also have distinct seats in the cerebral cortex? Was there any evidence in favour of such a supposition and, if so, what happened to it?

In 1888, a Swiss ophthalmologist from Neuchatel by the name of Louis Verrey (Figure 4.1) published a remarkable paper entitled *Hémi-achromatopsie droite absolue*.[1] The paper is remarkable both for the quality of evidence in it and for its subdued, modest, tone. In it he described the case of a sixty-year-old woman who had suffered a stroke affecting the occipital lobe of her left hemisphere. The main consequence was an inability to see the world in colour in the right half of her field of view, everything in that half now appearing to her in shades of grey. Colours could be seen normally in the other half. There was, probably to the relief of many sceptics, some diminution in acuity as well as a peripheral blindness (scotoma), largely restricted

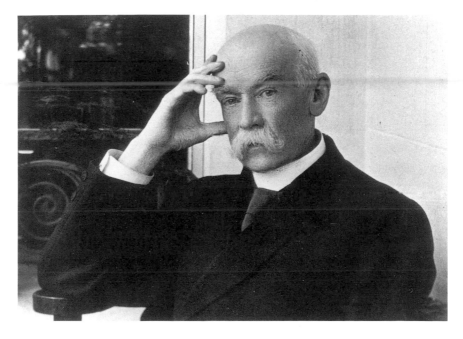

Fig. 4.1 Louis Verrey (1854–1916), Swiss ophthalmologist. He identified the centre for the colour sense in the human cerebral cortex but imagined it to be part of the primary visual cortex. He never pursued the logical consequence of his discovery, of why colour should be separately represented in the cortex. Instead, he opened up a clinic in Lausanne and, perhaps wisely, indulged his interest in French and Italian holidays. (Photograph courtesy of Dr. J.D. Verrey of Lausanne, ophthalmologist and great-grandson of Louis.)

to the upper quarter of the right half of the field of view. But her total inability to see in colour in one half of her field of view was by far the most striking phenomenon.

It was relatively easy, even then, to give a neurological explanation for why the defect was restricted to one side. The pathways from the retina to the brain which account for it are described in the previous chapter. More difficult to explain was the colour blindness resulting from the cerebral lesion, a syndrome known as *cerebral achromatopsia*. The fact that the achromatopsia was accompanied by a peripheral blindness suggested that the primary visual centre, which receives the retinal fibres through the lateral geniculate nucleus, must be damaged. This, together with the fact that there was a severe disturbance in colour vision, in a part of the field of view in which no other abnormality could be demonstrated, led Verrey to believe that within this primary visual centre there must be several subdivisions, one of which is devoted to colour. It was a reasonable conclusion for its time. The fact that the lesion in the brain was largely centred in a cortical area which, *we now know*, lies outside the primary visual cortex did not present a problem to Verrey. At that time, the primary visual cortex had not yet been definitively equated with an anatomical area of unique appearance, the striate cortex. Many considered that it included much more of the occipital lobe[2] (see Figure 4.2).

The implications of Verrey's conclusion were momentous, indeed so momentous that even he failed to see them.[3] For, if colour vision could be specifically and separately compromised, this would suggest that colour is separately represented in the brain. From this it would follow that functional specialization is a much more widespread phenomenon, extending to the submodalities of a modality, in this case the sensation of colour within vision. It would also follow that the cerebral processes involved in vision are not unitary, as our

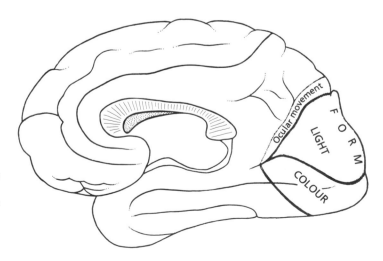

Fig. 4.2 The extent and subdivisions of the primary visual cortex, as depicted in 1906. (Reproduced from Mills C.K. (1906). In *The Eye and the Nervous System*, edited by W.C. Posey & W.G. Spiller. Lippincott, Philadelphia.)

unitary experience of the visual world might suggest. Many profound questions about the brain and about vision would have followed. It is no wonder that this finding was too revolutionary to many.

Verrey's was not the first description of cortical colour blindness. Others had reached similar conclusions about a colour centre in the brain from clinical examination, though most had not had the advantage of a post-mortem examination of their patients' brains. They were thus unable to determine the precise location and extent of the lesions.[2] One can, then, not only marvel at the vigour with which they put their case for a colour centre but also puzzle at how, having put their case, they did not proceed to enquire more deeply into why this should be so. Among these was Hermann Wilbrand, a German neurologist and ophthalmologist. He had supposed from his clinical studies that there are three separate visual centres in the cerebral cortex, one for the 'reception' of 'light impressions', another for 'form impressions' and a third for 'colour impressions', all being subdivisions of the primary visual receptive centre of the cerebral cortex.[4] To account for the fact that colour vision could be selectively compromised, Wilbrand had supposed that these three centres occupied different layers of the same cortical area such that damage sustained by one might spare the other two. Even more impressive was the conclusion of William Gowers (Figure 4.3), Professor of Medicine at University College London. In his book *Diseases of the Nervous System* he wrote that, '...the symptom [hemiachromatopsia] probably depends on disease of one part of the occipital lobe, and is proof of a separate centre for colour vision'.[5] But, unlike Wilbrand, he thought that the colour centre would be an area separate from the area for 'light impressions'. He wrote, 'It is, on the whole, probable that all impressions go first to the region of the apex of the occipital lobe, since disease here causes absolute hemianopia, and that a special half-vision centre for colour lies in front of this'.[6] Events have proved him right in his speculations. The only problem was that he did not have the evidence. His conclusion was based, as in a court of law, on the balance of probabilities.

Verrey had a distinct advantage. He had studied his patient and had been able to examine her brain after death. His conclusion bears the hallmark of authority. He wrote, 'The centre for the chromatic sense will be found in the most inferior part of the occipital lobe, probably in the posterior part of the lingual and fusiform gyri' (Figure 4.4). Unlike Wilbrand, Verrey thought that his 'centre for the chromatic sense' did not constitute a separate layer within the primary visual receptive centre. Instead, he considered it to be a separate part of one large cortical field, the primary visual receptive centre of the cerebral cortex, the remaining parts constituting a centre for 'light impressions' and a centre for 'form impressions'. Thus, to Verrey, the primary

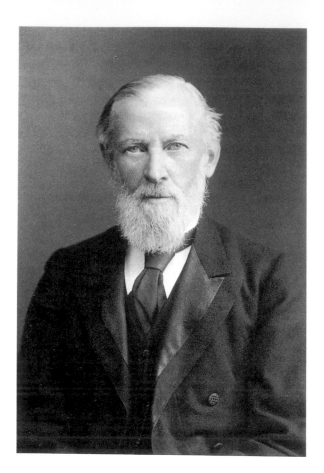

Fig. 4.3 Sir William Gowers (1845–1915), Professor of Medicine at University College London. He had a brilliant insight into the organization of the visual cortex which he never pursued. (Reproduced by permission of the President and Council of the Royal Society.)

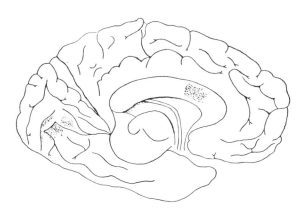

Fig. 4.4 The lesions in the brain examined by Louis Verrey, which led him to the conclusion that the colour centre is situated in the lingual and fusiform gyri. (Reproduced from Verrey, L. (1881). *Archs. Ophtalmol. (Paris)* **8**, 289–301.)

visual receptive area went beyond the confines of the striate cortex and included the cuneus dorsally and the lingual and fusiform gyri (see Figure 4.5). With such confidence in his conclusions, he could afford to be modest. He terminated his article thus: 'All this shows us how many questions about cerebral localization have yet to be settled and how uncertain we are of our grounds. Any new

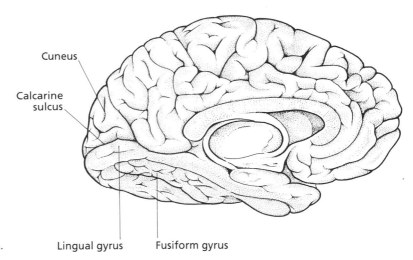

Fig. 4.5 The relationship of the lingual and fusiform gyri to the calcarine sulcus in the human brain.

contribution to this study nevertheless has its importance for the edification of this monument of which Charcot and his students were the founders, and it is this that has led me to publish my observations'.

It has never ceased to surprise me why Verrey, having come this far, could not go beyond and speculate as to why this should be so. He might have opened up a surprisingly fresh enquiry into the functions and functioning of the visual cortex and into the role of colour vision. As it is, there is no evidence that he ever returned to the subject, not even to defend his position against his detractors, although the fact that his paper was re-issued verbatim in 1893 implies that he had not lost faith in his findings.[3] Instead, he established a clinic in Lausanne and acquired a large and faithful clientele, giving his services freely to those in need and ignoring his detractors who began dismissing his evidence even in the year of its publication. In 1888, the very year in which Verrey published his article, Mackay questioned the evidence for a colour centre in the brain on a number of grounds.[7] Chief among these was his belief that the testing of achromatopsic patients had not been adequate and that post-mortem examinations had not been available. The post-mortem examination provided by Verrey did not impress Mackay. In a footnote he wrote that the study of Verrey, '. . . arrives most opportunely to support my contention for more careful clinical study, and affords the additional interest of a post-mortem examination'!

Verrey's observation is repeated . . .

But MacKay's scepticism was not to last long. Eleven years later[8] he had changed his mind following an examination of a single achromatopsic patient whose brain became available for post-mortem study. The patient must have been impressive enough for Mackay to lose sight of the detailed clinical examinations which he had demanded from others earlier. For the 'light sense' in this patient 'was not especially investigated for want of proper means at the patient's house'! But then MacKay's patient had complete colour blindness in his entire field of view, whereas Verrey's 'was one sided (only hemi-achromatopsia) and showed a more extensive lesion of the cerebrum' (though one could argue that Verrey's patient had the advantage, since one could control in the same patient for the absence of colour vision in one half field against its presence in the other). At any rate, Mackay and Dunlop became convinced enough to write that even though, 'one swallow does not make a summer...the facts in this remarkable case, the first, as far as we know, in which a *total* acquired colour blindness from a cerebral lesion has been supported by patho-logical examination, point strongly towards the conclusion that if there is a separate centre for colour, its seat is the grey matter of the fusiform convolution' since their lesion, 'being of still smaller dimen-sions [than Verrey's] carries the prediction a stage further' [original emphasis]. With such generosity was Verrey's primacy in the field acknowledged.

...but the notion of a colour centre is dismissed again

Here entered a problem of anatomy which was to lead to a great deal of confusion, especially when taken in conjunction with the prevalent concept of the day. If the cortical area leading to cortical colour blindness had been situated in the frontal lobes of the brain or at the tip of the temporal cortex, or in a region well removed from the occipital lobes, then the notion of a special colour centre in the brain would probably not have suffered so much. At any rate, it would have been more acceptable. But the area concerned, in the lingual and fusiform gyri, was situated in the occipital lobe (Figure 4.5), just next to what was beginning at the time to emerge, through the work of Henschen and of Flechsig, as the primary visual receptive centre (striate cortex) of the brain. Because vascular lesions do not respect the boundaries of functionally discrete territories in the cortex, it was common to find that lesions whose foci were outside the striate cortex nevertheless also involved the striate cortex as well, to a greater or lesser degree. Experience showed that such an involvement resulted in a scotoma or an area of blindness. With the knowledge derived from this experience it became easy to argue that the observed cerebral colour blindness was a result of the involvement of the striate cortex itself. Or, at any rate, of the involvement of the primary visual receptive centre itself, since not everyone at that time was in agreement with the notion that the primary visual cortex was limited to the striate area. Indeed, as we have seen, Verrey himself was of the opinion that his 'centre for the chromatic sense' was a mere subdivision of this primary visual receptive area. This notion, too, found little favour. Harris[9] wrote emphatically, 'That the cortical half vision centres are not subdivided into centres of light, form and colour respectively, and that hemiachromatopia may be due to a lesion anywhere in the visual path between the chiasm and the cortex'. Moreover, as we shall see, the close proximity of the two cortical zones, the striate cortex and the lingual and fusiform gyri, and the observed colour blindness following a lesion in the latter was an irritation to those who were trying to define the extent of the primary visual centre in the cerebral cortex and limit it to the striate cortex. An easy way around this awkward impasse was to dismiss the evidence purporting to show that there is a colour centre in the brain. Theories of cortical *visual* function of the day helped this process along. No one saw a hint of a similarity between the possible separate representation of colour and of other attributes of vision and the separate representation of different functions which had movement as a common denominator.

The lost opportunity

And a great opportunity was lost. The notion that there might be separate centres in the brain for colour vision, for form vision and for the imprecisely defined 'light' vision would, if pursued, have led to important questions about the visual cortex and about brain function. Why are these attributes of vision represented in separate areas? Are there any other attributes of vision which are separately mapped? Does the brain merely analyze, passively, the visual stimulus? If not, what does it do? How is the retina represented in these distinct visual centres? How is the information contained in them assembled to give us a coherent picture of the visual world? The answers to these questions would have given a new vision of the brain. But the existence of a separate colour centre was never truly established by the clinical evidence, and such evidence as the clinicians had assembled was quickly dismissed. The questions were therefore never asked. It was to be almost a century before neurobiologists began to find these questions interesting, in fact only after separate visual areas in the cortex outside the striate area were discovered experimentally in the monkey.

It would be true to say that the descriptions of Verrey and of Mackay and Dunlop marked the high point for a concept of a colour centre in the brain until the 1970s. Most of the later important papers on the visual cortex, if they dealt with the subject at all, dismissed the notion, even when the evidence they had seemed to speak in favour of such a supposition, as Lenz's evidence[10] did. The grounds on which they dismissed the evidence were not greatly different from those that Mackay had used before his conversion. The real reasons were much more profound, but they had little to do with colour vision itself.

References

1 Verrey, L. (1888). Hémiachromatopsie droite absolue. *Archs. Ophtalmol. (Paris)* **8**, 289−301.
2 Zeki, S. (1990). A century of cerebral achromatopsia. *Brain* **113**, 1721−1777.
3 Zeki, S. (1993). The mystery of Louis Verrey. *Gesnerus* (in press).
4 Wilbrand, H. (1884). *Ophthalmiatrische Beiträge zur Diagnostik der Gehirnkrankheiten.* J.F. Bergmann, Wiesbaden.
5 Gowers, W.R. (1888). *A Manual of Diseases of the Brain.* J. & A. Churchill, London.
6 Gowers, W.R. (1887). *Lectures on the Diagnosis of Diseases of the Brain.* J. & A. Churchill, London.
7 MacKay, G. (1888). A discussion on a contribution to the study of hemianopsia, with special reference to acquired colour-blindness. *Br. Med. J.* **2**, 1033−1037.
8 MacKay, G. & Dunlop, J.C. (1899). The cerebral lesions in a case of complete acquired colour-blindness. *Scot. Med. Surg. J.* **5**, 503−512.
9 Harris, W. (1897). Hemianopia, with especial reference to its transient varieties. *Brain* **20**, 308−364.
10 Lenz, G. (1921). Zwei Sektionsfälle doppelseitiger zentraler Farbenhemianopsie. *Z. Ges. Neurol. Psychiatr.* **71**, 135−186.

Chapter 5: The evidence against a colour centre in the cortex

Anyone looking at the evidence in favour of a separate colour centre in the brain around, say, 1900 could be forgiven for being sceptical but not for dismissing the notion. At a time when the dominant effort was to define the primary visual receptive area in the cerebral cortex, the area which neurologists believed was responsible for seeing, the evidence for a colour centre was weak. This was especially so since the putative centre was thought by its proponents to lie outside the area that was beginning to be defined as the one responsible for 'seeing', and within the territory of what was beginning to be considered as the cortex responsible for 'understanding' what was seen. In brief, not only was the evidence anatomically unpersuasive but it was also in conflict with concepts of the organization of visual cortex that were prevalent at the time, and these concepts explained much, or so it seemed.

The numbers game

Leading those who were trying to chart and define the primary visual receptive centre in the brain was Salomon Henschen. To do so, he had amassed a large number of cases of blindness due to cerebral lesions, boasting that, '...I have found in my hospital in Uppsala, nearly 40 hemianopic cases, supplemented in the post-mortem records; whilst Seguin, in 1886, could only discover about the same number in the whole of literature'.[1] He had concluded correctly from this mass of material that the primary visual receptive centre in the brain was co-extensive with the anatomically distinct striate cortex, and that adjacent retinal points are mapped in adjacent cortical points. This rigid point-to-point representation of the retina on the striate cortex led Henschen to conceive of the latter as the 'cortical retina',[2] a term not devoid of a theoretical implication and one which reflects well his view that it is with the striate area that the brain 'sees'. Henschen thus made an outstanding contribution to our understanding of the organization of the primary visual receptive centre in the brain. He was very proud of his discovery and became very irritated when he was not credited with it, chiding one author (Alouf) for naming all investigators, 'with the exception of the one who was the first to give a detailed description of the area, namely Henschen...my name does not even appear in the bibliography' when, in fact, 'By comparison with my photos...I find Alouf's descriptions not only useless, but incorrect throughout'.[3] Those today who find themselves unjustly not quoted for their discoveries will no doubt feel more sympathetic to Henschen than the habitual 'non-quoters'.

The topographic connections between the retina and the striate, or calcarine, cortex uncovered by Henschen and others explained a great deal. A lesion affecting the striate cortex would lead to a total (hemianopic) blindness in the opposite field of view, or to only a relatively small area of blindness — a scotoma. Patients were unable to see anything, including colours, in their scotomatous, or blind, fields. If the lesion was in the upper lip of the calcarine sulcus, where the upper retina is mapped, the area of blindness would be in the lower quadrant of the visual field because the upper retina 'sees' the lower part of the field of view. *If the lesions were in the lower lip of the calcarine sulcus, the area of blindness would be located in the upper quadrant of the field of view* (Figure 5.1), a critical point for understanding the arguments in favour of and against a separate colour

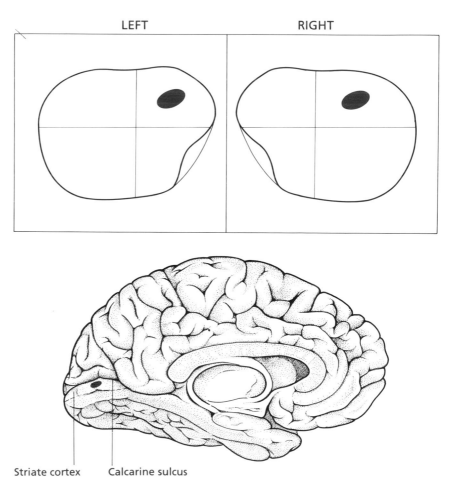

Fig. 5.1 Damage to the lower lip of the calcarine sulcus causes a scotoma in the contralateral upper retinal quadrant.

Striate cortex   Calcarine sulcus

centre in the brain. This rigid localization of the retinal surface on the primary visual receptive centre therefore accounted well for the mass of evidence showing the consequences of lesions in the striate cortex. Colour vision was not immune to the effects of such lesions, but was compromised along with every other attribute of vision. How natural then to suppose that colour 'impressions', along with other visual 'impressions', were received by the sole visual receptive centre in the brain, the striate cortex, and analyzed there. This seemed to correlate well with our unitary perception of the visual world.

By comparison, the evidence for a colour centre in the brain, lying outside the striate cortex, was derived from a few cases only. Of these, the most impressive, because they were accompanied by post-mortem studies, were those of Verrey,[4] of MacKay and Dunlop[5] and, much later, of Lenz.[6] The proponents of a colour centre had supposed that lesions in the neighbourhood of, but outside, the striate cortex would affect colour vision selectively. Yet, as von Monakow had emphasized, almost every case of achromatopsia was complicated by secondary disorders.[7] Most had an associated scotoma, as indeed did the patients of Verrey and Dunlop and MacKay. To many, this implied that a lesion in the striate cortex itself was the causative factor, since lesions here were known to produce blindness. They supposed, though without enquiring why, that colour vision was more susceptible to the effects of a lesion in the striate cortex and, hence, that it could be disturbed more or less selectively. This would explain, so they believed, the syndrome of cerebral colour blindness.

The repetition of tedious arguments

We find more or less the same argument used tediously at regular intervals over half a century. During the Great War, Marie and Chatelin, the French neurologists, argued that, 'It is in effect classical to consider hemiachromatopsia as resulting from a mild lesion of the visual sphere or radiation'.[8] Some half a century later, Teuber and his colleagues in America used much the same argument. They wrote, 'There is thus no evidence for a genuine dissociation of color and form vision... Seemingly selective impairment of one aspect of vision (e.g. color discrimination) reflects, we believe, a corresponding rank order in the vulnerability of different levels of function, in the presence of lesions in their common substrate'.[9] In between, in 1945, Holmes (Figure 5.2) had written somewhat dogmatically that, '... the striate area of visual cortex is merely a perceptive centre... the perception of colour also depends on [it]; mild lesions of the cortex which do not abolish perception of light frequently disturb colour vision; there is no evidence that this is subserved by any other region of the brain'.[10] Such a statement gained added authority from the fact that Holmes

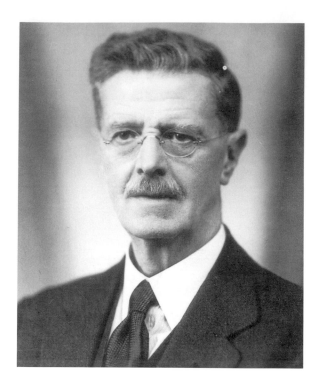

Fig. 5.2 Sir Gordon Holmes (1876–1965), the doyen of British neurologists during the first half of this century. He has been described as a man 'of strong likes and dislikes with little inclination to diplomacy or compromise'. One of the ideas which he disliked most, like the American psychologist Hans-Lucas Teuber (1916–1977), was the idea of a dissociation of visual functions following cerebral lesions. (Reproduced by permission of the President and Council of the Royal Society.)

had studied 'hundreds of cases' of brain injuries acquired in the Great War,[11] and was therefore to be trusted more than those who had tried to erect suspect and parvenu theories by studying a few isolated cases, or so neurologists believed. Much effort was expended, especially by Henschen in his eighth decade, in trying to prove that the striate cortex was also a centre for the reception of colour impressions and that no separate visual receptive centre existed outside it.

Thus, the presence of a scotoma in almost every reported case of achromatopsia argued strongly for involvement of the striate cortex. But the fact that the scotomas of achromatopsic patients invariably affected their peripheral vision and spared their central vision, as well as the fact that they always involved the upper part of their field of view, made little impression on Henschen. In fairness, it made no impression on anyone else either, until Meadows pointed it out in 1974.[12] If Henschen had taken the few available cases of achromatopsia seriously and studied the position of the scotomas, he would have found some evidence against his view of how central vision is represented in the primary visual cortex (see below). But there is no evidence that he took any of this seriously and the view among neurologists who considered the matter at all was that there just weren't enough cases from which to draw adequate conclusions.

Equally impressive was the fact that, in most cases of cerebral colour blindness, there were other associated disorders, chiefly an inability to recognize familiar faces, a syndrome known as *prosopagnosia*. We know that this is due to the fact that the area critical for the perception of familiar faces is also located in the fusiform gyrus, neighbouring the colour centre though distinct from it.[13] But before this was known the coincidence suggested to some, among them the American neuropsychologist Karl Lashley, that a defect in the perception of colours was the consequence of a more diffuse cortical involvement, resulting in its inability to undertake complex functions.[14] An alternative explanation might be that even small lesions in the association cortex have many effects. It was awkward to reach definite conclusions. Indeed, it may be said that the association of other disorders with the achromatopsia, along with the presence of the scotomas, constituted perhaps the most powerful grounds for doubting the presence of a separate colour centre in the brain.

But to dismiss the evidence was another matter. The rarity of cases has not prevented acceptance of conclusions about the brain, before or since. From more recent times one could give as an example the single case study of Zihl and his colleagues[15] on the motion-blind patient. This is particularly interesting, for its acceptance was immediate because, as I shall later show, it was not in contradiction to the concepts prevailing at the time it was made, as was the syndrome of cerebral achromatopsia when it was first described.[16] Moreover, even the presence of scotomas did not invalidate the case for a separate colour centre.

Achromatopsia is a defect of central vision

Because we see colour best with our central vision and poorly or not at all with our peripheral vision, it is obvious that the syndrome of cerebral colour blindness is one of central vision, in which patients complain of an inability to see colours in their central visual fields. Yet the scotomas accompanying the cerebral achromatopsias were commonly peripheral and always included the upper visual fields, though they were sometimes more extensive. This critical condition can be accounted for by the fact that the lingual and fusiform gyri lie ventral to the inferior limb of the calcarine sulcus, where the upper visual fields are mapped. In any case, the association of peripheral scotomas with a colour blindness in central visual fields should have made Henschen feel uncomfortable, and probably did so. If accepted it would reveal an inconsistency in the conclusions which he had reached regarding the nature of retinal representation in the striate cortex. He had supposed, wrongly as it turned out, that the centre of vision is represented anteriorly in the striate cortex, i.e. in the very anterior extremity of the calcarine sulcus, whereas it is actually represented posteriorly, at the convexity of the occipital pole (see Figure 5.3). That

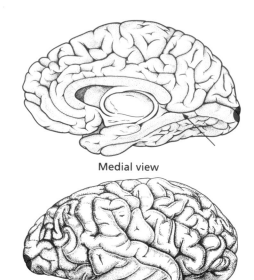

Medial view

Lateral view of right hemisphere

Fig. 5.3 Central vision (the vision used for seeing objects and details) is represented in the occipital pole (shown in red). Henschen thought that it was represented in the anterior part of the calcarine sulcus (arrow). He became very angry when his belief was questioned.

an anteriorly placed lesion should lead to a central defect was consistent with Henschen's erroneous view. That the defect should be more or less specific to colour vision could then be accounted for by supposing that colour is more vulnerable to cortical lesions, as many were to suppose later. But the presence of an absolute *peripheral* scotoma associated with a central defect for colour vision alone made the interpretation more awkward. It implied either that both the periphery and the centre are represented in the anterior portion of the calcarine sulcus, a notion that would put paid to Henschen's 'rigid localization', or that the periphery alone was represented there, which would be incompatible with Henschen's view that it is the centre that is represented there. Put more bluntly, Henschen found himself trapped. Perhaps because of this, he chose to ignore the evidence altogether. Von Monakow at least saw the contradiction and argued that the case of MacKay and Dunlop,[5] with a peripheral scotoma following an anteriorly situated lesion, was incompatible with Henschen's schema of the manner in which the retina is mapped in the calcarine or striate cortex.[17] He had seen the inconsistency but did not pursue it. He had his own views about macular representation in the cortex. These were even further removed from reality than Henschen's.

There had in fact been other cases, not themselves directly used as evidence for or against the notion of a colour centre, but nevertheless interesting in that if they had been more carefully considered, the case for a colour centre may have become more acceptable, or at least they would have added their weight to the scant evidence. One such case was Förster's.[18] His patient, following a successive double hemianopia which had spared his central vision, had suffered from loss of colour vision and spatial disorientation; he could not recognize large objects, but could read and recognize small ones. This patient had been autopsied by Sachs, who reported his findings to the International Medical Congress in Paris in 1900, perhaps not the most amicable meeting in the history of neurology. Sachs had found a large vascular damage involving the fusiform and lingual gyri of both hemispheres but not the pole of the occipital lobe, where central (macular) vision is represented. He concluded correctly that central vision is represented posteriorly in the occipital pole, and peripheral vision anteriorly in the limbs of the calcarine sulcus. In brief, he concluded that Henschen had been wrong in this respect. So here was a case which complemented previous cases of cerebral colour blindness. Central vision was spared, but colour vision was gone. The common feature was a lesion extending anteriorly and involving the lingual and fusiform gyri. Yet this aroused not a tremor of interest. Instead, Henschen denounced Sachs' findings hysterically, stating that, '...this case proves NOTHING on the subject of the localization of the macula'[19] [his emphasis] and insisting that the optic radiations must have been involved. As we shall see, the optic radiations and the white matter in general were to come to the rescue of many a faltering argument several times again in the future.

The post-mortem evidence is dismissed

Another argument used to dismiss the notion of a colour centre in the brain was that relating to post-mortem examination. The post-mortem evidence that Verrey and MacKay and Dunlop had provided, although far better than anything Broca could come up with in 1861 in relation to the localization of language, was judged not to be sufficient. A striking example of this can be found in the writings of Lenz.[6] Lenz's patient had developed an achromatopsia affecting, by definition, his central visual fields, coupled with a scotoma restricted to the upper contralateral, retinal quadrant. Lenz was determined to conduct a minute 'microscopic' post-mortem examination, considering that previous 'macroscopic' examinations showed nothing more than that a lesion anywhere in the visual pathway could lead to colour vision defects. He waxed eloquent about his own study, believing it to 'represent the beginning of systematic attempts to penetrate this great riddle of nature'. His examination showed a lesion in the fusiform gyrus and a more or less intact striate cortex. Incredibly, this led him inexorably in the direction of white matter, a favourite refuge and one used previously by von Monakow, among others. He concluded that the loss of colour vision had resulted from lesions in the white matter and the consequent interruption of impulse conduction, followed by some secondary atrophy and degeneration. The involvement of the fusiform gyrus made little impression on him. He wrote, 'the clinical demonstration of a far-reaching dissociation between spatial and colour perception led to the assumption of a special colour centre located in the fusiform gyrus...Wilbrand had previously pointed to physiological results and I have indicated the pathological anatomical findings which appear to render such an assumption untenable', although in his material the lesion in the fusiform gyrus had at least equal claim to have been the causative factor.

The domino of fragile concepts

It is therefore obvious that, however weak the evidence in favour of a colour centre in the brain outside the striate cortex may have been, the evidence against the notion was weaker still. That the notion of a colour centre was nevertheless dismissed was due to the powerful and pervasive concepts of the day, concepts which we shall discuss in the next few chapters. Central to these concepts, and the first among them, was the neurologists' philosophical view of vision and, indeed, of the brain, the supposition that cortical vision was a dual process consisting, first, of the reception and analysis of visual 'impressions' — the process which led to 'seeing' — and, next, of their 'association' with previous impressions — a process which led to 'understanding' what was seen, each process having a separate and anatomically distinct cortical seat. It followed from this that there is a single cortical area which uniquely receives and analyzes all visual 'impressions', including colour, and another, distinct area which makes sense of these impressions. This belief gained much from the third concept, that a distinctive cortical function such as 'seeing' should be reflected in a distinctive cortical architecture, while a function such as 'association' should be reflected in a different cortical architecture. It followed from this that an absence of architectonic differences implied an absence of functional differences. The fourth concept supposed that the sole strategy that the brain uses to analyze the visual environment is a hierarchical strategy, an analytic doctrine much aided by the fifth concept which supposed that the information in the visual environment is labelled and the function of the brain is merely to analyze that label. All these concepts were intertwined and there were solid reasons for adhering to them, or so people imagined. To overturn such concepts required a good deal more than a few cases of achromatopsia. But the fragility of these concepts was such that, apart from the third, once one of them was shown to be false the rest collapsed, as in a domino game.

References

1 Henschen, S.E. (1893). On the visual path and centre. *Brain* **16**, 170–180.

2 Henschen, S.E. (1894). Sur les centres optiques cérébraux. *Rev. Gén. Ophtal. (Paris)* **13**, 337–352.

3 Henschen, S.E. (1930). *Pathologie des Gehirns*, 8. I. *Lichtsinn–und Farbensinnzellen im Gehirn*. Verlag des Verfassers, Stockholm.

4 Verrey, L. (1888). Hémiachromatopsie droite absolue. *Archs. Ophtalmol. (Paris)* **8**, 289–301.

5 MacKay, G. & Dunlop, J.C. (1899). The cerebral lesions in a case of complete acquired colour-blindness. *Scot. Med. Surg. J.* **5**, 503–512.

6 Lenz, G. (1921). Zwei Sektionsfälle doppelseitiger zentraler Farbenhemianopsie. *Z. Ges. Neurol. Psychiatr.* **71**, 135–186.

7 Monakow, C. von (1914). *Die Lokalisation im Grosshirn*. (Quoted by K.S. Lashley (1948). The mechanism of vision. XVIII. Effects of destroying the visual 'associative areas' of the monkey. *Genet. Psychol. Monogr.* **37**, 107–166.)

8 Marie, P. & Chatelin, C. (1915). Les troubles visuels dus aux lésions des voies optiques intracérébrales et de la sphère visuelle corticale dans les blessures du crane par coup de feu. *Rev. Neurol. (Paris)* **22**, 882–925.

9 Teuber, H.-L., Battersby, W.S. & Bender, M.B. (1960). *Visual Field Defects After Penetrating Missile Wounds of the Brain*. Harvard University Press, Cambridge.

10 Holmes, G. (1945). The Ferrier Lecture: The organization of the visual cortex in man. *Proc. R. Soc. Lond.* B **132**, 348–361.

11 Holmes, G. (1931). A contribution to the cortical representation of vision. *Brain* **54**, 470–479.

12 Meadows, J.C. (1974). Disturbed perception of colours associated with localized cerebral lesions. *Brain* **97**, 615–632.

13 Meadows, J.C. (1974). The anatomical basis of prosopagnosia. *J. Neurol. Neurosurg. Psychiatr.* **37**, 489–501.

14 Lashley, K.S. (1948). loc. cit. [7].

15 Zihl, J., Cramon, D. von. & Mai, N. (1983). Selective disturbance of movement vision after bilateral brain damage. *Brain* **106**, 313–340.

16 Zeki, S. (1990). A century of cerebral achromatopsia. *Brain* **113**, 1721–1777.

17 Monakow, C. von (1905). *Gehirnpathologie*, Vol. 4, *Verstopfung der Hirnarterien*. Hölder, Vienna.

18 Förster, O. (1890). Ueber Rindenblindheit. *Albrecht v. Graefes Arch. Ophthal.* **36**, 94–108.

19 Henschen, S.E. (1900). Sur le centre cortical de la vision. In *XIII Congrés International de Médecine (Ophtalmologie), Paris*, edited by M. Rochon-Duvigneaud, pp. 232–245. Masson & Cie, Paris.

Chapter 6: The concept of the duality of the visual process

For nearly a century now, neurologists have been greatly influenced by the speculations of a German neurologist named Heinrich Lissauer and by the work of Hermann Munk before him. Munk had shown that, following certain cortical lesions, dogs could see but could not recognize objects in their visual world, although they recovered a few weeks after the lesions had been made. He called this phenomenon *Seelenblindheit*, or mind-blindness, an affliction that some of my friends diagnose in many of their colleagues, both ancient and modern! Based on clinical evidence and on the descriptions of Munk, Lissauer speculated that the cortical processes involved in vision were twofold.[1] The first consisted of the process of reception of 'visual impressions' and its conscious perception. This he designated as *apperception*, a term derived from Leibniz and popular among early psychologists, especially Wundt, and which, strangely enough, means perception. Lissauer defined apperception, '. . . as the highest degree of perception, in which the consciousness accepts the sensory impression with maximal intensity'. Next there followed the process of 'connecting other conceptions (ideas) with the content of the perceptions; this is an act of association' and which gave the perceptions their meaning. He considered mental blindness to be the consequence of an apperceptive disturbance and implied that it may be the result of a lesion in the primary visual receptive cortex. He wrote, 'Mental blindness accompanied by partial defects of the still perceived visual half field would be of cortical origin'. The white matter was ever ready to lend a helping hand around difficult impasses. For Lissauer considered that without these 'partial defects', mental blindness would be due to damage of 'transcortical origin'.[1]

The concept of association cortex and its implications

Soon these ideas were modified somewhat. The striate cortex came to be considered the 'perceptive' visual cortex and the cortex surrounding it, which includes the cortex of the lingual and fusiform gyri, came to be conceived of as 'association' cortex. This notion received powerful support from the brilliant myelogenetic work of the Professor of Psychiatry at Leipzig, Paul Flechsig.[2] Flechsig had found that certain areas of the cortex, which he called 'primordial' and among which he numbered the striate cortex, were myelinated at birth. In other words, the nerve fibres of the cells there, as well as the fibres reaching them, had acquired their coverings, or myelin sheaths, at birth. These areas were connected with the sense organs but not with each other. Interposed between the primordial areas were the 'intermediate' and 'terminal' zones which formed the association cortex (*Assoziationszentren*) and which became myelinated much later, as if maturing while the organism was acquiring its experience (Figure 6.1). The association centres were not connected with the sense organs, but received their inputs from the primordial areas. Flechsig thought that he had seen in this arrangement a fundamental insight into cortical function, dismissing other views about the causes of the differences in the pattern of myelination as 'totally useless from a scientific point of view'. He expounded his views in numerous articles, of which one was somewhat grandly entitled *Gehirnphysiologie und Willenstheorien*.[3] The term 'apperception' was not one that Flechsig felt comfortable with, writing that, 'on the one hand it explains too much and on the other hand too little'.[3] But he believed that association

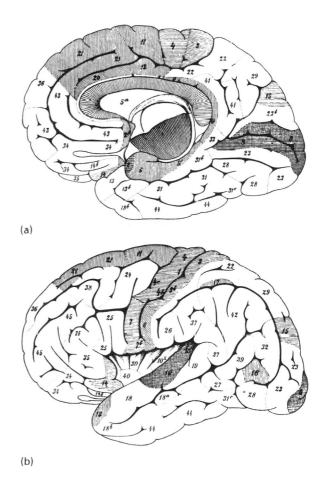

(a)

(b)

Fig. 6.1 The 'primordial' areas of the cortex (shaded), as charted by Paul Flechsig. (a) When one half is cut away (medial view). (b) Lateral view. (Reproduced from Flechsig, P. (1920). *Anatomie des menschlichen Gehirns und Rückenmarks*. Thieme, Leipzig.)

cortex was the repository of 'psychic' functions (*Cogitationszentren*), zones which play a fundamental role in the associative stage of Lissauer.

Gradually, these ideas gained prominence among visual neurologists, though in a distorted and simpler manner than intended by Flechsig and Lissauer. Historians of science may well claim with justice that the way in which the ideas of Flechsig and Lissauer were used by visual neurologists does an injustice to these ideas. This may well be so, but the important point is that it is these, possibly distorted, ideas that began to dominate thinking about the nature of visual representation in the brain. Neurologists began to consider that, in functional terms, the apperceptive stage corresponded to the activity of the striate, or primary visual, cortex which Holmes was later to qualify as the visual 'perceptive' cortex.[4] This would receive passively all the visual impressions formed on the retina and a defect in it would lead to a corresponding area of blindness or scotoma. Flechsig himself drew considerable satisfaction from the close correspondence between his 'primary' visual sphere, as myelogenetically defined, and the calcarine, or striate, cortex as defined by Henschen, whom he considered to be 'the most careful worker in the field'.[2] He wrote, 'We become more and more convinced that only the gyri on either side of the calcarine fissure...receive the visual radiation. No other part of the cortex leads with certainty at least in man to a defect in the visual field and...the region...shows absolutely sharp boundaries...If only this field represents the entering place of the visual radiation into the organ of psyche we can delimit the functional circumference of the primary visual sphere in a very sharp manner'.[3] The 'impressions' thus received would be passed on to the 'visuopsychic' cortex, there to be associated with previous visual 'impressions' of a similar kind, leading to recognition. These ideas are clearly summarized towards the beginning of this century, and were not to change much until the 1970s. Bolton[5] wrote, 'A general review...shows that cortical visual representation has been described as twofold, consisting of a primary region in each hemisphere for the reception of impressions passing from the corresponding halves of both eyes, and a secondary, possibly psychic centre in each hemisphere...'. Not much later Campbell[6] wrote in a similar vein of two areas, 'one specialized for the primary reception of visual sensations, the other constituted for the final elaboration and interpretation of these sensations' (Figure 6.2). The idea that colour, considered to be one of the primary visual 'impressions' formed in the retina to be transmitted to the cortex, should be received in an area outside the one devoted to the reception of all visual impressions and, moreover, that that area should be in what was considered then to be 'visuopsychic' or association cortex, was unpalatable. It ran counter to the knowledge that neurologists had derived from experience.

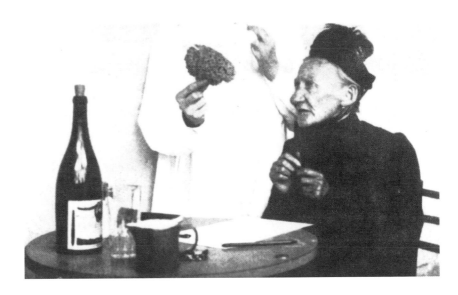

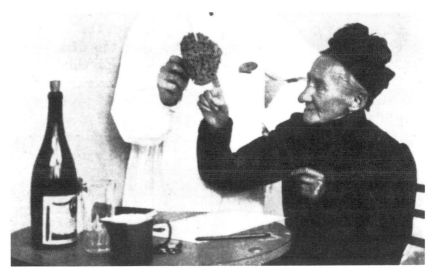

Fig. 6.2 This figure, of a lady who obviously 'sees' but cannot 'understand' what she sees unless she uses another sense, is a classic illustration of how neurologists believed the visual cortex is organized. (Reproduced from von Stauffenberg, F. (1914). *Arb. Hirnanat. Inst. Zurich* **8**, 1–212.)

If only neurologists had known about an alternative view of what colour vision is...

It is interesting to note that there was, at the time, an alternative view of colour vision and one which neurologists could plausibly be said to have been acquainted with. Others, less involved with the brain but experts on colour vision nevertheless, had considered that colour vision is an elaborate process, requiring the use of memory, learning and judgement — the very functions which neurologists had delegated to the visuo-psychic cortex. Helmholtz and Hering considered, at least implicitly, that colour vision involves knowledge and thus that higher processes must be involved, though they did not explicitly refer to the cortex or specify where in the cortex colour may be processed. They invoked these higher processes in order to be able to account for the phenomenon that psychologists have called, perhaps inappropriately, colour constancy. Helmholtz wrote, 'By seeing objects of the same colour under these various illuminations, in spite of the difference of illumination, we *learn* to form a correct idea of the colour of bodies, that is to *judge* how such a body would look in white light; and since we are only interested in the colour that the body retains permanently, we are not conscious at all of the separate sensations which contribute to form our *judgement*', since the determination of colour is, '...not due to an act of sensation *but to an act of judgement*'[7] [my emphasis]. Hering also postulated higher cortical factors. He wrote, 'All objects that are already known to us from *experience*, or that we regard as familiar by their color, we see through the spectacles of *memory* color, and on that account quite differently from the way we would otherwise see them'[8] [my emphasis]. In similar vein, Clerk Maxwell spoke of colour as being 'a mental science'.[9] Learning, judgement, knowledge, memory, experience — here was the stuff that would involve the visual association cortex, at least according to the concepts prevalent in those days. And here was another view of colour vision, from men with high positions in the world of learning, whose writings antedate the debate on the colour centre in the cerebral cortex by at least three decades. Were the neurologists aware of these views? If they were, they must have guarded the secret very closely, for it is difficult to find any discussion about the nature of colour vision in any of the neurological papers debating the issue of a colour centre in the brain. To those neurologists, and to others since, colour was a visual 'impression' like any other visual impression, and its 'analysis' had to involve the visual receptive centre in the cortex alone. This seemed logical enough. After all, all the fibres in the optic pathway terminate in the striate cortex and lesions there lead to absolute blindness, including a blindness for colour. What is perhaps more difficult to accept today, though comprehensible in the light of the then conceptual framework, is that, without exception, they were not prepared to entertain the notion that colour may involve the striate cortex *and* other specialized areas outside as well. Not entertaining such a notion, and aware of the evidence showing a dissociation of colour, they sought for a way of finding a specialization for colour within the striate cortex itself. Hence the view of Poppelreuter[10] that there must be a segregation for colour in the striate cortex. Henschen devoted a whole book, the last of his eight-volume *Pathologie des Gehirns*,[11] to the topic. The volume was written in his eighty-third year, obviously because '...the seemingly intractable problem of the anatomical cerebral organization of colour perception...which had been regarded as insoluble' was to haunt him to the end of his life and he considered it '. . .appropriate, especially in view of my age and my declining strength, to publish my studies at once'. His starting point is his discovery of 'the law of the size of cells' which states, 'the more peripheral the cells are situated in the visual centre, the larger are the cells. . .in order to be able to receive more light'. Since smaller cells are concerned with macular vision, they must therefore be the ones that are concerned with colour. There are plenty of small cells in layer 4 of the striate cortex, from which it follows that the colour centre is in the striate cortex. The argument is hardly worth developing further here. It is merely interesting to note that every item of evidence, however flimsy, was used to prove that 'the cortical retina is also a retina for colour impressions'.[12]

If neurologists were ignorant of what eminent scientists were saying about colour vision, the eminent scientists had little notion of what was happing in the clinical world, probably because of the unjustified contempt in which scientists usually hold the work of clinicians, believing their methods to be unscientific. Although the first edition of Helmholtz's great work was published before the debate on a colour centre in the cerebral cortex began, the 1911 edition, prepared by his disciples, contains no mention of cerebral achromatopsia. And, in general, I am not aware of any serious discussion, or indeed any discussion, of cerebral achromatopsia in relation to colour physiology in any scientific text of the relevant period. Had scientists taken the clinical evidence seriously, as indicative of complex processes occurring in the brain, they might have swayed the opinion of clinicians, ever respectful of scientists, and induced them to consider the clinical evidence more seriously. As it happens, the two groups remained unaware of each others ideas.

Hence the doctrine that vision is a dual process, of which the second phase is merely associational, prevented acceptance of evidence which implied that a visual 'impression', colour, should be 'received' by the associational cortex. To accept this evidence would have entailed changing one's view of how the brain works in vision. If only the early neurologists had grasped the notion that colour is much more than a mere visual 'impression', that indeed it involves a problem of knowledge by the brain, knowledge about certain properties of objects, then things might have been different.

References

1 Lissauer, H. (1890). Ein Fall von Seelenblindheit nebst einem Beitrage zur Theorie derselben. *Arch. Psychiatr. Nervenkr.* **21**, 222−270.

2 Flechsig, P. (1901). Developmental (myelogenetic) localisation of the cerebral cortex in the human subject. *Lancet* **ii**, 1027−1029.

3 Flechsig, P. (1905). Gehirnphysiologie und Willenstheorien. *Fifth International Psy-*

chology Congress, pp. 73–89. (Translated by G. von Bonin (1960). In *Some Papers on the Cerebral Cortex*. C.C. Thomas, Springfield.)

4 Holmes, G. (1945). The Ferrier Lecture: The organization of the visual cortex in man. *Proc. R. Soc. Lond.* B **132**, 348–361.

5 Bolton, J.S. (1900). The exact histological localisation of the visual area of the human cerebral cortex. *Philos. Trans. R. Soc. Lond.* **193**, 165–222.

6 Campbell, A.W. (1905). *Histological Studies on the Localisation of Cerebral Function*. Cambridge University Press, Cambridge.

7 Helmholtz, H. von (1911). *Handbuch der Physiologischen Optik*. Voss, Hamburg.

8 Hering, E. (1877). *Outlines of a Theory of the Light Sense*. (Translated by L.M. Hurvich & D. Jameson, 1964.) Harvard University Press, Cambridge.

9 Maxwell, J.C. (1872). On colour vision. *Proc. R. Instn. GB* **6**, 260–271.

10 Poppelreuter, W. (1923). Zur Psychologie und Pathologie der optischen Wahrnehmung. *Z. Ges. Neurol. Psychiatr.* **83**, 26–152.

11 Henschen, S.E. (1930). *Pathologie des Gehirns*, 8. I. *Lichtsinn–und Farbensinnzellen im Gehirn*. Verlag des Verfassers, Stockholm.

12 Henschen, S.E. (1894). Sur les centres optiques cérébraux. *Rev. Gén. Ophtal. (Paris)* **13**, 337–352.

Chapter 7: The extent of the visual receptive cortex

Given the concept of a separation between 'seeing' and 'understanding' what is seen, it is not surprising to find that much of the early work in support of this doctrine was devoted to charting the extent and precise location of the visual receptive centre responsible for seeing and to unravelling the nature of visual representation within it. One must not conclude that the concept came first and the search next. Rather, the two fed each other and seemed to be in perfect harmony, at least to neurologists. Verrey had implied that his colour centre was part of the primary visual receptive centre, though specialized for the reception of colour impressions. There were, however, other views about the position and extent of the cortex that 'received' the 'visual impressions'. The two views which commanded most attention, and which were antagonistic to each other, were those of von Monakow and of Henschen. These two neurologists disliked each other. Their views about the nervous system were so opposed that without total capitulation by one side or the other there could have been no meeting ground between them. They were nevertheless agreed on one point, that there is no colour centre outside the striate cortex. They therefore joined forces in burying this evidence.

Von Monakow's concept of a 'mobile retinal centre'...

Von Monakow had his own vision of the brain. He had been impressed by a recurrent feature occurring with scotomas and hemianopias due to lesions of the occipital cortex, namely, that central (macular) vision is commonly spared, a phenomenon known as *macular sparing* (Figure 7.1). Today we account for this in two ways. One is the dual blood supply to the occipital pole, which receives branches of both the middle and posterior cerebral arteries; an occlusion of one would still leave the other intact. Another explanation lies in the fact that, along the vertical meridian of the retina, are ganglion cells whose axons may cross over to the opposite side of the brain and others whose fibres remain uncrossed.[1] But this knowledge was not available at the time, the most exhaustive study of the blood supply of the occipital lobe having been published by Beevor in 1907.[2] Macular sparing made a deep impression on von Monakow. It fitted rather well with other views he entertained about the brain, namely its plasticity. He believed that, if a lesion destroyed some part of the brain, then impulses

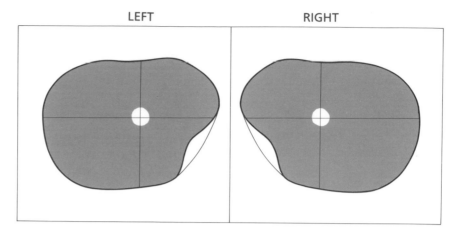

Fig. 7.1 Macular sparing is a condition in which, following extensive lesions of the striate cortex which lead to total blindness or to a hemianopia (red), central vision is spared so that the subject can still read and fixate objects.

could be routed to another part, which would then acquire the functions of the lost part. Such a view led him to the doctrine of a mobile retinal centre, in which central vision could be represented in a number of different positions in the occipital lobe. His view was summarized many years later by Henschen[3] who wrote, 'The famous brain scientist Constantine v. Monakow...learned that, when a lesion affects some cells in the geniculate or in the visual centre, the visual impulse from the eye can be transferred in the geniculate or the visual centre to adjacent cells. This theory completely dominated all his views on the operations of the brain. But if it is true that a sensory impulse can be transferred through an intermediary ganglion to several central organs, then there can be no distinct localization in the cerebral cortex. From this view he drew all the consequences and became so dominated by this new doctrine that, for the sake of theory, he denied even the most undeniable facts. This was the case particularly as regards the visual pathways and centre, whereby he came into contradictions with his own experience. This [v. Monakow's] doctrine was disastrous for the development of the theory of visual function, and during almost thirty years he persistently fought the present author [Henschen] who, on the basis of facts, advocated a strict localization' (see Figure 7.2).

There was much in favour of von Monakow's view, or so he imagined. Firstly, there was the phenomenon of macular sparing, repeatedly observed and beyond doubt. Förster's case, of a patient whose occipital lobe was damaged but whose occipital pole (where central vision is represented) was intact, provided a good example, and he used it. Explaining that little was known about the visual centre, 'in spite of the work of Henschen', he wrote that, 'it is only certain that this representation [of the macula] goes far beyond the area striata, for we know examples in which a man is deprived of both of his occipital lobes...who not only has light perception from the

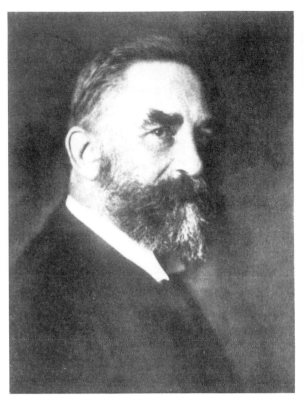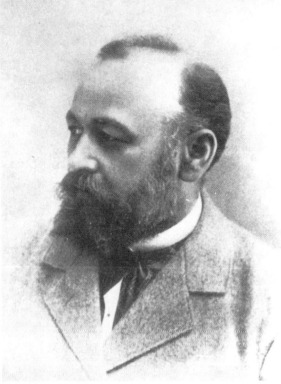

Fig. 7.2 The two deadly enemies who were united in their opposition to the idea of a colour centre in the cerebral cortex. Salomon Eberhard Henschen (1847–1930) (right), was a brilliant Swedish neuro-pathologist, consumed by his dislike for Constantine von Monakow (1853–1930) (left), the Russian born Swiss neurologist. On one occasion he is reputed to have broken the pointer during a lecture, at the mention of von Monakow's name, exclaiming '. . .Eine neue Dummheit von Monakow'. Von Monakow, on the other hand, thought that not much was known about the visual cortex 'in spite of the work of Henschen'. (Reproduced by permission from Polyak, S. (1957). *The Vertebrate Visual System.* University of Chicago Press, Chicago.)

smallest central field, but can even recognize objects. . .and can even read'.[4] Next there was anatomical evidence which showed, or so he believed, the powerful plasticity of the cortex. Referring to two cases of blindness, one acquired at birth through infection, von Monakow remarks on the 'sparse anatomical findings in the occipital lobe despite permanent abolition of both optic nerves and considerable atrophy of the optic radiations'.[5] This leads him to conclude that the occipital lobe must have compensated by taking over some other sensory function, thus supporting his view that there is no fixed localization in the cerebral cortex. Moreover, there was supporting anatomical evidence for a widespread cortical representation of macular vision, at least in the monkey. In 1889, Lannegrace had written that, 'The optic fibres. . .irradiate over a considerable extent of the cortical convexity, from the occiput behind to the motor region in front. . .the visual zone, *zone of hemianopia*, is thus very wide; but it has its principal residence in the occiput'[6] [his emphasis].

Thus, to postulate a separate colour centre, lying outside the striate cortex and dealing with colour alone, was not only unnecessary for von Monakow, it was also dangerous for his theory of a mobile representation of central vision in the cerebral cortex. It implied that the cortical representation of central vision was not so mobile after all. All the clinical evidence, including cerebral colour blindness, could be accounted for by the very large extent of the visual receptive centre which, in any case, went beyond the confines of the striate cortex and in which the centre of vision was widely represented.

...and Henschen's concept of a 'cortical retina'...

Henschen cared nothing for this view. He saw in it a threat to his own doctrine of a visual receptive centre confined to the striate cortex and in which the retina is rigidly mapped, his 'cortical retina'. The cortical zone lying outside.the striate area was also visual, but not visuo-sensory. Henschen believed that it was concerned with higher 'visuo-psychic' functions. This view, and the rigid map of the retina in the striate cortex proposed by Henschen, was much disliked by von Monakow and his followers. They referred to it as 'une localisation à outrance'.[7] Blindness, whether large (hemianopias) or small (scotomas), could only be produced by involvement of the striate cortex or of the optic radiations leading to it, so Henschen believed. He wrote, 'As to the perception of colours, the commonly received opinion that it is situated on the ventral surface will not admit of criticism. Some of my own cases prove positively that colour perception is also situated in the calcarine cortex'.[8] Henschen was master of all at this kind of assertion without proof, a vice which he was nevertheless quick to see and criticize in others. To him, the views of von Monakow concerning the extent of the visual receptive centre were, '...based on an assertion without proof. Science does not recognize assertions'.[9] The evidence of Verrey and of MacKay and Dunlop could also be dismissed by assertion. Henschen[9] wrote, 'The two cases of achromatopsia published by Verrier and Machay [*sic*] do not demonstrate, in my opinion, what these authors wanted to demonstrate'.

...left no room for a colour centre

Today, we know that Henschen was right in equating the primary visual receptive centre with the striate cortex and that von Monakow was wrong in supposing that it included almost the entire occipital lobe. Yet, from the point of view of a colour centre in the cortex, the two opposing views made little difference. They were both very hostile to the idea because it implied something which seemed conceptually unacceptable to both. The difference between von Monakow and Henschen related only to the extent of the visual receptive centre. To both, that visual receptive centre, whatever its extent, had to 'receive' *all* the 'visual impressions', including colour. For von Monakow to admit that there was a colour centre in which central or macular vision was represented, and specific damage to which could lead specifically to colour blindness, was to admit that the cortex was not so plastic after all and that the macular centre was not mobile. Moreover, it was to admit that one visual 'impression', colour, would be received separately from the other visual 'impressions', an idea he had not even entertained. He therefore dismissed the notion. For Henschen, on the other hand, to admit to a colour centre outside the striate cortex was to admit either of two unpalatable facts: that the visual receptive centre may be larger than the striate cortex or that one of the attributes of vision, colour, may be received separately, in another cortical area, an idea he had briefly entertained and found absurd. Henschen[9] wrote emphatically, 'the cortical retina is at the same time a retina for colour impressions'. To him, if it were true that there was a separate colour centre lying outside his cortical retina, then, 'with the calcarine cortex destroyed and the cortex of that other gyrus [lingual and fusiform] intact, a patient would have to be absolutely blind and yet be able to see colours, which makes no sense'.[10]

Henschen's work was extended by Holmes, and his mistakes were corrected. Holmes' equation of the striate, or calcarine, cortex with the perceptive visual cortex, the cortex with which one 'sees', was almost universally accepted. Indeed, until the early 1970s, whenever one spoke of other cortical areas as visual, one ran the serious risk of being misunderstood to mean the calcarine cortex or striate area alone. Holmes' 'visual cortex' replaced the more laborious 'visuo-sensory' cortex, prevalent earlier. But it meant the same thing. No one wished to deny that there may be other visual areas outside the striate cortex. But how many? Campbell[11] (Figure 7.3) provided an answer that the Oracle at Delphi would have approved of. He wrote that there may be 'one or more' areas. But the ever-cautious Campbell hedged even this Delphic wisdom with further doubt. Like Bolton,[12] he thought that a visual area outside the striate cortex was 'doubtfully existent and doubtfully located'. At any rate, whether one or many or none, all agreed that the cortical zone lying outside the striate cortex, if indeed it was visual in function, must have a higher, 'visuo-psychic' function. In the simple words of Henschen, one 'saw' with the visuo-sensory cortex and 'understood' with the visuo-psychic cortex. This notion, which represented in a sense a view of how the

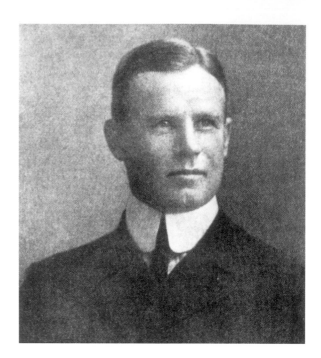

Fig. 7.3 A.W. Campbell (1868–1937), the British neuroanatomist with the Delphic wisdom. He thought that the prestriate visual cortex (his visuo-psychic cortex) might consist of 'one or more areas'. (Reproduced by permission from Polyak, S. (1957). *The Vertebrate Visual System.* University of Chicago Press, Chicago.)

brain works, at least in vision, was to have a deep influence on dismissing the evidence for a colour centre lying outside the striate cortex, which, in turn, led to an erroneous view of how the brain undertakes the task of constructing the visual image.

The determination of the precise limits of the visual receptive centre, which came to be referred to as the 'visuo-sensory' cortex, or area 17 of Brodmann, or the calcarine cortex, the demonstration that it is co-extensive with the striate area, as well as the demonstration that it has a rigid retinal map in it, finally put paid to all notions of a separate visual receptive centre devoted to receiving colour impressions. Monbrun[13] wrote in 1939, 'At present, all authors have rallied to the theory of a single cortical [visual] centre'. Using the occasion to take a direct hit at von Monakow, he added that '...the concept of a "fixed projection" of the retina on the cerebral cortex... was fought for a long time...and above all by von Monakow' but 'War veterans with partial hemianopias have not yet seen reappear the restitution of function so dear to Monakow'. Several years before, Gordon Holmes, the much admired and revered neuro-ophthalmologist, had sounded the final death knell. He wrote, 'My observations...tend to show that an isolated loss or dissociation of colour vision is not produced by cerebral lesions',[14] a view he put forward even more forcefully in 1945.[15] Indeed, the issue seems to have been dead during the Great War. Marie and Chatelin[16] could find only one case of cerebral colour blindness among their war-wounded patients, a rarity which spoke in favour of an absence of dissociation, or so they believed. Moreover, there was an awkward logical problem, demanding caution. It was well stated by Magitot and Hartmann[17] in 1926 in their massive review of cortical blindnesses. They wrote, 'In admitting a chromatic functional specialisation for the calcarine cells, should we admit equally the presence of specialised neurons in the optic pathways?'. Really, they had seen the point. Once a specialization in one centre was established, the logical conclusion would have been to postulate it for regions feeding that centre. Indeed, that is precisely what did happen later. But at the time at which Magitot and Hartmann were writing there was, alas, no evidence showing specialized neurons in the optic pathways.

The notion of a colour centre vanishes from the clinical literature

Now we can see how the notion of a separate colour centre in the cerebral cortex 'vanished'[18] from the literature. In his brief discussion Damasio holds Holmes a good deal more responsible for this than I do, writing that Holmes' '...authority and the importance of his other superb observations cast a shadow on the descriptions of acquired achromatopsia'. My view is that Holmes was a man of his time, subscribing fully to the then prevalent concepts without enquiring into their validity. The fact that Holmes himself never observed a case of cerebral colour blindness does not impress, especially since he does not cite the evidence of those who did while, at the same time, being emphatic in his denial.

But whatever Holmes may have thought, there remained the awkward problem of achromatopsia. How to deal with it? Walther Poppelreuter[19] (Figure 7.4) thought that it must be due to damage of the striate cortex. He wrote, 'There has been no evidence for an exact point-to-point co-ordination between the retina and the calcarine cortex.... There are several principles of topographic geometric projection [to the calcarine cortex], mainly these three: 1. We have a plurality of different systems, which are affected by defects in different ways and can also remain functional in different ways, i.e. the defect can show itself as specific for different systems. The latter are...1. Light-dark system; 2. Colour system; 3. Spatial (form) system; 4. Motion; 5. Orientation (or direction)'. Soon thereafter, Halpern and Hoff[20] speculated that colour vision is localized to layers 2 and 3 of the striate cortex. Poppelreuter's formulation was prophetic. There was only one thing missing — the evidence. Perhaps because of this, his formulations did not lead to the more searching questions of why there should be a separation in the representation of the different attributes of vision. It certainly did not lead to a new vision of how the brain sees.

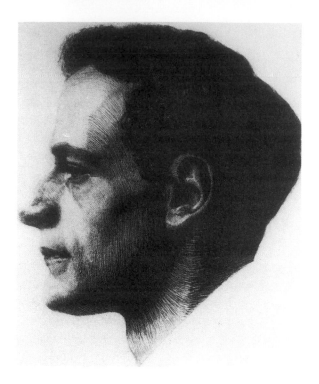

Fig. 7.4 Walther Poppelreuter (1886–1939), the German neurologist who was far ahead of his time in believing that there must be a separate representation of colour, motion, depth and form in the primary visual cortex (area V1), a notion which no one took seriously. (Reproduced by permission from Poppelreuter, W. 1990. *Disturbances of Lower and Higher Visual Capacities Caused by Occipital Damage.* Clarendon Press, Oxford.)

Hence the idea of a colour centre, separate from the primary visual receptive centre, was difficult to accept in a world which believed that an image of the visual world, including all its forms, motions and colours, would be 'impressed' on the retina and then transmitted to be received and analyzed by one visual centre in the brain, the 'cortical retina'.

References

1 Stone, J., Leicester, J. & Sherman, S.M. (1973). The naso-temporal division of the monkey's retina. *J. Comp. Neurol.* **150**, 333–348.
2 Beevor, C.E. (1907). The cerebral arterial supply. *Brain* **30**, 403–425.
3 Henschen, S.E. (1930). *Pathologie des Gehirns* 8. I. *Lichtsinn–und Farbensinnzellen im Gehirn.* Verlag des Verfassers, Stockholm.
4 Monakow, C. von (1900). Reply to Henschen. In *XIII Congrés International de Médecine (Ophtalmologie), Paris*, edited by M. Rochon-Duvigneaud, pp. 246–249. Masson & Cie, Paris.
5 Monakow, C. von (1900). Pathologische und anatomische Mittheilungen über die optischen Centren des Menschen. *Neurol. Zentralbl.* **19**, 680–681.
6 Lannegrace (1889). Influence des lésions corticale sur la vue. *Archs. Méd. Exp. Anatomie Pathol.* **1**, 289–324.
7 Vialet, M. (1894). Considérations sur le centre visuel cortical à propos de deux nouveaux cas d'hémianopsie suivis d'autopsie. *Archs. Ophtalmol. (Paris)* **14**, 422–426.
8 Henschen, S.E. (1983). On the visual path and centre. *Brain* **16**, 170–180.
9 Henschen, S.E. (1900). Sur le centre cortical de la vision. In *XIII Congrés Inter-*

nationale de Médecine (Ophtalmologie), Paris, edited by M. Rochon-Duvigneaud, pp. 232–245. Masson & Cie, Paris.

10 Henschen, S.E. (1910). Zentrale Sehstörungen. In *Handbuch der Neurologie, 2,* edited by M. Lewandowsky, pp. 891–918. Springer-Verlag, Berlin.

11 Campbell, A.W. (1905). *Histological Studies on the Localisation of Cerebral Function.* Cambridge University Press, Cambridge.

12 Bolton, J.S. (1900). The exact histological localisation of the visual area of the human cerebral cortex. *Philos. Trans. R. Soc. Lond.* B **193**, 165–222.

13 Monbrun, A. (1939). Les affections des voie optiques rétrochiasmatiques et de l'écorce visuelle. In *Traité d'Ophtalmologie*, Vol. 6, edited by P. Baillart, C. Contela, E. Redslob & E. Velter, pp. 903–905. Société Française d'Ophtalmologie, Masson, Paris.

14 Holmes, G. (1918). Disturbances of vision by cerebral lesions. *Br. J. Ophthalmol.* **2**, 353–384.

15 Holmes, G. (1945). The Ferrier Lecture: The organization of the visual cortex in man. *Proc. R. Soc. Lond.* B **132**, 348–361.

16 Marie, P. & Chatelin, C. (1915). Les troubles visuels due aux lésions des voies optiques intracérébrales et de la sphère visuelle corticale dans les blessures du crane par coup de feu. *Rev. Neurol. (Paris)* **22**, 882–925.

17 Magitot, A. & Hartmann, E. (1926). La cécité corticale. *Bull. Soc. Ophtalmol. (Paris)* **38**, 427–546.

18 Damasio, A.R. (1985). Disorders of complex visual processing. In *Principles of Behavioral Neurology*, edited by M.-Marsel Mesulam, pp. 259–288. F.A. Davis, Philadelphia.

19 Poppelreuter, W. (1923). Zur Psychologie und Pathologie der optischen Wahrnehmung. *Z. Ges. Neurol Psychiatr.* **83**, 26–152.

20 Halpern, F. & Hoff, H. (1929). Kasuistiche Beiträge zur Frage der cerebralen Farbenblindheit. *Z. Ges. Neurol. Psychiatr.* **122**, 575–586.

Chapter 8: The spell of cortical architecture

The cerebral cortex is a multi-layered structure consisting of cells and their processes, including the nerve fibres (Figure 8.1). It is traditional to consider it as being essentially composed of six layers, with subdivisions within them. This derives from the speculations of the German anatomist, Korbinian Brodmann, who provided one of the most widely used charts of the brain, based on his histological studies. Brodmann believed that, developmentally, the primitive condition was that of six layers, from which other subdivisions arose. Whatever the merits of his case, this subdivision has worked well in practice and there is no reason not to adhere to it.

A popular method for revealing cortical architecture: the cytoarchitectonic method

The layers of the cortex are perhaps best visualized when the brain is sectioned and stained with an agent that reveals the cell bodies, for example, one of the many Nissl methods that stain the ribonucleic acids within them. This reveals the cytoarchitecture of the cortex, that is, how cells are stacked together in the cortex (Figure 8.1). The

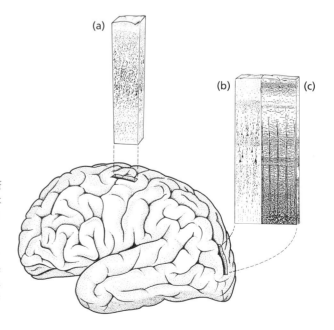

Fig. 8.1 Two methods for studying the architecture of the cerebral cortex. The cytoarchitecture of the cortex is revealed by treating the cortex with a method that stains the cells' bodies, thus showing how they are arranged in layers. (a) The cytoarchitecture of the motor cortex. (b) The cytoarchitecture of the primary visual cortex, area V1. (c) The myeloarchitecture of the cortex (for V1), is revealed by staining the cortex by a method which shows the myelin sheaths covering the nerve fibres.

cerebral cortex consists essentially of two categories of cell, with subdivisions within each. One category is the pyramidal cell and the other is the star-shaped or granule cell. When sections through the cortex are stained to display these cells and then examined, two facts emerge. One is that large regions of the cortex have essentially the same six-layered structure, in which layer 4 consists mainly of granule cells and the layers above and below it mainly of pyramidal cells (Figure 8.1a). The second striking feature is that there are some regions of the cortex which have a cytoarchitecture that is so radically different from this apparently uniform cytoarchitecture of large expanses of cortex that they can be demarcated at a glance. Chief among these is the motor cortex lying in the frontal lobes. It can be readily distinguished because of the absence of granule cells in it. It is therefore known as the frontal agranular cortex. Equally striking is the richly layered primary visual cortex which has a stripe running through its larger than usual layer 4 — hence the term striate cortex (Figure 8.1b).

Other methods for revealing cortical architecture

The cytoarchitectonic method is not the only one with which to study the architecture of the cerebral cortex. There are other techniques and more are becoming available as work progresses. Each method reveals a different aspect of cortical architecture. The nerve fibres of cells are commonly covered with a sheath known as myelin, which varies in thickness. One can therefore study the pattern of myelination in the cerebral cortex, and thus chart cerebral areas according to myeloarchitecture (Figure 8.1c), a procedure which has turned out to be more reliable than the cytoarchitectonic approach in indicating functional boundaries between areas. Or one can stain the same cortical area histochemically to reveal areas of high metabolic activity. One such method, introduced recently and highly successful in revealing a novel pattern of architecture, is the cytochrome oxidase method.[1] This stains for the metabolic enzyme cytochrome oxidase, which is found in the mitochondria of cells. The architecture of the striate cortex that it reveals, its cytochrome oxidase architecture, is much more elaborate than the one revealed by the cytoarchitectonic method (Figure 8.2). While with the cytoarchitectonic method one can distinguish between the cortical layers of V1, with the cytochrome oxidase method one can distinguish further features, such as subregions of high metabolic activity.[2] This metabolic, cytochrome oxidase, architecture has assumed a great significance in our current understanding of the functional organization of the striate cortex and we shall return to it later. Here it is important to emphasize that other visual areas, such as V2, also have a characteristic cytochrome oxidase architecture.

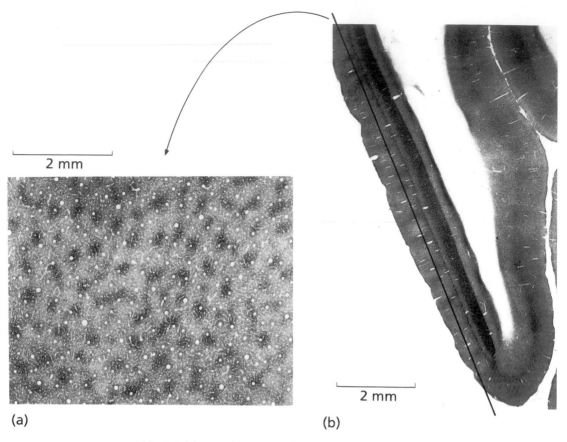

Fig. 8.2 (a) Part of a section through layers 2 and 3 of area V1, cut parallel to the cortical surface (along the line shown in (b), and stained for cytochrome oxidase to reveal one aspect of the characteristic cytochrome oxidase architecture of this visual area.

An axiom of neurology...

Ever since the beginning of neurology as a discipline, neurologists have supposed that cortical areas that differ in their function will also differ in their architecture and, conversely, that areas which are uniform in architecture are also uniform in function. This is undoubtedly so. But the preferred method used in the past to reveal differences in architecture, the cytoarchitectonic method, was not always equal to the task. While it revealed readily the distinction between the striate cortex and that surrounding it, it was very difficult to find further subdivisions within the 'visual association' cortex itself. This led Brodmann to subdivide the 'visual association' cortex into two more or less concentric zones which he called areas 18 and 19[3] (Figure 8.3), these being the eighteenth and nineteenth areas, respectively, that he studied. Others (e.g., von Bonin and Bailey[4]) have encountered equal difficulties with the 'visual association' cortex of man. This did not inhibit them from subdividing it into more or less the same zones,

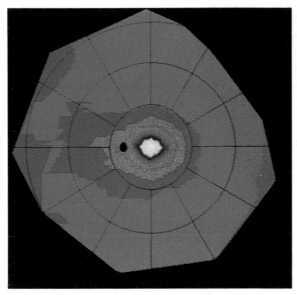

(a)

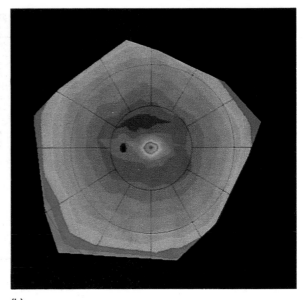

(b)

Plate 1 The change in the densities of (a) cones and of (b) rods from the central retina outwards. Highest densities are shown in white and red and lowest densities in blues (black indicates ~ zero density). Note the very high density of cones in the fovea (white in (a)) and the rapid decline at more peripheral retinal positions. The density of rods shows a reciprocal picture, with a rod free area in the centre (fovea, black) and an increasing density at more peripheral positions. The black dot to the left in both (a) and (b) marks the position of entry of retinal blood vessels (blind spot). (Reproduced by permission from Curcio C.A. *et al.* (1990). *J. Comp. Neurol.* **292**, 497–523.) (c) The central retina is the part with which one fixates, while the peripheral retina captures signals from more peripheral parts of the field of view.

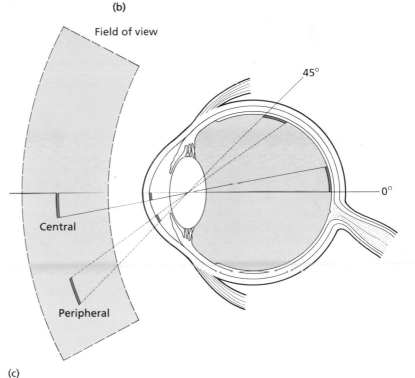

(c)

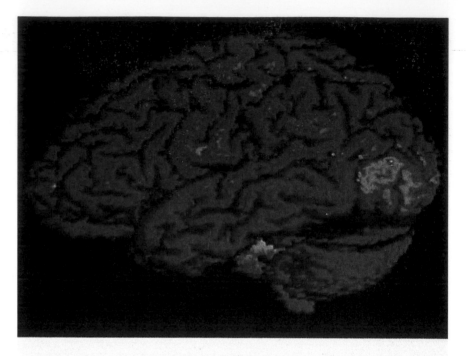

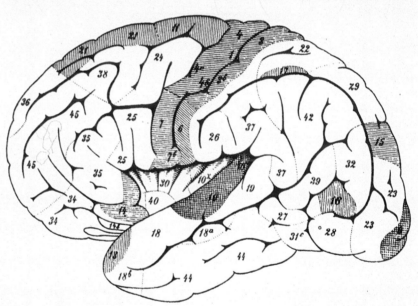

Plate 2 (above) The location of the cerebral area which is active when human subjects perceive visual motion, determined from studies using positron emission tomography. The area is similar in location to the area defined as Feld 16, which Flechsig found to be myelinated at birth (below). This area was damaged in the patient described in Chapter 10.

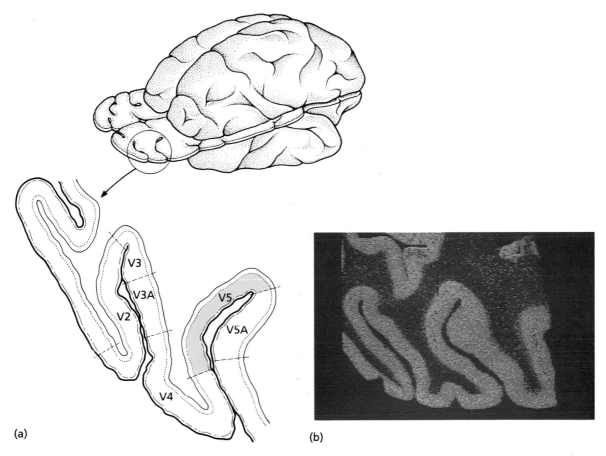

(a)

(b)

Plate 3 (a) The position of area V5 is shown in a horizontal section taken through the brain of the macaque monkey. (b) When such a section is stained for the enzyme cytochrome oxidase and then imaged through a computer, area V5 and the adjoining area V5A (the V5 complex) are shown to be cytochrome oxidase rich (appearing reddish in colour).

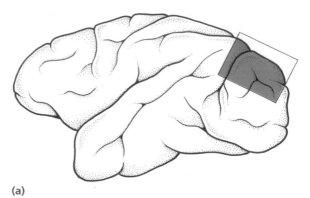

(a)

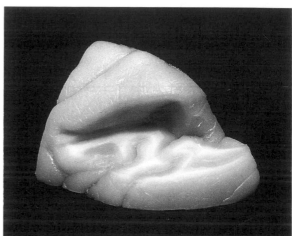

(b)

Plate 4 An example of a three-dimensional computer reconstruction of a region of the brain, in this case the dorsal region of the parietal lobe of the left hemisphere. (a) The boxed area of the brain shows the region reconstructed, from which much of the lateral part (shaded zone), including the occipital operculum, has been removed. The three-dimensional reconstruction in (c) is of the region shown in (b) (although on the computer any part can be removed at will, and then put back). In this particular reconstruction, part of the cortex of area V6 has been injected with horseradish peroxidase (dotted zones) and the distribution of labelled cells traced to adjoining zones. The latter form long narrow bands. The advantage of such reconstructions is that they can be rotated on the computer in any desired way and do not involve much distortion, except that resulting from perspective viewing. However, only limited parts of the cerebral cortex can be viewed in any one reconstruction. Viewing figure (c) with a green filter over the right eye and a red filter over the left eye, will produce an impression of depth.

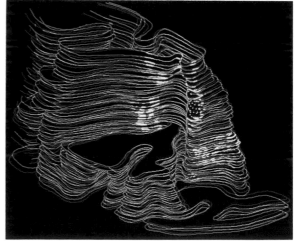

(c)

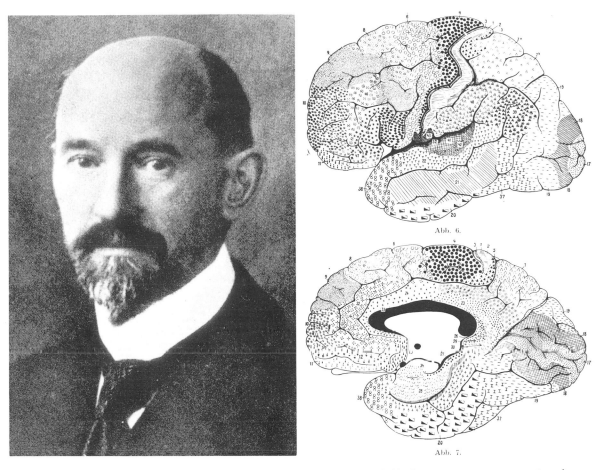

Abb. 6.

Abb. 7.

Fig. 8.3 Korbinian Brodmann (1868–1918) (left), the German neuroanatomist whose work was to have a lasting influence in brain studies, and his cytoarchitectonic chart of the brain (right). Brodmann settled on as effective a terminology for the cortical areas as any ever invented — he numbered them according to the sequence in which he studied them. (Reproduced by permission from Polyak, S. (1957). *The Vertebrate Visual System*. University of Chicago Press, Chicago.)

which they called areas OA and OB instead, using merging colours to indicate the uncertain boundary between the two areas.

...and the dilemmas it created

Here was a dilemma for those who proposed a colour centre in the cortex lying outside the striate cortex. If this were a separate cortical area, then, theoretically at least, it should have a distinctive architecture; on this basis one should thus be able to distinguish it from surrounding cortical regions. But the method of *cyto*architecture, the most widely used method in earlier times, did not reveal a corresponding zone with an architecture different from that of areas 18 and 19, themselves difficult to tell apart on *cyto*architectonic criteria.

Instead, areas 18 and 19 cut across the lingual and fusiform gyri, where the putative colour centre was supposed to lie, so that part of each gyrus was characteristic of area 18 while the other was characteristic of area 19. It was difficult to justify the notion of a separate colour centre without some anatomical, i.e. cytoarchitectonic, evidence to its identity and its borders. In fact, another architectonic method, the method of myeloarchitecture, did suggest that these cytoarchitectonic areas could be further subdivided. In particular, Lungwitz[5] had undertaken a tedious study to try and differentiate subregions within this zone on the basis of myeloarchitecture. He proposed an elaborate subdivision, which included the delineation of the lingual gyrus and subdivisions within the fusiform gyrus. But Lungwitz despised his own work. He doubted the validity of subdivisions based on myeloarchitectonic criteria, and pleaded in vain for functional studies. He didn't take his subdivisions seriously, nor did anyone else. He made no allusion to the fact that clinical evidence had proposed a special function for the lingual and fusiform gyri. Nor did any clinician refer to his work. There was no need to. At the time that Lungwitz was writing, the evidence for a colour centre in the human cortex had been dead for at least thirty years.

In fact, even the modest subdivision into areas 18 and 19 was not universally accepted. Lashley and Clark[6] in particular experienced a greater difficulty in seeing the distinction between the areas than others had. Their experience with this, as with other proposed cytoarchitectonic boundaries, led them to question the validity of the cytoarchitectonic method and, along with it, the modest subdivisions proposed for the 'visual association' cortex by Brodmann and others. Instead, they proposed that areas 18 and 19, along with Brodmann's area 7 which lies in the parietal lobe, should be considered as a 'single unit'.

Lashley's hostility

What Lashley meant by a 'single unit' was not made explicit, but the terminology corresponded rather neatly to his theory of cerebral mass action which supposed that all parts of the cerebral cortex contributed equally to the execution of complex tasks. Colour vision was, to him, just such a task.[7] The difficulty of subdividing the cortex on architectonic criteria was therefore much to his liking. He believed it to be the anatomical reflection of his view. Indeed, the title of his paper is instructive, for it betrays something about his thinking. It is entitled, *The cytoarchitecture of the cerebral cortex of Ateles: A critical examination of architectonic studies*. He had studied the *cytoarchitecture* of the cerebral cortex but he proceeded to generalize from this to all *architectonic* studies. It reflects his contempt not only for cytoarchitectonic studies, but for all architectonic studies. As well, he cared nothing for the evidence which purported to show specific visual defects following specific lesions. Quoting approvingly von Monakow's statement that, 'I do not know of a single case in which a purely traumatic lesion in the occipital lobes of an otherwise sound brain resulted in a persistent visual agnosia', he argued that, 'Dissociation of functions, as in isolated loss of color vision...are less clearly referable to injury in any specific region' and considered that the clinical evidence was so 'confusing and inconclusive' that there seemed little reason to ascribe 'such secondary disorders...to lesions in the cortex adjacent to the striate cortex'.[7] Quoting Alder,[8] he believed rather that, 'The development of agnosia in toxic conditions...points to diffuse damage and disorganization rather than to focal lesions'.[7] The reference to Alder was unfortunate. One of the most remarkable features of Alder's paper was that, after carbon monoxide poisoning, her patient's colour vision was remarkably accurate, while vision for other attributes was severely impaired. This constituted a sort of negative evidence in favour of the separation of visual functions in the brain, but Lashley chose not to refer to it. We shall return to it later.

This was not the last time that a specialization for colour vision was to be dismissed because of negative architectonic evidence. Many years later, in a repeat of history, the physiological evidence for a colour specialization within the primary visual cortex itself was to be dismissed by Hubel and Wiesel,[9] partly at least because there seemed to be no architectonic subregions containing high concentrations of wavelength-selective cells.[2] The discovery that the striate cortex has a more elaborate architecture than is revealed by the cytoarchitectonic method led to a re-examination of the physiological evidence and to the subsequent demonstration of small subregions within it which are specialized for colour.[2]

The cytoarchitectonic method, then, did not reveal an area with clear boundaries within the lingual and fusiform gyri, where some clinicians had supposed the colour centre to be located. This made it improbable that there would be a distinct area there. Logical considerations, and the then prevalent concepts of vision as a process, made it even more improbable that a cytoarchitectonically non-existent area should be a colour area. It did not make sense. Not every one thought in this way. Von Monakow cared nothing for cortical subdivisions, whether demonstrable by cytoarchitectonic methods or not. To him, the function of cortical areas was interchangeable, which is presumably why Lashley quoted him so approvingly. And the retinal centre or macula was, in any case, widely represented in the cortex, indeed in cortical areas which differed in their cytoarchitecture, or so he imagined. Von Monakow's views, therefore, did not depend upon cortical architecture but rather upon other theoretical considerations which he was much attached to.

It is not unlikely that the mistake of supposing that an area, or a region of an area, has a uniform function because of its uniform architecture will be repeated in the future. In general, the search for functional subdivisions is undertaken only after the demonstration of anatomical subdivisions. The demonstration of ocular dominance columns in the striate cortex[9] and the delimitation of distinct areas within the prestriate cortex[10] constitute two rare exceptions, although both were greatly strengthened by the subsequent demonstration of their anatomical bases. This perhaps gives substance to the aphorism of Gudden that, 'Anatomy first and then physiology; but if physiology first, then not without anatomy'. Much of the cerebral cortex remains to be charted and it seems likely that the kind of subdivisions found in areas V1 or V2 will also be found elsewhere. The mistake would be to suppose that the anatomical subdivisions in these uncharted areas will be the same, or revealable by the same methods. It is only the general principle of subdivisions which will probably be found to hold true. The details will inevitably vary.

References

1 Wong-Riley, M.T.T. (1979). Changes in the visual system of monocularly sutured or enucleated cats demonstrable with cytochrome oxidase histochemistry. *Brain Res.* **171**, 11–28.

2 Livingstone, M.S. & Hubel, D.H. (1984). Anatomy and physiology of a color system in primate visual cortex. *J. Neurosci.* **4**, 309–356.

3 Brodmann, K. (1905). Beiträge zur histologischen Lokalisation der Grosshirnrinde. Dritte Mitteilung: Die Rindenfelder der niederen Affen. *J. Psychol. Neurol. Lpz.* **4**, 177–226.

4 Bonin, G. von & Bailey, P. (1951). *The Isocortex of Man.* University of Illinois Press, Urbana.

5 Lungwitz, W. (1937). Zur myeloarchitektonischen Untergliederung der menschlischen Area praeoccipitalis (Area 19 Brodmann). *J. Psychol. Neurol. Lpz.* **47**, 607–638.

6 Lashley, K.S. & Clark, G. (1946). The cytoarchitecture of the cerebral cortex of Ateles: A critical examination of architectonic studies. *J. Comp. Neurol.* **85**, 223–305.

7 Lashley, K.S. (1948). The mechanism of vision. XVIII. Effects of destroying the visual 'associative areas' of the monkey. *Genet. Psychol. Monogr.* **37**, 107–166.

8 Adler, A. (1944). Disintegration and restoration of optic recognition in visual agnosia. *Arch. Neurol. Psychiatr.* **51**, 243–259.

9 Hubel, D.H. & Wiesel, T.N. (1977). The Ferrier Lecture: Functional architecture of macaque monkey visual cortex. *Proc. R. Soc. Lond.* B **198**, 1–59.

10 Zeki, S.M. (1978). Functional specialization in the visual cortex of the rhesus monkey. *Nature* **274**, 423–428.

Chapter 9: Hierarchies in the visual system

The notion of hierarchies in the visual system was to have a powerful negative influence in questioning the doctrine of functional specialization in visual cortex, and hence of separate pathways and areas for colour vision. This is surprising, because nowhere is the doctrine of hierarchies adequately formulated in physiological terms. It nevertheless permeated thinking and created an attitude of mind that was prevalent among many physiologists, at least for a time. Its influence has been due not so much to dismissing the evidence in favour of functional specialization but rather to ignoring it, and supposing thereby that the hierarchical strategy is the sole strategy that can account for the operations of the visual system. But an exclusively hierarchical strategy, which implies that the visual areas are connected strictly serially with each other, is incompatible with the observation of specific visual defects which affect selectively certain attributes of vision, e.g. colour vision or depth perception, since a lesion in any visual area should compromise all the attributes of vision more or less equally, because all the attributes of vision would be expected to be represented in each visual area. This consideration did not present a problem. Such observations had been successfully dismissed and did not therefore pose a serious obstacle, assuming anyone to have been aware of them in the 1950s. Moreover, there were excellent reasons for supposing that the hierarchical strategy may be the sole one that the brain uses to analyze the visual environment.

The origins of the hierarchical concept

As with so much else that was to mould the thinking of neurologists, it is difficult to trace the origins of the concept of hierarchies in vision. But central to it is the usually unspoken assumption that objects in the visual world are conveniently labelled and that all that the visual system has to do is to analyze that label. The analysis can then be undertaken hierarchically, with each level of the visual pathways undertaking an analysis at a certain level of complexity and leaving it to subsequent stages to continue the analysis at a more complex level, or at least to analyze more of the label. No one should underrate the importance of unspoken assumptions. They are often the most powerful because they are part of the scientific culture, and therefore remain unquestioned, though they get perpetuated. Moreover, with an attribute such as colour, there was at least a plausible reason for supposing that there is a convenient label, rooted in the belief that colour of an object is determined by the excess of any given wavelength (the code) reflected from that object, that a green object looks green because it reflects more green light. And, to repeat, it is useless to plead that there were some who had seen that colour is a vastly more complex problem than such a naive view would suggest. Those who had seen the mysteries of colour vision had been remarkably inarticulate in communicating their enlightenment to others, even in the scientific community.

The notion of hierarchies derived at least partial support from the organization of the visual system from retina to the primary visual cortex, with one centre feeding into another, and higher, centre. It is also implicit in early doctrines of vision which supposed that, by some unknown mechanism, a picture of the visual world was first 'impressed' upon the retina, then 'received' by the primary visual cortex and finally 'associated' with previous visual 'impressions' to lead to recognition, vague notations which are explicit only in suggesting a greater degree of complexity. All manner of visual disturbances of cerebral origin came to be referred to the 'visual association' or 'visuo-psychic' cortex, and chief among them were the visual agnosias, that is to say, syndromes in which visual stimuli are perceived but are not recognized, or so neurologists imagined. Holmes, who believed that colour vision, relative localization of objects in space and the recognition of form all depended on the striate cortex alone, nevertheless thought that, 'The visual cortex is not...concerned in more highly evolved functions which are developed by the integration of visual with other sensory impressions', citing object agnosia as well as colour agnosia as functions of the surrounding, ill-defined, cortex.[1] Once associated with previous impressions, the present impression would be transferred to a repository in the inferior temporal cortex, where an engram or memory trace would be formed. The sequence constituted what one may call a hierarchical chain of increasing complexity.

The idea of complexity, and of hierarchy, is also implicit in much of psychophysics and in introspective psychology which supposes that, much as a visual stimulus can be broken down into its elements, so the nervous system builds up an image of the stimulus by analyzing its components first, and then assembling these components, building-block fashion, at successive stages of the visual pathways. The latter, at any rate, came to be the view of hierarchy propounded by physiological studies, and in particular by those of David Hubel and Torsten Wiesel.

The physiological evidence for hierarchies

Using the cat and the monkey, Hubel and Wiesel had been studying the physiological properties of cells in the primary visual cortex which, for simplicity, we can refer to henceforth as V1. This can be done by recording the electrical activity of cells by means of electrodes inserted in their close neighbourhood. Cells in the nervous system increase or decrease their on-going electrical discharges in response to the appropriate stimulation. These changes can be picked up by an electrode and fed into an oscilloscope and an audio-monitor. Visual stimuli are usually flashed on a screen facing the animal, and the part of the screen which, when so stimulated, yields a response from the cell is called its *receptive field* (Figure 9.1). Once the receptive field is plotted, one can study in greater detail the kind of visual stimuli which, when flashed into the receptive field of the cell, give the best response. Hubel and Wiesel were not the only ones to undertake such studies. Others had been there before. But the others had laboured under the common, but understandable, misapprehension that the

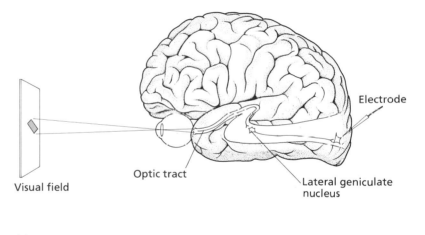

(a)

Fig. 9.1 The receptive field of a cell is that part of the field of view which, when stimulated, yields a reaction from the cell, measured as a change in its electrical discharge. (a) An electrode is placed in the vicinity of a cell in the visual cortex and the receptive field (RF) of the cell is plotted on a screen (in red). Once the receptive field is defined, its characteristics can be studied in greater detail. In this instance (b) the cell is found to be orientation selective, responding to an obliquely oriented line and being unresponsive to the orthogonal orientation.

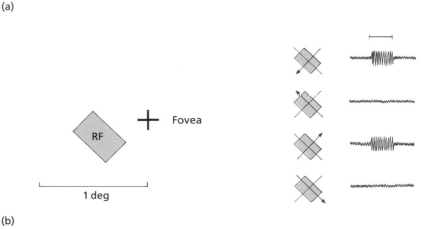

(b)

cells of the visual cortex would naturally respond to light as such. They had therefore illuminated the entire screen facing the animal with diffuse light. Indeed, in Germany, Richard Jung had developed in the 1950s one of the most advanced systems then available for recording from cells in the visual cortex. But because he used diffuse illumination to activate his cells, he obtained little response from them. Technologically, his approach was powerful; conceptually it was weak. Later in life, Jung was to blame others and his administrative duties for not realizing that his stimuli were conceptually ineffective, advising young scientists that one should 'not leave the laboratory during a productive period of research'.[2] But he also had this important advice to give, '...that a field should first be explored by simple qualitative pilot studies to find out the most rewarding approach, before experiments are reduced to quantification with a single method'.[2] He recounts how Hartline had told him that he had searched for the frog's 'off' neurons by moving a stick through diffuse light and that when he (Jung) had proposed this simple 'shadow search' approach to his colleagues, the latter had objected to doing such 'sloppy experiments, but planned to construct a rather complicated machine...When I was asked later why we missed the orientation specificity during five years' work on cortical neurons, I used to tell this story and remark that we might have found them in one experiment if we had used the stick with its easy movements in all orientations instead of the quantifying machine'.[2]

Quick to spot an important finding, Hubel and Wiesel needed no such lessons. There are interesting stories, well recounted by Hubel, to explain how they settled on such stimuli after the chance appearance of an oriented crack in a slide which drove a single cell in the cat's visual cortex wild. Without recourse to any complicated machinery, they exploited this finding by shining lights of different orientation on the screen facing the animal. At any rate, during the course of their studies, they discovered that all cells in V1 had very small receptive fields and that all cells outside the layer that receives the predominant input from the lateral geniculate nucleus (i.e. layer 4) were orientation selective.[3] Such cells do not respond to diffuse light and respond only weakly to spots of light. To obtain an optimal response from them, the activating stimulus must be a line of the right orientation and must fall within the right (excitatory) part of the cell's receptive field (Figure 9.2). The simplest of such cells were called, appropriately enough, simple cells. Different cells had different orientational preferences. To give an optimal response the appropriately oriented line had to extend the whole length of the cell's receptive field; halving the length of the line falling within the cell's receptive field halved the response. On the other hand, extending the appropriately oriented line beyond the boundaries of the receptive field did not alter the vigour of the response. In addition, there were distinct subcomponents of these receptive fields. In particular, when a line of the appropriate orientation was flashed in a given region of the cell's receptive field, the cell gave an ON response. But flashing the same light in flanking regions not only inhibited the cell, there was a response when the stimulus was taken off (an OFF response, itself the direct consequence of the preceding inhibition)[4] (Figure 9.2).

This was epoch-making work. It showed, first, that light was a necessary, but not a sufficient, condition for activating all cells of the visual system. This may seem obvious now; it was not so obvious before. Next, it showed, even if indirectly, that an image of the visual world is not 'impressed' upon the retina as was commonly supposed (those who commonly used this term were never explicit as to what it meant in physiological terms). Instead, such analysis as is carried out by the retina was now known to be relatively simple and, it turned out, that of the striate cortex was not that much more sophisticated either. And it served, lastly, to underline the important hierarchical principle in operation. For the properties of such cells could be accounted for, so Hubel and Wiesel believed, by supposing that each simple cell receives a convergent input from several lateral geniculate cells, which would constitute the building blocks from which the responses of simple cells could be built up.[4]

The most common feature of geniculate cells, like that of the retinal ganglion cells, is a centre–surround receptive field (Figure 9.3). Light falling in the centre of the receptive field excites the cell,

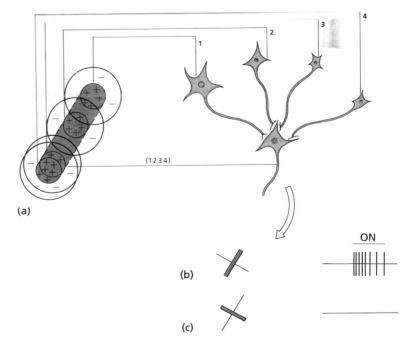

Fig. 9.2 A simple orientation selective cell behaves as if it receives input from several centre-surround antagonistic cells of the lateral geniculate nucleus (a). Flashing a line with an orientation that stimulates more of the excitatory centres (+) will stimulate the cell (b). Changing the orientation so that more of the inhibitory (−) surrounds are stimulated will diminish the cell's response. An orthogonal orientation to the one shown in (a) will yield no response from the cell (c), since it will invade both excitatory and inhibitory regions, which will therefore cancel out. (Redrawn from Hubel, D.H. & Wiesel, T.N. (1962). *J. Physiol. (Lond.)* **160**, 106–154).

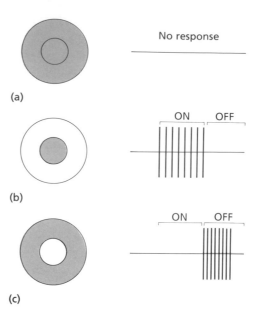

No response

(a)

ON   OFF

(b)

ON   OFF

(c)

Fig. 9.3 The cells of the inner layer of the retina (whose fibres project to the brain), and the cells of the lateral geniculate nucleus, do not respond to light as such. Rather they respond to a difference in the intensity of light between one part of their receptive fields and another part. Thus, stimulating such cells with diffuse light (a) is ineffective in eliciting a response; flashing a light in the centre of the receptive fields yields an ON response (b); while in the surround a response is obtained only when the light is switched OFF (c). The cell is therefore said to have an antagonistic 'centre–surround', or a concentric, receptive field.

thus increasing its electrical discharge rate. Light falling in the surround inhibits the cell, the cell now increasing its discharge rate only when the light is flashed OFF. Such cells are also common in the retina, where they were first discovered by Barlow and by Kuffler, both in 1953.[5,6] We shall call them the Kuffler–Barlow cells. The important point here is that their receptive field structure is such that they could be said to constitute the very elements from which simple cells in V1 could be built up, thus reinforcing the hierarchical doctrine (Figure 9.2).[4]

Hubel and Wiesel called such cells the simple cells of V1 to distinguish them from functionally more elaborate cells which they called the complex cells, and which they supposed received their inputs from the simple cells. Complex cells are orientation selective, like the simple cells, but can be distinguished from the latter by two features: they have larger receptive fields and, instead of having discrete regions from which one can obtain ON and OFF responses, both types of response can be obtained from every part of the receptive field (Figure 9.4). The characteristics of these cells could be accounted for, so they believed, by supposing that several simple cells excited one complex cell, again in building-block fashion.[4]

And this was not the end of the story. Even more complicated cells were seen, first referred to as hypercomplex cells and found in visual cortical areas lying outside the striate cortex, that is, in visual 'association' cortex.[7] Like simple and complex cells, these responded to lines of specific orientation. Unlike them, the length of the line was critical. They behaved then as if they received an input from two

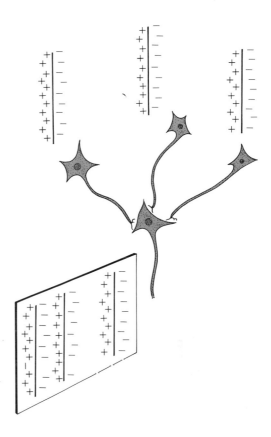

Fig. 9.4 The receptive field organization of a complex cell (below left) in the primary visual cortex. These complex cells are also responsive to lines of specific orientation (+) and behave as if they receive an excitatory input from several simple cells with oriented receptive fields (above). (Redrawn from Hubel, D.H. & Wiesel, T.N. (1962). *J. Physiol. (Lond.)* **160**, 106–154.)

or more complex cells, but this time using both excitatory and inhibitory inputs (Figure 9.5). For example, if three complex cells with the same orientational preferences were to connect with one hypercomplex cell, and the input from one were to be excitatory and from the other two inhibitory, then the hypercomplex cell would respond to a line that is stopped at both ends. If, on the other hand, it were to receive an input from two complex cells, of which only one is inhibitory, then extending the line in one direction would not affect the response of the cell, but extending it in the other direction would. It all seemed very much in accord with a building-block, hierarchical, model.

The fact that the hypercomplex cells were originally found in cortical areas lying outside what was then thought to be the primary visual cortex in the cat encouraged an extension of the notion of hierarchies to areas outside the striate cortex. The fact that the receptive fields of cells in visual areas lying outside the striate cortex were larger than those inside the striate cortex and the 'higher' the visual area, the larger the receptive fields of single cells in it, naturally encouraged the 'building block' doctrine.[7] Finally, the fact that the hierarchical strategy could be used to account for the properties of cells from the retina to the visual 'association' cortex seemed to suggest that it is the sole strategy in operation. Hubel and Wiesel[8]

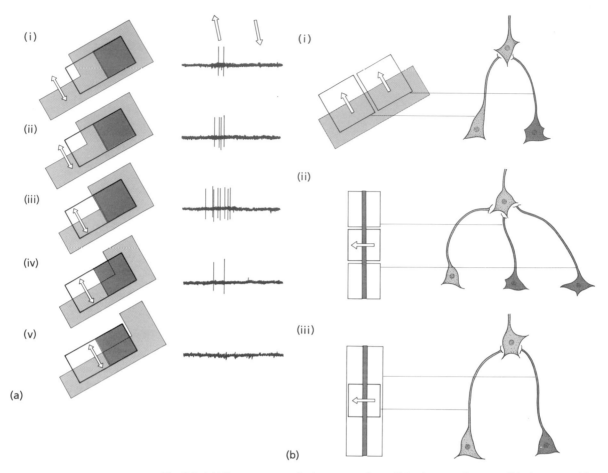

Fig. 9.5 (a) The responses of a hypercomplex cell in the visual cortex. (b) Three possible combinations which could lead to the emergence of cells with hypercomplex properties. In (i) two cells of the same orientation connect with a third cell, though one with an inhibitory (red) and the other with an excitatory input. The consequence is that the cell will only react if the length of the exciting line is limited to the receptive field of the exciting cell. (ii) and (iii) show other possible combinations. (Redrawn from Hubel, D.H. & Wiesel, T.N. (1965). *J. Neurophysiol.* **28**, 229–289.)

had found that even cells which were wavelength selective were also orientation selective, suggesting an additive, building-block mechanism in accord with the hierarchical strategy. Theirs were not of course the only studies. Other studies, notably those of Poggio and his colleagues,[9] suggested that many cells in the primary visual cortex of the monkey are not orientation selective. But such studies made little impression and had little influence. The overriding influence was that of Hubel and Wiesel and their studies, however carefully couched in descriptions, strongly suggested that the hierarchical strategy was the sole strategy in operation.

The concept of hierarchies nevertheless remains a powerful and useful one even today. The difference is that instead of thinking of an exclusively hierarchical strategy, with visual areas being connected serially with each other and each analyzing all the attributes of vision but at a more complex level than its predecessor, we think of each of the specialized visual areas, and of the separate but parallel visual pathways leading to it, as consisting of a hierarchical chain. But the switch from a single hierarchical chain to multiple pathways, each with its own hierarchical organization, is not a subtle extension of the concept of hierarchies. It is a fundamentally different concept of the organization of the visual cortex.

References

1 Holmes, G. (1945). The Ferrier Lecture: The organization of the visual cortex in man. *Proc. R. Soc. Lond.* B **132**, 348–361.
2 Jung, R. (1975). Some European neuroscientists: A personal tribute. In *Neurosciences: Paths of Discovery*, edited by F.G. Worden, J.P. Swazey & G. Adelman, pp. 477–511. MIT Press, Cambridge.
3 Hubel, D.H. & Wiesel, T.N. (1977). The Ferrier Lecture: Functional architecture of macaque monkey visual cortex. *Proc. R. Soc. Lond.* B **198**, 1–59.
4 Hubel, D.H. & Wiesel, T.N. (1962). Receptive fields, binocular interaction and functional architecture in the cat's visual cortex. *J. Physiol. (Lond.)* **160**, 106–154.
5 Kuffler, S.W. (1953). Discharge patterns and functional organization of mammalian retina. *J. Neurophysiol.* **16**, 37–63.
6 Barlow, H.B. (1953). Summation and inhibition in the frog's retina *J. Physiol. (Lond.)* **119**, 69–88.
7 Hubel, D.H. & Wiesel, T.N. (1965). Receptive fields and functional architecture in two non striate visual areas (18 and 19) of the cat. *J. Neurophysiol.* **28**, 299–289.
8 Hubel, D.H. & Wiesel, T.N. (1968). Receptive fields and functional architecture of monkey striate cortex. *J. Physiol. (Lond.)* **195**, 215–243.
9 Poggio, G.F., Baker, F.H., Mansfield R.J.W., Sillito, A. & Grigg, P. (1975). Spatial and chromatic properties of neurons subserving foveal and parafoveal vision in rhesus monkey. *Brain Res.* **100**, 25–29.

Chapter 10: A motion-blind patient

In 1983 a miracle happened. A single-case clinical paper was published[1] and immediately accepted by the clinical and scientific community. The paper was by Zihl and his collaborators in Munich, and it described some very interesting results. These were derived from a forty-three-year-old female patient who had suffered a vascular disorder of the brain, with a consequent lesion in a specific part of the cortex outside the striate area (see Plate 2, facing p. 68). This had led to several problems, including a difficulty with calculations and a mild aphasia. But the most striking observation by far was the patient's inability to see objects in motion. So severe was this that, 'She had difficulty, for example, in pouring tea or coffee into a cup because the fluid appeared to be frozen, like a glacier. In addition, she could not stop pouring at the right time since she was unable to perceive the movement in the cup (or a pot) when the fluid rose. The patient also complained of difficulties in following a dialogue because she could not see the movements of...the mouth of the speaker'. She had difficulty in crossing roads because of the cars whose exact position was difficult for her to judge — 'When I'm looking at the car first, it seems far away. But then, when I want to cross the road, suddenly the car is very near' — she could not see the position of the car in between. In brief, she had no knowledge of visual movement and little knowledge of the visual world when it was set in motion.

This was not a defect in the appreciation of movement as such, because the perception of movement elicited by auditory or tactile stimulation was unaffected. The defect was very selective to visual motion perception. She had no scotoma and her perception of the other attributes of the visual scene was apparently normal. Brain scans revealed bilateral damage, more extensive in the right hemisphere. But, although there had been involvement of the white matter, the calcarine or striate cortex itself was apparently unaffected on either side. The authors concluded that their result '...supports the idea that movement vision is a separate visual function depending on neuronal mechanisms beyond the primary visual cortex'. I refer to the syndrome in which a patient is specifically unable to perceive objects in motion as akinetopsia.[2]

In the clinical, though not in the neurobiological, world this idea was nothing if not novel. It is true that the notion of defects in motion perception had been mooted in the past, based on altogether indifferent evidence. Best,[3] in a work which with justice is rarely cited, had suggested that the perception of movement and of space may be the function of areas outside the striate cortex. But then Best had no evidence to support his claim, and his ideas on the organization of the visual cortex were themselves a trifle bizarre. He had imagined that the sole function of the striate cortex was that of the fusion of the images from the two eyes. This theory was not very different from that of Ewens[4] which Henschen[5] was to qualify as 'a theory in the air'. There were two other papers which described akinetopsic symptoms, but the akinetopsia was part of a more general disturbance and the absence of a post-mortem verification of the position and the extent of the lesion rendered the evidence useless.[2] One of these patients, that of Goldstein and Gelb, was re-examined many years later by Richard Jung in Freiburg. He concluded that the patient was able to see both shapes and movements and was therefore not akinetopsic.[6] Jung stressed, 'The importance of elaborated [sic] investigations in single cases of brain injury'. This was not vastly different from the cautionary remarks about achromatopsia made by MacKay almost half a century earlier, when he had urged, '...the desirability of investigating cases of hemianopsia with more thoroughness than is usually shown'.[7]

The first suggestion that movement may be represented separately in the *striate* had in fact been made by Riddoch in 1917[8] (Figure 10.1). He had been studying the visual fields of those who had received gunshot wounds during the Great War. He had found that patients could commonly see movements in their blind (scotomatous) fields, though they were unable to appreciate the other attributes of the moving stimulus. Unlike other descriptions, his conclusions were based, not on the loss of visual motion perception, but on its presence in an otherwise blind field. These findings led him to consider that, 'Movement may be recognized as a special visual perception', separate and in addition to the perceptions '...of light, of form, and of colour'.

Riddoch tried to ascertain the lesions in the brain by means of X-ray examinations. But the localization was very poor. He nevertheless interpreted his phenomenon conservatively in terms of the striate cortex alone. But his conclusions were immediately challenged by Holmes[9] and then relegated to oblivion. Holmes was a man in whom '...there was more than a streak of austerity with strong likes and dislikes and no pretence of diplomacy or compromise'.[10] One of the ideas which he much disliked, and with which he had little inclination to compromise, was that of the dissociation of functions following lesions in the visual cortex. The equal of Henschen in the use of assertive phrases to dismiss uncomfortable facts, he wrote that Riddoch's statements were 'certainly incorrect' since in 'all my cases...the blindness was total...neither the presence nor the

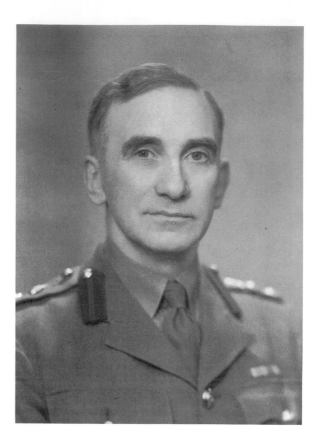

Fig. 10.1 George Riddoch (1888–1947), the British neurologist who, as a temporary Captain with the Royal Army Medical Corps during the Great War, described how patients blinded by damage to their area V1 could still perceive motion. His findings were dismissed by Gordon Holmes and have only assumed significance in recent years. (Photograph courtesy of Dr. Jane Riddoch, neuropsychologist and grand-daughter of George.)

movement of any object of reasonable size could be recognized', a statement which would seem to leave out of account Holmes' own case 11 in the same paper. This latter patient had been examined three months after sustaining his injuries, when it was found that, '. . .he was generally conscious only of the movement of the white test object'.[9] Echoing his words about the dissociation of colour vision, Holmes wrote impatiently, '. . . that the condition described by Riddoch should not be spoken of as a dissociation of the elements of visual sensation' since '. . . occipital lesions do not produce true dissociations of function with intact retinal sensibility'. Holmes was probably correct in doubting whether Riddoch's phenomenon could be accounted for in terms of the striate cortex, though wrong in dismissing the phenomenon.[2] At any rate, apart from very similar conclusions reached by Poppelreuter in 1923,[11] and also interpreted in terms of the striate cortex alone, neurologists did not take much note of Riddoch's findings. It would be difficult to find a reference to him in most textbooks of neurology, at least those published before 1974, some of which otherwise make a point of dismissing the notion of a colour centre in the brain. There is no reference to the topic, for example, in Duke-Elder's monumental book which covers almost every other aspect of vision.[10] Riddoch did not even figure in the denial of the phenomenon. Perhaps the only person, apart from Holmes, to deny such a dissociation emphatically was Teuber[12] and he did so without reference to Riddoch, who appears to have been truly dead by then, at least in terms of any influence he may have had on the subject. In 1960 Teuber wrote, 'It is commonly thought that cerebral lesions implicating central visual pathways tend to produce greater impairment for pattern than for motion perception. The evidence for such a statement is, however, unconvincing. It is not unexpected to find areas in defective visual fields where targets are perceived when they are in motion but not when they are stationary. The movement takes the target over a wider angular extent in the field and thus produces more stimulation'. Returning to the topic after a period of fourteen years, during which not much had happened, Koerner and Teuber[13] wrote that, '...we could not find any dissociation between detection of a moving and a stationary target'. This was almost identical to the earlier statement of Teuber et al.[14] that, 'There is thus no evidence for a genuine dissociation...of colour and form vision', also made without reference to authors like Verrey or MacKay and Dunlop, or even Lenz, though quoting approvingly Holmes' earlier, and identical, views.

Yet, the paper by Zihl and his colleagues was immediately accepted. There was not a murmur of dissent. This is in spite of the fact that it was a single case and was not free from association with other defects, although these were relatively mild. The position of the lesion was, it is true, determined by brain scans. But the precise extent had nevertheless been difficult to chart accurately, and there was a heavy involvement of white matter — just the kind of involvement which was used to explain away the syndrome of achromatopsia earlier. Yet this time there was no resistance. There was no MacKay[7] to complain, 'that the cases are very few in number', no Poppelreuter[11] to encourage colleagues to regard '...it as more important to present in the first place the mass of new material in its purely factual aspects and to postpone the theoretical elaboration', no Henschen[15] to say that the 'cortical retina is also a retina for [movement] impressions', no Critchley[16] to write of '...a mere handful of instances of alleged [motion] agnosia, most of which are unconvincing'. It is not to the clinical world that one looks for a reason behind this almost miraculous change of attitude, but to the scientific discoveries that finally changed the concepts which were to dominate facts in the world of visual neurology.

There is an important lesson to be drawn from this brief history. Clinical studies have consistently come up with syndromes which, in the light of the prevailing knowledge, seemed bizarre. They will no doubt continue to do so in the future. In the past, the temptation has commonly been to try to account for these syndromes in the context of known facts and concepts. If these syndromes were difficult to account for in these terms, the temptation was to dismiss them, sometimes successfully. Aphasia, colour anomia, achromatopsia have all been questioned. Neurologists have been highly successful in dismissing achromatopsia until, in the words of one of them, it 'vanished' from the clinical literature.[17] Maybe the history of neurology teaches us to ask whether the concepts that we have are broad enough to accommodate the new facts that are constantly emerging and questioning our deeply held beliefs about the brain.

References

1 Zihl, J., Cramon, D. von & Mai, N. (1983). Selective disturbance of movement vision after bilateral brain damage. *Brain* **106**, 313–340.
2 Zeki, S. (1991). Cerebral akinetopsia (cerebral visual motion blindness). *Brain* **114**, 811–824.
3 Best, F. (1919). Zur Theorie der Hemianopsie und der Höheren Sehzentren. *Albrecht v. Graefes Arch. Ophthal.* **100**, 1–31.
4 Ewens, G.F.W. (1893). A theory of cortical visual representation. *Brain* **16**, 475–491.
5 Henschen, S.E. (1894). Sur les centres optiques cérébraux. *Rev. Gén. Ophtal. (Paris)* **13**, 337–352.
6 Jung, R. (1949). Über eine Nachuntersuchung des Falles Schn...von Goldstein und Gelb. *Psychiatr. Neurol. Med. Psychol.* **12**, 353–362.
7 MacKay, G. (1888). A discussion on a contribution to the study of hemianopsia, with special reference to acquired colour blindness. *Br. Med. J.* **2**, 1033–1037.
8 Riddoch, G. (1917). Dissociation of visual perception due to occipital injuries, with especial reference to appreciation of movement. *Brain* **40**, 15–57.
9 Holmes, G. (1918). Disturbances of vision by cerebral lesions. *Br. J. Ophthalmol.* **2**, 353–384.
10 Duke-Elder, S. (1971). *A System of Ophthalmology* J. & A. Churchill, London.
11 Poppelreuter, W. (1923). Zur Psychologie und Pathologie der optischen Wahrnehmung. *Z. Ges. Neurol. Psychiatr.* **83**, 26–152.
12 Teuber, H.-L. (1960). Perception. In *Handbook of Physiology*, 3(1), edited by J. Field, H.W. Magoun & V.E. Hall, pp. 1595–1668. American Physiological Society, Washington DC.
13 Koerner, J. & Teuber, H.-L. (1973). Visual defects after missile injuries to the geniculo-striate pathways in man. *Exp. Brain Res.* **18**, 88–113.
14 Teuber, H.-L., Battersby, W.S. & Bender, M.B. (1960). *Visual Field Defects After Penetrating Missile Wounds of the Brain.* Harvard University Press, Cambridge.
15 Henschen, S.E. (1910). Zentrale Sehstörungen. In *Handbuch der Neurologie*, 2, edited by M. Lewandowsky, pp. 891–918. Springer-Verlag, Berlin.
16 Critchley, M. (1965). Acquired anomalies of colour perception of central origin. *Brain* **88**, 711–724.
17 Damasio, A.R. (1985). Disorders of complex visual processing. In *Principles of Behavioural Neurology*, edited by M.-Marsel Mesulam, pp. 259–288. F.A. Davis, Philadelphia.

Chapter 11: The multiple visual areas of the cerebral cortex

The concept of a visual image formed in the retina and then transmitted to be 'received' by the 'cortical retina' before being 'associated' with previous visual, and other, 'impressions' seemed to correlate well with the known anatomy of the visual pathways and of the cortical areas. It also seemed to correlate well with a hierarchical doctrine of visual processing. Between them, such concepts left little room for supposing that there is a separate cortical area for colour vision, and therefore that there may be a functional specialization in the visual cortex for colour vision, from which it would follow that there must be a specialization for other visual attributes as well. Acceptance of such a doctrine would entail rejection of the earlier concepts one after another. It would also lead to the awkward question of why separate attributes of vision should be separately mapped in the cerebral cortex. The best way around the impasse, and around the awkward questions, was to ignore altogether any evidence which may suggest a functional specialization in the visual cortex, whether for colour or motion or any other attribute. In this respect, the conduct of scientists was not greatly different from that of other groups of men. When confronted with a difficult problem which goes against their way of thinking, scientists often begin by shutting their eyes firmly to the evidence and pretending that it does not exist. The next stage consists of accepting the evidence but pretending that it is not important or that it can be adequately explained by the known facts. The third and final stage consists of admitting the evidence and its significance but pretending that it has all been said before. Something much like this has happened to the evidence relating to colour specialization in the cerebral cortex.

A major turning point in our knowledge of how the cortex handles visual information was provided by the discovery of multiple visual areas that are functionally specialized to undertake different visual tasks. This may seem surprising. Scientists and laymen often believe that scientific problems must be tackled systematically, that unless one understands the characteristics of the first stage of a complex system one cannot hope to understand those of the next stage, and cannot therefore understand how the system functions. There are many instances in which this is true. Perception in general, and vision in particular, are not among them. Indeed, the study of the visual system has proved to be a precarious occupation. Powerful clues to understanding important aspects of its organization and functioning were first obtained by studying cortical visual areas, in particular the 'higher ones', not the retina or the lateral geniculate nucleus (LGN). This is in spite of the fact that the number of studies on the latter outnumber by far those on the former. Moreover, we perhaps understand much better the functions of area V1 or of area V5 than we do those of the LGN. At least, we understand the organization of these visual areas sufficiently well to be able to account for much that is interesting and important in vision. By contrast, the equally minutely studied LGN has told us very little that is of interest about vision as a process, beyond the vague statement that it may act as 'a sharpener' of the retinal image',[1] a surprisingly banal function for so large and complex a structure. All of which shows that it is a mistake to avoid studying the apparently more 'complex' areas of the cerebral cortex simply because one has failed to understand the seemingly more 'simple' structures. Nowhere is this better illustrated than in the doctrine of functional specialization in the visual system, derived first from studies of the 'higher' cortical areas and, over a decade later, found to be true of the retina as well.

That there are visual areas outside the primary visual cortex has been known for at least thirty years. But it is only in the last decade that their presence has started to overturn deeply held concepts of the cerebral processes underlying vision. One of the earliest papers was by Clare and Bishop,[2] appropriately entitled *Responses from an association area secondarily activated from optic cortex*. There is much that is of interest in this title, which, in a sense, betrays a mode of thinking. Though situated well outside the territory which was then considered to be the primary visual cortex in the cat, the area that they described was nevertheless a visual area, and defined by the use of visual stimuli. Yet it is deprived of this status, which is invested on the 'optic' cortex alone, by which they meant the primary visual cortex. The 'new' area is, instead, considered to be an 'association' area, although no associational activity was studied there. Indeed, the area was 'inferred to comprise an association area relating optic and acoustic activity', because, 'It is usually taken for granted that impulses are propagated from an active projection area of cortex, for instance a sensory projection area such as primary optic cortex, to surrounding "association" areas'.[2]

Not long after the discovery by Clare and Bishop, two further visual areas were charted in cat cortex on the basis of cytoarchitectonic differences in cortical appearance and referred to as areas 18 and 19.[3] Hubel and Wiesel[4] recorded from these areas and found that most cells in them display some very specific features, being of either the complex or the hypercomplex variety. This seemed to perpetuate the chain of hierarchies into 'association' cortex. Indeed, no further significance, beyond that of associating and elaborating the responses of visual cells in previous areas, was attached to these areas. Nevertheless, to anyone thinking of this new evidence in terms of older concepts of 'association' cortex — indeed the concept of association cortex used by Clare and Bishop only years before — the function of association cortex must have undergone a subtle change since the type of association occurring here was now considered to be between visual signals, rather than between visual and other signals or between past and present visual signals. But this new view of association cortex is not discussed in any of the papers and there is no evidence that anyone was particularly thinking of what the new evidence meant.

In the late 1960s and early 1970s an increasingly large number of visual areas in the so-called visual association cortex of the monkey were described (Figure 11.1a). The evidence came principally from two species of monkey, the Old World macaque[5] and the New World owl monkey.[6] In the Old World monkey the evidence was anatomical in nature at first, and consisted of demonstrating the regions of the 'visual association' cortex to which the primary visual cortex sends connections. It was found that the primary visual cortex,

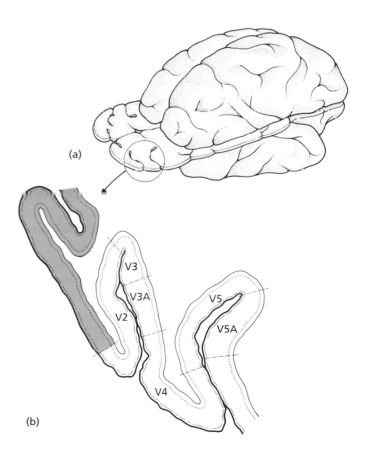

Fig. 11.1 The visual cortex of the macaque monkey is very extensive and much of it is buried in sulci. Its extent is best appreciated when the brain is cut horizontally (a). In the section shown in (b), the primary visual cortex at the back is shown in grey. Lying in front of the primary visual cortex are several visual areas, each one of which undertakes a different task.

which has a detailed map of the retina in it, in turn projects in a detailed, point-to-point manner to some regions of the visual 'association' cortex, implying that the detailed retinal map is reproduced independently in these regions. By contrast, the projections to other regions of this 'association' cortex were found to be far less precise, with adjacent points in the primary visual cortex projecting in a convergent, overlapping, way to them and implying that the retinal topography thus created in them is less precise. In the owl monkey the evidence came from physiological 'mapping' studies. Such studies make the assumption that it is the retina that is mapped in the cortical areas concerned with vision and, consequently, do not concern themselves with the functional properties of cells in the visual areas. Instead, they study the nature of the retinal representation in cortex outside the striate area by stimulating large groups of cells with spots of light, based on the assumption that if they are visual areas they will respond to light. Whatever the assumptions behind these studies, they also showed, like the anatomical studies, that *there are multiple areas outside the primary visual cortex, that the retina is independently represented in each and that the nature of retinal representation differs from area to area*. Thus, in neither of these studies were the areas characterized functionally by studying the specific visual stimuli to which the cells in each area would be most responsive. Nevertheless, the demonstration of multiple visual areas outside the striate cortex suggested, at the very least, that vision cannot be the simple dual process that neurologists had believed it to be, thus destabilizing the first chip in this domino game. It was, however, to be many years before the full impact filtered through, and there remain quarters where its impact has yet to be felt, even today.

In addition to showing that there are several visual areas in the cortex, besides the primary visual cortex, the studies in the macaque monkey also showed that these areas co-exist in cortical regions of uniform *cyto*architecture. For example, four separate visual areas are known to exist within the cytoarchitectonic area 18 of Brodmann (Figure 11.2b). Among other things, this evidence showed that cyto-architectonic uniformity is not necessarily a guide to functional uniformity in the cortex, thus leading to the downfall of the next chip in the domino game. This is not to say that there are no *architectonic* differences between these areas. Indeed, present evidence shows that the use of techniques other than the cytoarchitectonic technique reveals remarkable differences, at least between some of the areas. Had such studies been available at a time when the presence of a colour centre in the human visual cortex outside the striate cortex was being debated, they would almost certainly have rendered the suggestive evidence of the clinicians more palatable, or so one might hope with hindsight. But they were not.

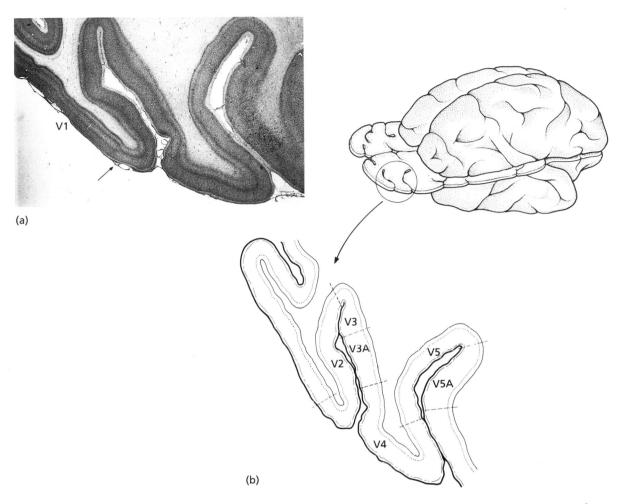

(a)

(b)

Fig. 11.2 A horizontal section through the posterior part of the brain is here stained to show the cytoarchitecture of the cortex (a). The part of the cortex lying at the back (to the left) is known as the striate cortex (area V1). It has a uniform cytoarchitecture which is distinctly different from the uniform cytoarchitecture of the part lying more anteriorly (to the right), the prestriate cortex. The arrow marks the transition between striate and prestriate cortex. In spite of its uniform cytoarchitecture, the prestriate cortex consists of several distinct visual areas (b). This shows that cytoarchitectural uniformity is not a good guide to functional uniformity.

The studies of the visual areas in the association cortex showed that the retina is 'mapped' independently in each of the visual areas but in a different way than it is in the primary visual cortex, that the receptive fields of cells in them are larger and that the areas themselves are consequently smaller in size than the primary visual cortex (Figure 11.3). Superficially, then, this seemed to agree with the concept of hierarchies, which supposed that cells in increasingly higher areas collect information from increasingly larger parts of the field of view. It is not surprising, then, that these studies did not call into question

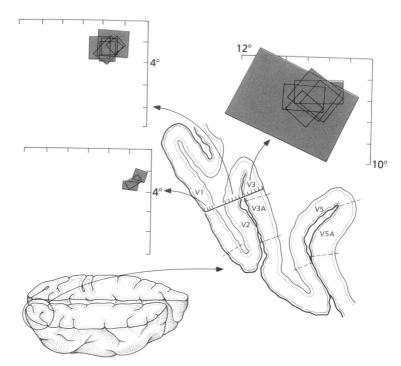

Fig. 11.3 The change in receptive field size of cells in three visual areas of monkey cortex. Receptive fields are smallest in area V1 and larger in area V3, with those in area V2 having intermediate sizes. Cells in the parietal and temporal visual areas (not shown) have even larger receptive fields.

the concept of association cortex as then formulated, i.e. of cortex in which received visual impressions are associated with previous visual impressions of a similar kind, resulting in recognition. Indeed, the language used by many, including myself, in the description of these areas was obviously strongly influenced by doctrines of the past. It was, in brief, the knowledge derived from experience that was holding sway. The retina, or the visual field, was thought to be independently 'represented' or 're-represented' in these areas, the topography was thought to be 'cruder'. This latter term is one which I used to describe one of the areas (V5) and then rapidly abandoned it, only to discover that others have started using it. For it is quite absurd to think that there is such a thing as a 'crude' representation in the brain. The representation of any function in any area of the brain is as precise as it needs to be for the area to execute its function. The mistake lies only in supposing that it is the retina that is represented in these areas, a common error which we shall discuss below. At any rate, apart from destabilizing the first chip in the domino game, the one that supposed that vision is a dual cortical process, and compromising the second, the notion that an area of uniform cytoarchitecture is necessarily a single cortical area, the discovery of many independent visual areas did little to overturn the concepts of the past. It merely seemed to emphasize a continuing process, easily interpretable as being 'hierarchical' in nature. But the concept of hierarchy as an exclusive strategy had no solid foundations. It was sufficient to show that each of the specialized visual areas receives an independent input from V1 for it to collapse too. And this evidence was already there in the anatomical studies on the macaque monkey visual cortex.[7]

References

1 Levick, W.R., Oyster, C.W. & Takahashi, E. (1969). Rabbit lateral geniculate nucleus: sharpener of directional information. *Science* **165**, 712–714.

2 Clare, M.H. & Bishop, G.H. (1954). Responses from an association area secondarily activated from optic cortex. *J. Neurophysiol.* **17**, 271–277.

3 Otsuka, R. & Hassler, R. (1962). Über Abfau und Gliederung der corticalen Sehsphäre bei der Katze. *Arch. Psychiatr. Nervenkr.* **203**, 212–234.

4 Hubel, D.H. & Wiesel, T.N. (1965). Receptive fields and functional architecture in two non-striate visual areas (18 and 19) of the cat. *J. Neurophysiol.* **28**, 299–289.

5 Zeki, S.M. (1969). Representation of central visual fields in prestriate cortex of monkey. *Brain Res.* **14**, 271–291; Cragg, B.G. (1969). The topography of the afferent projections in the circumstriate visual cortex of the monkey studied by the Nauta method. *Vision Res.* **9**, 733–747; Zeki, S.M. (1971). Cortical projections from two prestriate areas in the monkey. *Brain Res.* **34**, 19–35; Zeki, S.M. (1971). Convergent input from the striate cortex (area 17) to the cortex of the superior temporal sulcus in the rhesus monkey. *Brain Res.* **28**, 338–340.

6 Allman, J.M. & Kaas, J.H. (1971). A representation of the visual field in the caudal third of the middle temporal gyrus of the owl monkey (*Aotus trivirgatus*). *Brain Res.* **31**, 85–105; Allman, J.M. & Kaas, J.H. (1971). Representation of the visual field in striate and adjoining cortex of the owl monkey (*Aotus trivirgatus*). *Brain Res.* **35**, 89–106.

7 Zeki, S.M. (1975). The functional organization of projections from striate to prestriate visual cortex in the rhesus monkey. *Cold Spring Harb. Symp. Quant. Biol.* **40**, 591–600.

Chapter 12: The basic anatomy of the visual areas

Before discussing the functional implications of these discoveries, it is desirable to familiarize oneself with the basic anatomy of the visual areas. This will in any case facilitate the descriptions to follow.

Basic techniques for studying anatomical connections

There are several ways of studying the anatomical organization of cortical areas. The simplest is to try and determine their location and extent. This can be done by studying their architecture, since an architecture characteristic of an area will define its borders. Unfortunately, there isn't a single architectural method that reveals the characteristic architecture of each area. With the presently available methods some areas have been discovered to have a characteristic architecture and others not.

Another way is to define their connections and in this description we are only concerned with one set of connections, those comprising the forward input to the visual areas; we can defer a discussion of other connections to a later chapter. There are at least three relatively modern methods for studying the connections of cerebral areas. One is to make a small cortical lesion. The consequence is that the fibres of cells destroyed by such a lesion will degenerate. This renders the fibres more argyrophilic (i.e. more ready to take up silver). Consequently, if sections taken through such a brain are stained for silver, the degenerated fibres can be readily seen. Areas showing such (silver) degeneration are the ones that receive fibres from the lesioned cortical zone, and hence are connected with it (Figure 12.1).

Another approach is to inject very small quantities of a radioactive amino acid into the cortex. The amino acids are taken up by the cells of the injected area, and are then transported down the axons to their terminals. Because they are radioactive, the terminals can then be shown up by suitable treatment (Figure 12.1). In addition to showing which areas are connected with which, these techniques also reveal the layer of the cortex in which the axon terminals (from the lesioned or injected area) terminate. The most recent of these techniques demonstrates these connections in the reverse direction and reveals features not shown by the first two methods. This technique depends upon injecting the enzyme horseradish peroxidase (HRP) into the regions where axons from a given source are suspected of terminating.

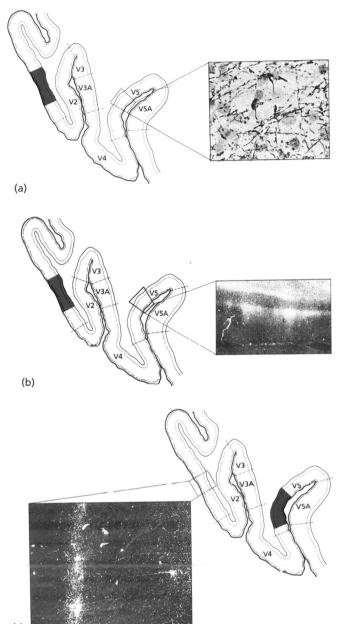

Fig. 12.1 Three methods of studying connectivities in the cerebral cortex. In each case, the example given relates to the connections between areas V1 and V5. (a) A small lesion is made in V1 and the degenerated fibres traced to V5. (b) A radioactively labelled amino acid is injected into V1 and the distribution of label is traced to V5. (c) Horse-radish peroxidase is injected into V5 and the cells in V1 projecting to the injected area are labelled.

The enzyme is taken up by the axon terminals and transported retro gradely, back to the cell body. The latter can be visualized by suitable treatment of the brain sections. This technique has the advantage of revealing in which layers the cells sending their axons to the injected area are located (Figure 12.1). The HRP can be combined with the lectin wheatgerm agglutinin (WGA) which binds to membranes, and can thus label the axons of cells emanating from an area. Thus, the injection of a combination of HRP–WGA into a cortical area is an ideal way of studying not only the positions of cells in other areas that send their axons to the injected area, but also the distribution of fibres emanating from the injected area. Cortical areas are usually reciprocally connected with each other, i.e. where area A sends an output to area B, it receives in turn a return output (from B to A). By injecting HRP–WGA one can therefore study the distribution of both the prograde (forward) and retrograde (backward) projections to and from an area. There is of course no reason why the three techniques should not be combined in a single preparation, and this has been commonly done.

Location and architecture of cortical areas

The visual cortex occupies the occipital lobe of the brain, although there are areas outside the occipital lobe which have functions related to vision in one way or another. Good examples are the frontal lobes, where the frontal eye fields are prominently involved in controlling eye movements; the parietal lobes, which contain several distinct areas, some of them being more obviously visual than others; and the inferior convexity of the temporal lobes which also contain several distinct visual areas (Figure 12.2). But, in general, areas which are predominantly and overwhelmingly visual in function are concentrated in the occipital lobe.

The occipital lobe is traditionally subdivided into two parts on anatomical grounds. The largest subdivision is area V1, which has a very distinctive cytoarchitecture and is therefore commonly referred to as the striate cortex (see Chapter 3). It differs sharply in its cytoarchitecture from the area surrounding it. Because it lies largely in front of the striate cortex, the area surrounding it is commonly known as the prestriate cortex. The prestriate cortex differs from the striate cortex in that it contains many visual areas, whereas the striate cortex is co-extensive with a single visual area, area V1 (Figure 12.3).

The visual areas of the prestriate cortex can be seen in a horizontal section through the brain, taken at the level indicated in Figure 12.3.

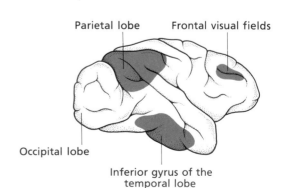

Fig. 12.2 The posterior quarter of the brain is visual in function. But there are many other parts which have some visual functions. Among these are the parietal cortex, the temporal cortex and the frontal cortex.

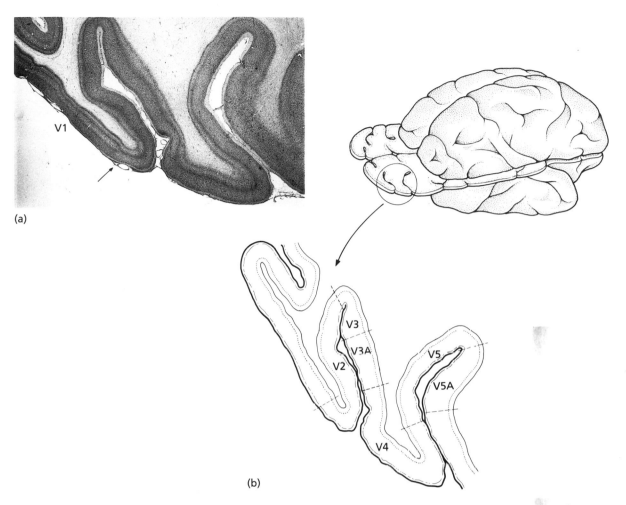

Fig. 12.3 (a) The cytoarchitecture of the striate cortex (area V1) and the cortex lying in front of it, the prestriate cortex (arrow marks transition), shown in this horizontal section taken through the back of the brain of a macaque monkey. (b) The visual areas of the prestriate cortex.

Of these, the one immediately surrounding area V1 is known as area V2. In the macaque monkey V2 is only just visible on the surface of the brain, most of it lying within the lunate and inferior occipital sulci (Figure 12.4a). Just as adjacent retinal points connect with adjacent cortical points in V1, with the consequence that the retina is topographically mapped in the latter, so adjacent points in V1 connect with adjacent points in V2, once again resulting in a detailed topographic map of the retina in area V2[1] (Figure 12.5). The retinal map in V2 is, however, somewhat strange. The representation of the horizontal meridian of the retina, which in V1 separates the representation of the upper retinal quadrant from the lower retinal quadrant, splits to form the anterior border of area V2. Why this

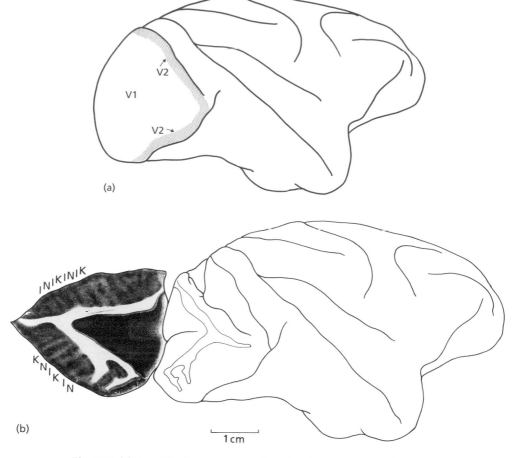

(a)

(b)

INIKINIK

KNIKIN

1 cm

Fig. 12.4 (a) Area V2 of macaque monkey visual cortex surrounds area V1 and most of it lies buried within sulci. It is best seen when the back of the brain is opened up (b). The characteristic architecture of area V2 revealed by staining it for the metabolic enzyme cytochrome oxidase. The back part of the brain has been opened up to reveal area V2 (a). Sections through area V2 taken in the plane of the paper are stained for cytochrome oxidase and reveal the characteristic thick (K) and thin stripes (N), which are separated from each other by the more lightly staining interstripes (I).

should be so is still not clear. The consequence of these connections is that the lower contralateral retinal quadrant (upper field of view) is mapped in the lower part of V2, and the upper contralateral quadrant (lower field of view) is mapped in its upper part. Although it was anatomical studies[1] which led to these strange conclusions, they have nevertheless been fully confirmed by subsequent electrophysiological studies.[2]

Area V2 is situated within a cytoarchitectonically uniform area, area 18 of Brodmann. It is not, therefore, distinguishable on this basis from the other areas lying within the same cytoarchitectonic area (18). But it can be distinguished from other visual areas by staining the brain for metabolic activity with the enzyme cytochrome oxidase,

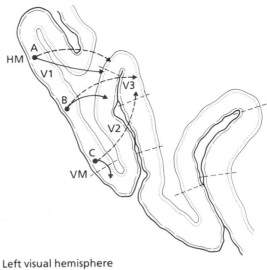

Left visual hemisphere

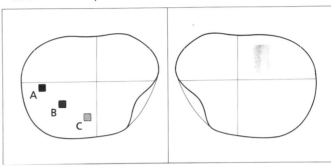

Fig. 12.5 The systematic connections between area V1 and areas V2 and V3, shown schematically. The retina is topographically represented in area V1, with the horizontal (HM) and vertical (VM) meridian representations occupying distinct zones. The systematic, point-to-point, connections between area V1 and areas V2 and V3 means that the retina (and hence the visual field, below) is also topographically represented in the latter areas.

and thus revealing its metabolic or cytochrome oxidase architecture. The metabolic architecture of V2 is very distinctive. It consists of a set of dark stripes running from the cortical surface to white matter, and separated from each other by lightly staining stripes (Figure 12.4b). These stripes are not very obvious in horizontal sections but are well seen in sections which are parallel to the cortical surface. The dark stripes are then found to be of two kinds, thick and thin. Thus, if one were to survey area V2 in a direction parallel to the cortical surface, one would encounter cycles consisting of a thick stripe, interstripe, thin stripe, interstripe, following which the cycle repeats itself.[3] In a macaque monkey, an entire cycle consisting of a thick stripe, thin stripe and two interstripes is about 4.5−5 mm. Even though the pattern is not always as clear as the one shown in Figure 12.4b, the architecture is nevertheless unique to area V2. Moreover, this metabolic architecture correlates well with a functional architecture since, as we shall see, different stripes of V2 appear to undertake different tasks and to have distinct cortical destinations.

The metabolic architecture of V2 differs profoundly from that of V1. Unlike V2, area V1 is also cytoarchitecturally distinct, but its metabolic architecture reveals further features which are not evident from examining its cytoarchitecture. Chief among these is a more darkly staining layer 4C, a lightly staining layer 4B and a row of darkly staining patches constituting layer 4A (Figure 12.6). Perhaps more significant from a functional point of view is another set of columns extending from surface to white matter and intersecting the tangential pattern at right angles. These 'columns' of darkly staining tissue are most evident in the upper cortical layers (layers 2 and 3) where they constitute the cytochrome oxidase blobs or puffs.[4] The blobs are best seen when sections parallel to the cortical surface are taken through layers 2 and 3 and stained for metabolic activity. When such sections are viewed, they are found to consist of a pattern of darkly staining regions, about 300 µm in diameter, and giving rise to what has been called a 'polka dot' pattern. The blobs are separated from each other by more lightly staining regions known as the inter-blobs. Functional studies, to be reviewed later, again show that this metabolic architecture correlates with a functional architecture, in that the cells within the blobs and those between them have different functional properties and project to different destinations in the cortex.

Although the description given above is for the macaque monkey, it applies equally well to the human brain.[5] Human V1 thus has a metabolic architecture which is similar to that of the monkey except that the dimensions of the blobs are different. Surrounding human striate cortex is an area with a metabolic architecture which consists of a set of thick and thin stripes which are separated from each other by more lightly staining interstripes, in other words, a pattern which is identical to that of monkey V2. In the human brain, much of area V2 must lie on the medial surface, surrounding the striate cortex. The part of V2 representing the upper retina (lower visual field) should thus lie in the cuneus, bordering the upper lip of the calcarine sulcus, while the part of V2 representing the lower retina (upper visual field) should lie in the lingual gyrus (see Figure 12.7).[6]

A distinctive metabolic architecture is not characteristic of other visual areas in the prestriate cortex, which is not to suggest that they may not have a very distinctive architecture, revealable by other methods. A good example is area V3 (Figure 12.8). This lies next to V2, is located within Brodmann's area 18 and receives a direct, point-to-point input from V1 with the consequence that the retina is also topographically mapped in it.[7] The retinal representation in area V3 is a mirror image of its representation in area V2, so that the representation of the horizontal meridian forms the common boundary between V2 and V3, while it is the vertical meridian that is represented at the anterior border of V3 (Figure 12.4b). Like V2, V3 can be subdivided into a dorsal and a ventral part, each representing a different retinal quadrant. It is therefore common to speak of V3d (dorsal) and V3v

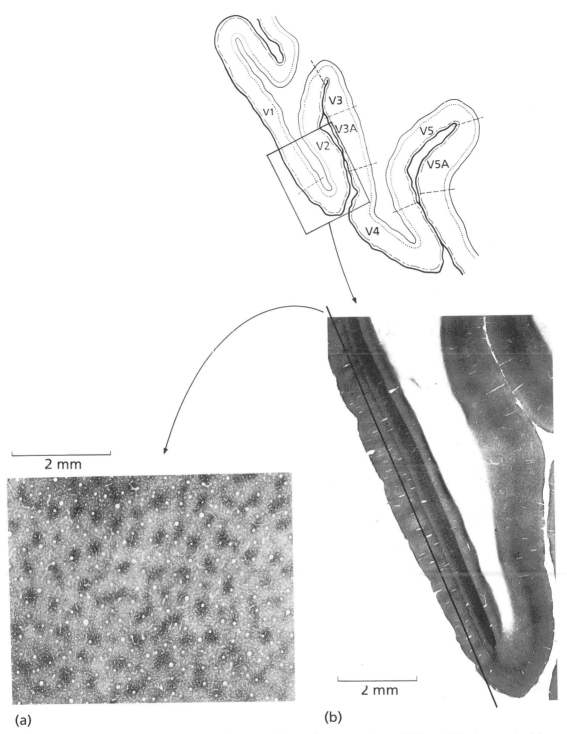

(a)

(b)

Fig. 12.6 The cytochrome oxidase architecture of area V1 (boxed) is characterized by a set of densely staining layers intersected by fairly densely staining columns extending from the surface to the white matter (b). These columns are especially prominent in layers 2 and 3. A section through the latter layers, taken parallel to the cortical surface (along the line in (b)) and stained for cytochrome oxidase, reveals the columns as blobs or puffs (a).

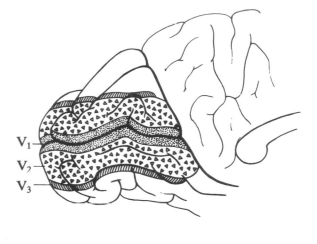

Fig. 12.7 The inferred position of area V3 in the human brain, lying on the medial side of the brain and surrounding area V2. (Reproduced by permission from Horton, J.C. & Hoyt, W.F. (1991). *Brain* **114**, 1703–1718.)

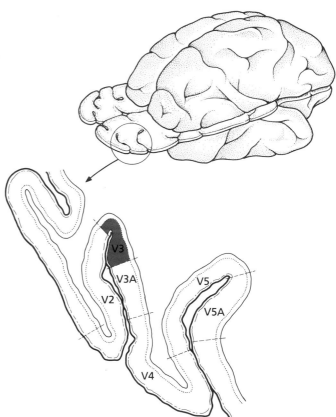

Fig. 12.8 Area V3 of macaque monkey visual cortex, seen in a horizontal section through the brain. Like area V2, it is connected in a point-to-point manner with area V1, and hence the retina is topographically mapped in it (see Figure 12.5). The arrangement of the connections between these areas is such that the retinal representation in area V2 is a mirror image of its representation in V1 and that of V3 is a mirror image of V2, with the representation of the upper and lower quadrants being neatly separated from each other.

(ventral). One study[8] claims that the subdivisions of V3 are sufficiently different from each other to constitute two different areas, but not all workers seem to be in agreement with such a further subdivision. Beyond a dense cytochrome oxidase content,[9] V3 does not have a discernible metabolic architecture, though future studies may well show that it has a characteristic architecture revealable by a method yet to be described. If the similarity between macaque and human brain extends to V3, then V3 should also be found to lie in both the cuneus and the lingual gyrus, with the former part representing the lower visual field and the latter part the upper visual field[6] (Figure 12.7).

Next to area V3 lies area V3A[10] (Figure 12.9). This shares certain functional characteristics with V3 but, except for the peripheral retinal representation within it, does not receive a direct input from V1.[11] Rather, it receives a strong input from V3. Area V3A is rather strange; it extends dorsally across the brain, on to its medial side, and seems to have central vision represented twice in it, for reasons yet to be determined. Like V2 and V3, it also lies within Brodmann's area 18 and to date no one has described a unique architecture characteristic of it. Because of the similarity that V3 shares with V3A in its functional properties, we speak of the V3 complex, though distinguishing the areas within this complex. We still do not know whether there is a human V3A, nor where it may be situated.

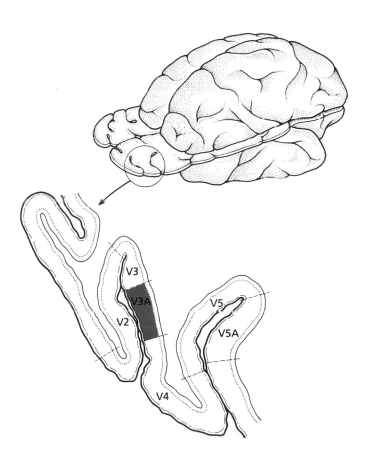

Fig. 12.9 The position of area V3A, as it appears in a horizontal section through macaque monkey visual cortex.

On the lateral side of the brain, area V3A is bordered by area V4 anteriorly[12] (Figure 12.10). V4 receives an input from the region of central (foveal) representation in V1, but its more prominent input is from V2.[13] Visual fields are not so neatly represented in V4, although there is a semblance of topography in that the receptive fields of cells in any given part of V4 are usually located in the same rough part of the visual field. There is a heavy emphasis on colour vision in this area. Lying in front of V4 is area V4A. This receives only a meagre input from V2, and almost none from V1. Instead, it receives a substantial input from V4 itself.[14] The properties of cells within it are very similar to those within V4. We therefore speak of the V4 complex, distinguishing its components nevertheless. It is possible that there are more subdivisions within V4 than this brief description suggests, but no one has given an adequate definition yet. There have been several attempts to characterize V4 architecturally, usually based on the technique of myeloarchitecture. The results have not been anywhere near as satisfactory in revealing a distinct architecture as the cytochrome oxidase technique has been in revealing a distinctive metabolic architecture for V1 and V2.

On the medial side of the brain, in a region which some may consider to constitute a part of the parietal cortex, area V3A is bordered

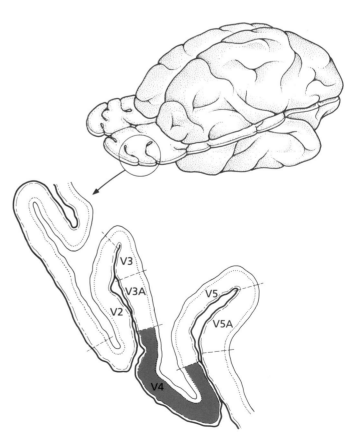

Fig. 12.10 The position of area V4 (the V4 complex) seen in a horizontal section taken through the posterior end of the macaque monkey brain. V4 consists of at least two, possibly more, subdivisions, but these are not shown here.

by area V6 anteriorly (see Figure 12.11).[15] The area has basic similarities in broad organization to the ones which are mentioned above. Thus, it receives an input from V2 — an area in which all the submodalities of vision are represented — and appears to have a central area and satellite areas, so that we may speak of the V6 complex. It has a very unconventional retinal map in it, assuming that the kind of map it contains can be said to be retinal at all. Recent physiological evidence suggests that among its functions must be that of space representation in the brain.[16]

Returning once again to the lateral side of the brain, lying more anteriorly to the V4 complex (anteriorly to V4A), is area V5[17] (Plate 3, facing p. 68). This area lies buried within the superior temporal sulcus. It is rich in cytochrome oxidase and is heavily myelinated,[18] though it does not possess a distinctive cytochrome oxidase architecture. It receives a direct input from V1. Anteriorly and inferiorly it is bounded by several other areas.[19] These do not receive a direct input from V1, but receive their input from V5 itself. They nevertheless share certain physiological characteristics with V5, in that the cells in them are selectively responsive to different kinds of motion.[20,21] We hence speak of the V5 complex.

All the visual areas described above have multiple cortical outputs. They all project to more than two other cortical areas and each has subcortical projections, often to the same structures. The significance of this is taken up below.

The total extent of the visual areas in reconstructions of the brain

It is obviously desirable to see the total extent of these areas and learn more precisely how they are disposed in relation to each other. But this is no simple task. The brain of the macaque monkey, like that of

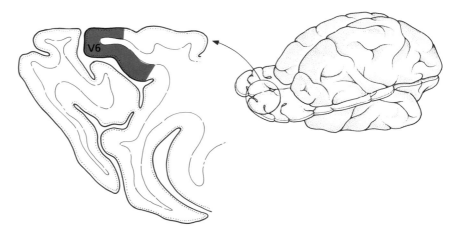

Fig. 12.11 The position of area V6 lying on the medial side of the brain, seen in a horizontal section through the macaque monkey brain.

man, is highly folded and an area of the cortex may be entirely buried within a sulcus, as is area V3, or, like V4, it may lie partially on a gyrus and partially within a sulcus. Moreover, the arrangement of the areas, and indeed the sulci, is not symmetrical with respect to a given co-ordinate. A sulcus or an area may have an antero-posterior inclination or a medio-lateral one. There may be, and commonly are, secondary foldings within a sulcus and one sulcus may open up into another. Alternatively, part of an area may lie on one surface of a sulcus and another part on another surface, a good example being area V1. Two areas which abut one another at one level may find a third area interposed between them at another level. This creates serious problems for studying an area, for two reasons. First, many interesting features of a cortical area, for example the pattern of distribution of inputs to it from other areas, commonly occur in a plane parallel to the cortical surface, with the consequence that one wishes to view an area in its entirety *en face*, as if one were flying over it. But, second, owing to the complex folding of the brain, it is in practice impossible to section all cortical areas in a single brain, or even a single cortical area, entirely in a plane parallel to the cortical surface, since one can only section the brain in one plane. Hence the need to reconstruct an area from many sections. Perhaps the simplest way of understanding this complex problem is to look at a Swiss roll, one created by a master chef. Let us suppose that, instead of using only jam, the chef decides to use both strawberry jam and chocolate cream in his Swiss roll, so that the roll, viewed from the outside, has alternate brown and red bands, corresponding to the chocolate cream and the strawberry jam respectively (Figure 12.12b). But viewed in this way, we have no means of knowing whether the bands are merely the ends of columns extending right along the long axis of the roll, whether they are elongated stripes, though not continuous from one end of the roll to the other, or whether they are merely small circular areas, perhaps blobs, forming some kind of jig-saw within the roll. It is even conceivable that the chef might have created whorls with complicated patterns, not visible from the outside. We could, of course, take another section somewhere through the middle of the roll. But if we find the same pattern, we would still not be certain whether the bands in the first 'section' are continuous with those in the second. We can, however, take many sections through the roll, trace a contour line along the jam and the cream, flatten each contour line, and then align them with respect to one another (Figure 12.12c). Such a simple reconstruction reveals that what the chef did, before rolling up the sponge, was to prepare elongated bands of filling on the sponge, one filling (jam) alternating with another (chocolate) (Figure 12.12a). We have, in brief, a reconstruction of the Swiss roll. An example of a relatively simple cortical reconstruction, perhaps the first of its kind,[14] is shown in Figure 12.13. The aim here is to reconstruct the pattern of distribution of fibres connecting area V5 of one hemisphere with the opposite side of the brain. The fibres connecting the two hemispheres distribute mainly in layer 4 of the cortex, though not with equal density throughout the extent of layer 4; some regions have a high

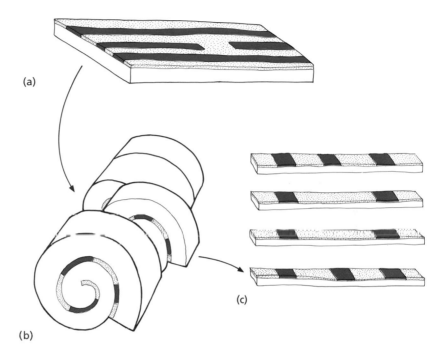

(a)

(c)

Fig. 12.12 The Swiss roll.   (b)

Fig. 12.13 An early two-dimensional map of a small region of the cortex. The aim was to reconstruct the pattern of distribution of the fibres that connect this area with its counterpart in the opposite hemisphere. A contour line (red) through the region of interest is drawn through each section and relevant details (in this case the distribution of fibres linking this zone with the opposite hemisphere; black dots) are entered. The contour lines are next aligned with respect to one another, thus giving a two-dimensional reconstruction of the area and the distribution of the fibres in it. (Redrawn from Zeki, S. (1977). *Proc. R. Soc. Lond.* B **197**, 195–223.)

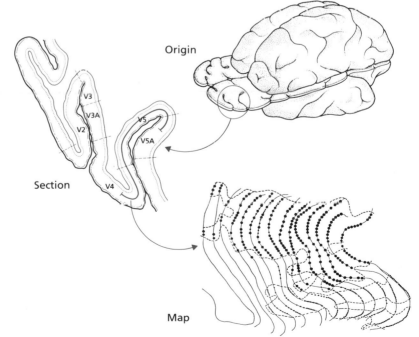

Origin

Section

Map

V3
V3A
V2
V5
V5A
V4

density of fibres connecting the two hemispheres, others a much lower density, and yet others none at all. All this information can be entered onto a contour line of the cortex, drawn through layer 4 of several contiguous sections. If one were then to align the individual contour lines with respect to one another, each contour line belonging to a different section, one would obtain a two-dimensional reconstruction of the area as if it were being viewed from the surface. There are, of course, any number of interesting anatomical features of an area which one can reconstruct in this manner and the example given above is but one. Moreover, if the sections from which the contour lines are taken are stained in such a way as to reveal a feature which is characteristic of an area, or unique to it, one can even determine the boundaries of an area and therefore its total extent.

The relationship of the areas with respect to one another in a highly folded brain requires a more elaborate reconstruction of large parts of the brain and the 'opening up' of regions which lie buried inside sulci, but the general principle is the same. In other words, one has to draw contour lines through sections of the brain taken at regular intervals and align these sections with respect to one another, using suitable markers such as the depth of a sulcus or the foldings of a gyrus. The alignment procedure is easy in those regions where the contour lines themselves are relatively straight but is much more difficult in regions of high curvature. The difficulty is compounded by the fact that the depth of a sulcus is never constant, with the consequence that contour lines may cross over. This makes it necessary to straighten out regions of high curvature, a procedure that introduces an error since straightening out a curved surface involves stretching it. Nevertheless, using this approach, one can obtain good two-dimensional reconstructions of large parts of the brain. Figure 12.14 shows the first such reconstruction to be done[22] and many others have been made since,[23] including ones for the human brain.[24] The advantages and the disadvantages of the method are evident at a glance. One disadvantage is that areas of the brain which are contiguous 'as the crow flies' are no longer contiguous on the reconstruction itself. For example, an electrode track in the posterior bank of the lunate sulcus (dark red line of Figure 12.14a), would, if pushed anteriorly, hit the anterior bank of the same sulcus (light red line of Figure 12.14a), whereas in the reconstruction itself it looks as if the anterior bank is separated from the posterior bank by other parts of the brain. In reality, the region of the brain intervening between the dark red and light red lines on the reconstructions should be conceived of as the two faces of the valley which one would have to descend and then ascend if, instead of flying, one were walking from the posterior bank to the anterior bank of the sulcus. This introduces the second disadvantage of the method, which is that the reconstructions are

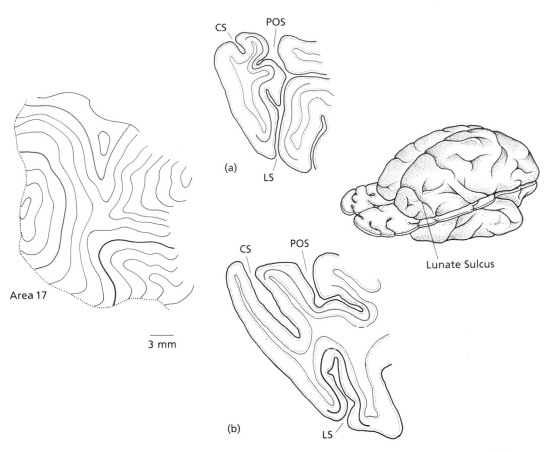

Fig. 12.14 An example of a two-dimensional reconstruction of a large part of the occipital lobe of the monkey brain. The reconstruction is made by drawing contour lines through successive sections and aligning them with respect to one another. It is commonly necessary to unfold the lines so that they do not cross each other and so that they can be better aligned with respect to one another. (Redrawn from Van Essen, D.C. & Zeki, S. (1978). *J. Physiol. (Lond.)* **277**, 193–226.)

difficult, even for specialists, to relate directly to the anatomy of the brain. The advantages are that large areas of the brain can be reconstructed in this way and the precise position and extent of one area, with respect to another, can be correctly determined.

The disadvantages can be overcome partly by the most recent method which we have developed for reconstructing areas of the brain.[25] This is the technique of rotatable three-dimensional reconstructions, which is achieved by a complicated computerized process. Like the first two methods described above, the input to the computer program consists of contour lines drawn through the appropriate layer of the cortex, taken from successive sections. The computer stacks the sections above each other serially and then plots them on a TV screen. A hidden line removal technique is added to simplify the resulting image, which, when viewed with red–green anaglyphs (red to the left), gives a good impression of the three-dimensional configuration of the cortex (Plate 4, facing p. 68). Entire regions of the brain can be 'removed' on the computer, and one can then view a sulcus which lies buried deep inside the brain, or one which extends to the surface, from almost any angle. This, in turn, allows one to study the tangential distribution of label within it, or some other aspect of its architecture. The advantage of the method is that the amount of distortion is much less, since there is no unbending of curved lines and therefore no stretching. Moreover, the reconstructions are easier to understand and, indeed, can even be understood by the non-specialist. The disadvantage is that, unlike the two-dimensional reconstructions, large parts of the brain cannot be viewed simultaneously in a single diagram. Both types of reconstruction are therefore useful.

From the two-dimensional reconstructions one can tell that the largest of the visual areas of the prestriate cortex is area V2 and the smallest is V5 (Figure 12.15), with areas V4 and V3A occupying an intermediate position between V3 and V2, and areas V3 and V6 occupying an intermediate position between V4 and V5. In the past few years, a part of area V3A has been partitioned off into other areas, which would make area V3A smaller than envisaged here, but the results of these studies have not been published in sufficient detail for one to be able to reach adequate conclusions. There are additional areas in the prestriate cortex, but these are not shown in the reconstruction given here. No doubt even more areas will be described in

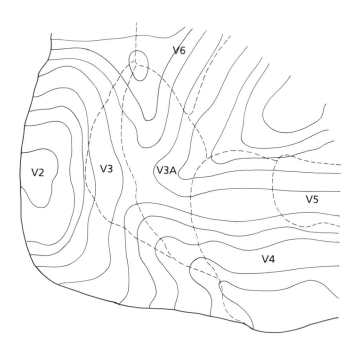

Fig. 12.15 The relative sizes of the prestriate areas, superimposed on a two-dimensional reconstruction of a part of the prestriate cortex, like the one shown in Figure 12.14.

the future and will find their appropriate positions in reconstructions such as the one shown in Figure 12.15.[26]

From the general description of the areas given above, several facts emerge:

1 Several areas may reside in a cortical region of uniform cytoarchitecture. Consequently, cytoarchitecture may not be a good guide to the presence and extent of cortical areas. This is not to say that different cortical areas residing in a cortical region of uniform cytoarchitecture will not be found to have other architectonic differences.

2 The definition of a cortical area must rely on a number of factors. These include: (a) a functional characteristic that differentiates it from other cortical areas; (b) a specific set of inputs and outputs that differs from the input and output of other cortical areas; and (c) a unique architecture. In the case of the visual areas, another important feature is an independent representation of the retina or of the visual field, or of a visual function (see below).

3 The visual areas vary in size. If the same extent of the field of view is represented in each area, it follows that the receptive fields of cells in the smaller areas must be larger, to accommodate the same extent of representation. On the other hand, different extents of the field of view may be represented in different areas. We shall see that both conditions obtain.

4 Each of the specialized visual areas has one or more satellite areas attached to it, undertaking functions belonging to the same attribute of vision as the core area.

5 Each of the areas listed above receives an input from either V1 or V2 and commonly from both. V1 and V2 are to be distinguished from other visual cortical areas in that all the submodalities of vision are represented in them. In other words, both contain cells which are selective for motion, orientation, wavelength and also depth.

6 Area V1 has an output to areas V2, V3, V4 and V5. The output to V4 is from the part of V1 representing the most central part of the retina only, the remaining output to V4 being channelled through V2. The output to V3A is from the parts of V1 representing the peripheral retina. Thus, the main output from V1 is mainly to the core areas; there is a far less prominent output to the satellite areas, or none at all.

7 As we shall see, the specialized visual areas differ profoundly from each other in their functional properties. It follows that they must be receiving different kinds of signals from the primary visual cortex, area V1. It follows from this that V1 must act as a segregator, parcelling out different signals to the different specialized visual areas.

8 Each of the specialized areas, V3, V4, V5 and V6, also receives a direct input from area V2. V2 also has an output to some of the satellite areas, for example to those of the V5 complex and the V4 complex. By the same argument given in (7), it follows that V2, like V1, must segregate signals before parcelling them out to the specialized visual areas.

This brief description has not exhausted all the visual areas which have been described. But they are pivotal areas for the specialization of function that is so prominent a feature of the primate visual cortex. Moreover, together with their anatomical connections and functional properties, they illustrate well the more general principles of multiple areas devoted to a single modality, of parallelism, functional specialization and cortical integration, principles which are applicable to the cortex at large. Indeed, when one comes to study uncharted regions of the cerebral cortex, one will be able to predict a good deal by using the general rules which we can derive from studying the anatomical connections and functional organization of the specialized visual areas described here.

Notes and references

1 Zeki, S.M. (1969). Representation of central visual fields in prestriate cortex of monkey. *Brain Res.* **14**, 271–291; Cragg, B.G. (1969). The topography of the afferent projections in the circumstriate visual cortex of the monkey studied by the Nauta method. *Vision Res.* **9**, 733–747.

2 Zeki, S.M. & Sandeman, D.R. (1976). Combined anatomical and electrophysiological studies on the boundary between the second and third visual areas of rhesus monkey visual cortex. *Proc. R. Soc. Lond.* B **194**, 555–562; Van Essen, D.C. & Zeki, S.M. (1978). The topographic organization of rhesus monkey prestriate cortex. *J. Physiol. (Lond.)* **277**, 193–226.

3 Livingstone, M.S. & Hubel, D.H. (1982). Thalamic inputs to cytochrome-rich regions in monkey visual cortex. *Proc. Natl. Acad. Sci. USA* **79**, 6098–6101; Tootell, R.B.H., Silverman, M.S., De Valois, R.L. & Jacobs, G.H. (1983). Functional organization of the second cortical visual area in primates. *Science* **220**, 737–739; Shipp, S. & Zeki, S. (1989). The organization of connections between areas V5 and V2 in macaque monkey visual cortex. *Eur. J. Neurosci.* **1**, 333–354.

4 Horton, J.C. (1984). Cytochrome oxidase patches: a new cytoarchitectonic feature of monkey visual cortex. *Philos. Trans. R. Soc. Lond.* B **304**, 199–253; Livingstone, M.S. & Hubel, D.H. (1984). Anatomy and physiology of a color system in the primate visual cortex. *J. Neurosci.* **4**, 309–356; Tootell, R.B.H. *et al.* (1988). Functional anatomy of monkey striate cortex. *J. Neurosci.* **8**, 1500–1624.

5 Horton, J.C. & Hedley-Whyte, E.T. (1984). Mapping of cytochrome oxidase patches and ocular dominance columns in human visual cortex. *Philos. Trans. R. Soc. Lond.* B **304**, 255–272; Burkhalter, A. & Bernardo, K.L. (1989). Organization of cortico-cortical connections in human visual cortex. *Proc. Natl. Acad. Sci. USA* **86**, 1071–1075.

6 Clarke, S. & Miklossy, J. (1990). Occipital cortex in man: Organization of callosal connections, related myelo- and cytoarchitecture, and putative boundaries of functional visual areas. *J. Comp. Neurol.* **298**, 188–214; Horton, J.C. & Hoyt, W.F. (1991). Quadrantic visual field defects. A hallmark of lesions in extrastriate (V2/V3) cortex. *Brain* **114**, 1703–1718.

7 Zeki, S.M. (1969), Cragg, B.G. (1969), loc. cit. [1]; Zeki, S.M. & Sandeman, D.R. (1976), Van Essen, D.C. & Zeki, S.M. (1978), loc. cit. [2]; Zeki, S.M. (1978). The third

visual complex of rhesus monkey prestriate cortex. *J. Physiol. (Lond.)* **277**, 245−277.

8 Burkhalter, A., Felleman, D.J., Newsome, W.T. & Van Essen, D.C. (1986). Anatomical and physiological asymmetries related to visual areas V3 and VP in macaque extrastriate cortex. *Vision Res.* **26**, 63−80.

9 Unpublished observations from this laboratory.

10 Van Essen, D.C. & Zeki, S.M. (1978), loc. cit. [2]; Zeki, S.M. (1978), loc. cit. [7].

11 Zeki, S. (1980). A direct projection from area V1 to area V3A of rhesus monkey visual cortex. *Proc. R. Soc. Lond.* B **207**, 499−506.

12 Zeki, S.M. (1971). Cortical projections from two prestriate areas in the monkey. *Brain Res.* **34**, 19−35.

13 Zeki, S.M. (1978). The cortical projections of foveal striate cortex in the rhesus monkey. *J. Physiol. (Lond.)* **277**, 227−244; Zeki, S.M. (1971), loc. cit. [12]; Zeki, S. & Shipp, S. (1989). Modular connections between areas V2 and V4 of macaque monkey visual cortex. *Eur. J. Neurosci.* **1**, 494−506. [Note that the definition of area V4A is slightly altered from the one given in Zeki (1971), loc. cit. [12].]

14 Zeki, S.M. (1977). Colour coding in the superior temporal sulcus of rhesus monkey visual cortex. *Proc. R. Soc. Lond.* B **197**, 195−223.

15 Zeki, S. (1986). The anatomy and physiology of area V6 of macaque monkey visual cortex. *J. Physiol. (Lond.)* **381**, 62P; Unpublished results from this laboratory; Area V6 may coincide in part with area PO described by Colby, C.L., Gattass, R., Olson, C.R. & Gross, C.G. (1988). Topographical organization of cortical afferents to extrastriate visual area PO in the macaque: a dual tracer study. *J. Comp. Neurol.* **269**, 392−413.

16 Galletti, C., Battaglini, P.P. & Fattori, P. (1991). Functional properties of neurons in the anterior bank of the parieto-occipital sulcus of the macaque monkey. *Eur. J. Neurosci.* **3**, 452−461; Battaglini, P.P., Fattori, P., Galletti, C. & Zeki, S. (1990). The physiology of area V6 in the awake, behaving monkey. *J. Physiol. (Lond.)* **423**, 100P.

17 Zeki, S.M. (1974). Functional organization of a visual area in the posterior bank of the superior temporal sulcus of the rhesus monkey. *J. Physiol. (Lond.)* **236**, 549−573.

18 Jen, L.S. & Zeki, S. (1983). High cytochrome oxidase content of the V5 complex of macaque monkey visual cortex. *J. Physiol. (Lond.)* **348**, 23P; Van Essen, D.C., Maunsell, J.H.R. & Bixby, J.L. (1981). The middle temporal visual area in the macaque monkey: myeloarchitecture, connections, functional properties and topographic organization. *J. Comp. Neurol.* **199**, 293−326.

19 Zeki, S. (1980). The response of cells in the anterior bank of the superior temporal sulcus in macaque monkeys. *J. Physiol. (Lond.)* **308**, 85P; Desimone, R. & Ungerleider, L.G. (1986). Multiple visual areas in the caudal superior temporal sulcus of the macaque. *J. Comp. Neurol.* **248**, 164−189.

20 Wurtz, R.H., Yamasaki, D.S., Duffy, C.J. & Roy, J.-P. (1991). Functional specialization for visual motion processing in primate cerebral cortex. *Cold Spring Harb. Symp. Quant. Biol.* **55**, 717−727.

21 Tanaka, K., Hikosaka, K., Saito, H. *et al.* (1986). Analysis of local and wide-field movements in the superior temporal visual areas of the macaque monkey. *J. Neurosci.* **6**, 134−144; Komatsu, H. & Wurtz, R.H. (1988). Relation of cortical areas MT and MST to pursuit eye movements. I. Localization and visual properties of neurons. *J. Neurophysiol.* **60**, 580−603.

22 Van Essen, D.C. & Zeki, S.M. (1978), loc. cit. [2].

23 Van Essen, D.C. & Maunsell, J.H.R. (1980). Two-dimensional maps of the cerebral cortex. *J. Comp. Neurol.* **191**, 255−281; Desimone, R. & Ungerleider, L.G. (1986), loc. cit. [19]; Andersen, R.A., Asanuma, C. & Cowan, W.M. (1985). Callosal and prefrontal associational projecting cell populations in area 7A of the macaque monkey: a study using retrogradely transported fluorescent dyes. *J. Comp. Neurol.* **232**, 443−455.

24 Jouandet, M.L., Tramo, M.J., Herron, D.M. *et al.* (1989). Brainprints: computer-generated two-dimensional maps of the human cerebral cortex in vivo. *J. Cog. Neurosci.* **1**, 88−117.

25 Romaya, J. & Zeki, S. (1986). Rotatable, three-dimensional computer reconstruction of the macaque monkey brain. *J. Physiol. (Lond.)* **371**, 25P.

26 For a more extensive two-dimensional map, based on the system developed here (Van Essen, D.C. & Zeki, S.M. loc. cit. [2]) and described above, see Felleman, D.J. & Van Essen, D.C. (1991). Distributed hierarchical processing in the primate cerebral cortex. *Cerebral Cortex* **1**, 1–47.

Chapter 13: Parallelism in the visual cortex

The demonstration of multiple visual areas in the cerebral cortex naturally suggests that vision is a much more complex process than was envisaged in the early theories of vision developed by neurologists. But, in itself, the presence of multiple visual areas is compatible with a hierarchical doctrine. All that one would need to suppose is that the visual areas are connected serially with each other, with one area feeding into the next. But, early on, anatomical studies showed that this was not so. Instead, the connections to the visual areas were found to be in parallel, although serial connections between them exist also.

The overwhelming visual input to the specialized areas of the prestriate cortex (previously known as visual 'association' cortex) does not come directly from the retina via the lateral geniculate nucleus. Instead it comes from V1. The arrangement of these connections is compelling. Each millimetre of V1, which represents a particular, small region of visual space, sends separate anatomical fibres to the different visual areas of the prestriate cortex (Figure 13.1). It would be difficult to imagine that the same small region of V1 sends identical signals to these different, functionally specialized, visual areas in these independent and parallel pathways. This is especially so since even the calibre of the fibres destined for the different areas differs, some areas receiving large-diameter, fast-conducting fibres, and others receiving smaller ones. This anatomical fact implies that signals reach some areas faster than others, as indeed has since been found to be the case.[1] It was therefore argued that each small region of V1 segregates signals related to different attributes of the visual scene, such as colour, form and motion, and distributes them out to different areas of the visual association cortex for further, independent, but parallel, processing.[2] In addition to suggesting strongly the presence of segregation within V1, the demonstration of the multiple, parallel outputs from each millimetre of V1 established the principle of parallelism in the visual cortex, and now, more generally, in the cortex at large. For parallelism is not unique to the visual cortex but is a feature of all cortical connections.[3]

It is to be noted that the logic used to predict a segregatory role for V1 is not greatly different from that employed by Magitot and Hartmann[4] in a very similar context, though they did so in a somewhat negative mode. They doubted whether there could be any

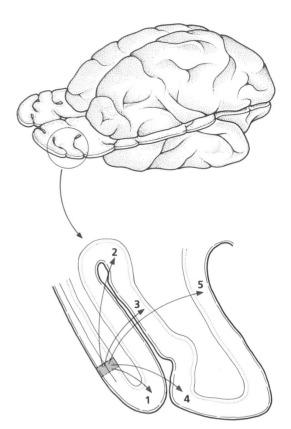

Fig. 13.1 The parallel anatomical outputs from a given small region of the primary visual cortex (area V1), which receives an input from a corresponding part of the retina and thus has all the visual information registered by that part of the retina represented in it. (Redrawn from Zeki, S. (1975). *Cold Spring Harb. Symp. Quant. Biol.* **40**, 591–600.)

specialization for colour in the striate cortex, since no one had then demonstrated the presence of 'specialized neurons in the optic pathways'.[4] By the same logic, once a specialization is demonstrated among a group of areas, it is logical enough to conclude that the area feeding those specialized areas must itself show some segregation of the specialized signals that it parcels to the different areas. This has indeed been found to be true for areas V1 and V2. More recent work, to be reviewed later, has shown that V1 and V2 have distinctive architectures consisting of repetitive sets of compartments, that different sets of compartments have different functional properties and different inputs and outputs.

That the prediction of a segregatory function for V1 should have been made by observing the parallel outputs from it to the specialized visual areas, and that it should have come several years before the actual demonstration of the functional segregation within it, augurs well for cortical studies. It provides a predictive lesson in the study of uncharted cortical regions because parallel outputs appear to be so ubiquitous a feature of cortical connectivity.[5] First, if in studying the anatomy of an uncharted cortical area one were to find that it has parallel outputs to several different areas (a very likely result), then it is almost certain that, sooner or later, it will be found to contain functionally segregated groups of cells within it. Next, if an area has a distinctive architecture consisting of several repetitive compartments, it is almost certain that it will be found to have multiple parallel outputs to different cortical areas, and that the output from each compartment will be found to differ from those in other compartments. It is also almost certain to show a functional segregation which correlates with the modular compartmentalization, when it is eventually studied physiologically. Finally, if an area is studied physiologically first and found to contain functional groupings of cells which are segregated from each other by other functional groupings, it is almost certain that the area will eventually be found to have a distinctive architecture and multiple outputs. Thus, the presence of one of the criteria given above is a certain guide to the presence of the others. As an example, take area V5. Although this is an area heavily concerned with motion processing, at the time I first wrote this chapter there had been no convincing demonstration of further functional sub-compartmentalization within it. Yet it was sufficient to learn of its multiple outputs to other cortical areas[5] to realize that it is only a matter of time before this functional segregation within V5 will be found. Because of this, we wrote in 1988 that, 'The functional logic of cortical connections therefore predicts that V5 is also a segregator, with functionally distinct groups of cells occupying anatomically distinct subdivisions'.[5] It did not take that long for our prediction to come true. In 1992, it was found that cells dealing with local and global motion processing are anatomically segregated there.[6] Nor are the lessons learnt from studying the visual areas applicable to uncharted visual areas only. On the contrary, they apply with equal vigour to all cortical areas, which is one further reason why the study of the visual cortex gives so powerful a vision of the brain.

Parallelism and its implications

All areas of the cerebral cortex send outputs to more than one area, from which it follows that there are parallel outputs from all cortical areas. These parallel outputs are not just to other cortical areas, but to subcortical centres as well. For example, all visual areas send fibres to the superior colliculus, a midbrain structure, and to the pulvinar, a subdivision of the thalamus. It implies that the signals emanating from a cortical area are of interest to several other cortical areas, and to several subcortical stations as well. Parallelism also implies a distribution and since all cortical areas have parallel outputs, it follows that each distributes its signals to several other areas and, hence, it is common to speak of the cerebral cortex as consisting of several parallel-distributed systems, a concept which computational neuro-biologists in particular are much attached to. Once again, it would be hard to imagine that each area distributes identical signals to the areas with which it connects. By analogy with V1, it is easier to suppose that each area distributes different signals to the areas with which it connects. From this it follows, again by analogy with V1, that all cortical areas are segregators. This in itself implies that each area undertakes multiple operations. Parallelism is therefore of profound significance for understanding the workings of the cerebral cortex, and increases by several orders of magnitude the enormity of the task needed to understand the workings of the brain.

Parallelism, computational neurobiology and neural networks

'Computational neurobiology' has been all the rage for some years and many consider that this approach is fundamental in any effort to unravel the intricacies of the brain. The general argument in favour of a strong computational approach in neurobiological studies is this: The brain is much too complicated an organ to be studied without some guiding theory. Because computers also undertake complex tasks, including that of 'seeing' (robotics), they are the natural source for such guiding theories, which can then be tested by direct experimentation. The argument is not without considerable merits. Theory has always been of importance in the collection of facts, including even the mere anatomical facts. After all, collection of the voluminous facts on the structure of the nervous system by Ramon y Cajal was not done in the void, but with the specific aim of proving the neuron doctrine, the one which supposed that the nervous system was not made of a continuous sheet but of discontinuous elements, the neurons, which connected with each other. It is likely that theory will be much more important in the future, particularly in studies of the higher functions of the brain, which includes the function of seeing. But does the experimental neurobiologist have to rely on the computational neurobiologist for his theory and, if so, to what extent?

In trying to formulate an answer, it is as well to record the striking fact that the principle of parallelism in the cerebral cortex at large, and in the visual cortex in particular, not only antedates the current conversion of computational neurobiologists to the idea, but was derived from what many would regard as pedestrian anatomical studies, not from computational theories or from neural networks, even though the latter might have been the natural source for such an idea. One looks in vain through the pre-1975 computational literature for a clear and explicit statement of the principle of parallelism in the visual cortex. Even after the anatomical demonstration of parallel connections in the visual cortex, and the demonstration of multiple, specialized visual areas, computational neurobiologists spoke in very vague terms about these concepts, if they spoke about them at all.

David Marr's book, *Vision*,[7] the Bible of visual computational neuro-biology and one which everyone admires yet few understand, makes no mention of the subject of parallelism or of the separate visual areas or of the specializations in the visual cortex, all demonstrated years before he published his book. It is a curious fact that computational neurobiologists should have been so late in seeing the significance of parallelism in vision, even though they now try to make out that they had been there all along. This may be due in part to the prevalence of serial, rather than parallel, computers until relatively recently; it may be due to a relative ignorance among computational scientists about the precise characteristics and capabilities of parallel computers.[8] Whatever the real reasons, it should make us all a little careful in accepting cortical theories derived from those whose tools are mathematics and computers rather than brains. The proper way of understanding the brain is to study the brain.[9]

This is not to say that neural networks and computational neuro-biology will not have an important role in cortical studies of the future. There is no doubt that they will and the relationship between brain studies, computational neurobiology and neural networks is therefore worth investigating briefly. One problem with computational neurobiologists is that they are far ahead of their time and yet far behind the times. They are far ahead in believing that neurobiology will have to depend upon theories generated by studying how the nervous system might undertake a task, which implies defining the task precisely, something which neurobiologists haven't been particularly good at. But they are far behind the times in believing that computational neurobiology can come up with theories that are of direct relevance to the neurobiologist, one which may be put to the experimental test, by ignoring the facts of the nervous system. Marr's book illustrates this perfectly. It is rightly prized for introducing a new way of looking at what the nervous system does, of defining its tasks. But at the same time, by ignoring the facts of the visual cortex, it renders the book of very limited value to anyone who might want to understand how the cerebral visual cortex might be undertaking the tasks thus defined, how it may be functioning. This ignorance derives in part from the profound contempt with which computational neurobiologists regard the experimental neurobiologist — well illustrated in Marr's ignorance of what has come to be one of the most powerful doctrines dictating work on the visual cortex — and in part from the fact that not nearly enough is known about the brain. To be of use to the neurobiologist, a computational approach has to rely on the facts of the nervous system. When Marr wrote his work even less was known about the visual cortex than is known today. His book is therefore of little use to the experimental neurobiologist investigating the cortical mechanisms of vision, although it is of fundamental importance in pinpointing a new approach to the problem of what the visual cortex does. Equally, a book on the same topic written today will probably be of little use to an investigator in twenty years' time. The point is that, to become meaningful to the experimental neurobiologist, the computational neurobiologist needs the facts of the nervous system even more than the experimental neurobiologist needs the theory generated by computational neurobiologists. Successful applications of computational neurobiology to experimental studies of how the brain undertakes particular tasks in colour and motion vision are to be found in those studies which have made as heavy a use of the knowledge derived from experimental studies as of that derived from defining the tasks computationally.[10]

The other problem with the application of computational neurobiology to nervous studies derives from the problem of implementation. It is one thing to identify the task that has to be implemented, another to identify how it might be implemented and a third to learn how the nervous system undertakes the implementation. Colour vision provides a good example. The task for the nervous system here is to 'discount the illuminant', since surfaces retain their colour when viewed in different lighting conditions, a problem recognized by many, including Helmholtz and in particular Land, neither of them a computational neurobiologist. One can then think about how that task can be implemented. But it does not follow that the nervous system will use the approach decided upon. Another example is the problem of integration, of how the specialized visual areas interact with each other to construct the integrated visual image. Marr refers to this as the addressing problem in a cursory conversation in his book. To have recognized that there is such a problem, as he and others[11] have done, is no mean achievement, particularly given the fact that most neurobiologists of vision never addressed the problem, even hypothetically, until very recently. But the manner in which the problem is posed by Marr and other computational neurobiologists is much too vague for the real neurobiologist, the one whose concern is to understand how a real nervous system undertakes such tasks. What does it mean in neurological terms? What kind of anatomical connections does it envisage? What kind of physiological mechanisms does it entail? Indeed, one might well use the language of the computational neurobiologist and ask, 'Within what anatomical constraints must the addressing procedure operate?' The answer to that derives from anatomy alone, not from mathematical models of the brain. A neurobiologist pondering these problems might well put his time to better use by studying the connections of the visual cortex — which also has a theory behind it — and thus help define the addressing problem in neurological terms far more sharply than any computational neurobiologist ever did. All of this emphasizes the point that, while the achievements of experimental neurobiology will be greatly enhanced by an appeal to the computational approach, the latter is lost without the facts generated by experimental neurobiology, at least as far as understanding the workings of the brain is involved.

But, to return to the main point, whatever parallel outputs from the striate cortex to the specialized visual areas of the prestriate cortex may have implied, it made little impact for a long time. It merely prepared the ground for what was to come later. The turning point came only with the direct demonstration of functional specialization in the visual association cortex of the macaque monkey.[12] With that, the final chip in the domino game, the one which was the case of much of the turbulent history of the visual process, finally collapsed.

References

1 Raiguel, S.E., Lagae, L., Gulyas, B. & Orban, G.A. (1989). Response latencies of visual cells in macaque areas V1, V2 and V5. *Brain Res.* **493**, 155–159.

2 Zeki, S.M. (1975). The functional organization of projections from striate to prestriate visual cortex in the rhesus monkey. *Cold Spring Harb. Symp. Quant. Biol.* **40**, 591–600.

3 See, for example, Goldman-Rakic, P. (1984). Modular organization of prefrontal cortex. *Trends Neurosci.* **7**, 419–429.

4 Magitot, A. & Hartmann, E. (1926). La cécité corticale. *Bull. Soc. Ophtalmol. (Paris)* **38**, 427–546.

5 Zeki, S. & Ship, S. (1988). The functional logic of cortical connections. *Nature* **335**, 311–316; Zeki, S. (1990). The motion pathways of the visual cortex. In *Vision: Coding and Efficiency*, edited by C. Blakemore, pp. 321–345. Cambridge University Press, Cambridge.

6 Born, R.T. & Tootell, R.B.H. (1992). Segregation of global and local motion processing in primate middle temporal visual area. *Nature* **357**, 497–499.

7 Marr, D. (1982). *Vision.* MIT Press, Cambridge.

8 Minsky, M. & Papert, S. (1988). *Perceptrons.* MIT Press, Cambridge.

9 See also, Crick, F. (1989). The recent excitement about neural networks. *Nature* **337**, 129–132.

10 Zeki, S. (1983). Colour coding in the cerebral cortex: the reaction of cells in monkey visual cortex to wavelengths and colours. *Neuroscience* **9**, 741–765; Movshon, J.A., Adelson, E.H., Gizzi, M.S. & Newsome, W.T. (1985). The analysis of moving visual patterns. In *Pattern Recognition Mechanisms*, edited by C. Chagas, R. Gattass & C.G. Gross, pp. 117–151. Pontifical Academy, Vatican City.

11 Milner, P.M. (1974). A model for visual shape recognition. *Psychol. Rev.* **81**, 521–535; Malsburg, C. von der & Schneider, W. (1986). A neural cocktail-party processor. *Biol. Cybern* **54**, 29–40.

12 Zeki, S.M. (1974). The mosaic organization of the visual cortex in the monkey. In *Essays on the Nervous System: A Festschrift for Professor J.Z. Young*, edited by R. Bellairs & E.G. Gray, pp. 327–343. Clarendon Press, Oxford; Zeki, S.M. (1978). Functional specialisation in the visual cortex of the rhesus monkey. *Nature* **274**, 423–428.

Chapter 14: Functional specialization in the visual cortex

What would be the reason for having so many visual areas? One might be tempted to suppose that they are needed for a process of increasing elaboration, of rendering the response properties of cells more and more complex, and thus enabling them to respond to more and more complex and specific stimuli, as envisaged by the hierarchical model. Such a process, which schematically resembles a sort of pyramid, could obviously not go on indefinitely. Logically, its end result would be one or, more realistically, a small number of 'pontifical' cells. These would have enormously complex properties, enabling them to respond to enormously complex stimuli — such as fire engines or grandmothers. Indeed, these were the very objects used to describe such cells, and 'fire engine' or 'grandmother' cells came to be popular terms to represent the end result of a hierarchical process, approvingly by some and disapprovingly of by others.

To those disapproving of a doctrine which endowed cells of the visual cortex with such high degrees of specificity, the improbability of having one or a small number of cells coding for one's grandmother was not the only problem, though it obviously was one. For how would an individual recognize his grandmother if such cells were to be knocked out of action by some kind of vascular accident, a common occurrence? One could of course assume that such specific cells are widely distributed throughout the cortex, an assumption for which there is no evidence. But there was another problem. If the cells in one area 'report' to the ones in the next and so on, in a chain, until the report is to the 'grandmother' cell, who does the 'grandmother' cell report to? Which cell in what area, or who is it in the end who knows what the stimulus is? This introduces the problem of knowledge and of consciousness, a problem which visual neurophysiologists have not, in general, been concerned with, though it is one of primordial interest. Allied to this is the problem of constancy or invariancy, the ability to classify a stimulus as a grandmother, or a fire engine, or any other form for that matter, in a variety of different viewing conditions. How does the nervous system achieve this feat? If visual neuro-biologists, assuming them to have thought about the subject at all, had an answer to the problem, they were remarkably quiet about it. Indeed, the best that can be said about those visual neurobiologists who disapproved of the concept of grandmother and fire engine cells is that they were for a long time remarkably inarticulate in making their opposition known. No matter that the concept may have been discussed in detail by psychologists and philosophers. It made little impact on the hard-nosed visual neurobiologists.

There was yet another problem which began gradually to unfold in the last decade. This was a problem of cortical connections. One would have supposed from the doctrine of exclusive hierarchies that the connections between the visual areas would be exclusively serial, with one area connecting to the other in a chain, culminating in what might be called a master area. But such a pattern of connections is not characteristic of visual areas or indeed of other cortical areas, which are instead connected in parallel,[1] although serial connections also exist within a given pathway. Indeed, anatomical studies have yet to reveal a single cortical area to which all the visual areas connect exclusively. Instead, each cortical area, whether visual or not, has multiple outputs. The consequence of this is that the results of the operations performed in any single cortical area are relayed to several other cortical areas through these connections. This is not to suggest that the same operation is relayed to different areas. Any given cortical area may undertake several operations simultaneously and distribute the results of its operations to several different cortical areas.

Such difficulties were resolved to some degree in the early 1970s by the discovery that different visual areas of the macaque monkey prestriate visual cortex undertake different visual tasks,[2] thus ushering in the concept of functional specialization in the visual cortex. The first area to be studied functionally in detail was area V5.[3] The studies consisted of isolating single cells with a micro-electrode inserted into the area and studying their responses to different stimuli flashed on a screen facing the animal, rather like the visual experiments on area V1 described earlier. The surprising finding in this area was that all its cells are sensitive to motion, and over 90% are directionally selective. In other words, they respond to motion of a visual stimulus in one direction but not in the opposite, null, direction (see Figure 14.1). Most cells responded to spots of light moving in one direction, although some preferred oriented lines. The interesting point was that none of the cells was concerned with the colour of the stimulus. Thus, if a cell could be driven by a spot moving from right to left within its receptive field, that spot could be black or white or any other colour and presented against a background of any other colour. Because all cells in V5 respond to moving stimuli, I initially called this area the motion area of the visual cortex, thus attaching a function to it unambiguously.[3]

It is interesting to note here that, historically, V5 was not the first area with a high concentration of direction-selective cells to be studied, although it was the first to be considered as a specialized visual area.

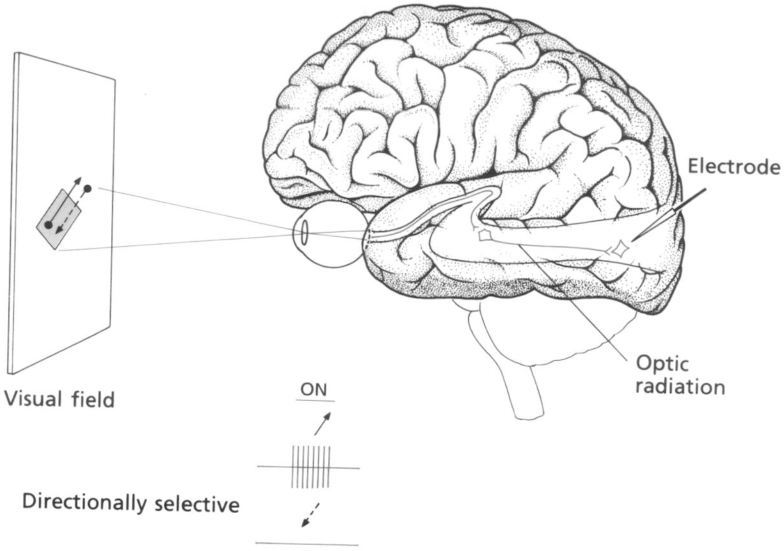

Fig. 14.1 The responses of a directionally selective cell in area V5. The cell responds to motion in one direction but not in the opposite, null, direction. Such cells commonly prefer small spots to oriented bars of light. For simplicity, the detailed connections linking the retina to the cortical recording site are omitted.

Hubel and Wiesel had recorded from an area outside the striate cortex in the cat, the Clare–Bishop area referred to earlier, and had found that most cells in it are directionally selective.[4] But they did not interpret this to mean a specialization for motion. Instead, they had supposed from their previous work[5] that the visual areas lying outside the primary visual cortex in the cat merely continued the process of analysis which starts at the retina, the higher the area, the more complex the analysis. Adherence to this concept of an exclusive hierarchical strategy was to confuse them when they found that most cells in the visual area defined by Clare and Bishop are directionally selective. They thought of it as executing 'the same processes' as earlier areas 'but with different degrees of refinement', leaving them '. . . with the puzzling prospect of an area for which we can. . . assign no obvious function'.[4]

Of course, to convince oneself that functional specialization is a feature of the prestriate visual cortex it was important to show that another, distinct, visual area is specialized for another, distinct, visual function, just as the doctrine of functional specialization in the cortex gained enormously when, after Broca's studies, those of Fritsch and Hitzig showed that movement is localized in a separate area. But, in a sense, the physiology of area V5 gave the game on functional specialization away. The macaque monkey has good colour vision. But here was an area in which all the cells responded to visual stimulation and shared the common property of being responsive to motion; yet none was interested in the colour of the stimulus. It was obvious that, if colour is processed in the cortex, it must be processed elsewhere. One could naturally suppose that it was not processed in the cortex at all.

William Rushton once told me that, by reference to the mentality of those who worked on colour vision rather than by reference to the published evidence, he had reached the conclusion that colour vision must be a subcortical phenomenon!

V5 is not the only area in which cells are not concerned with colour. Recordings from areas V3 and V3A showed that the great majority of cells in them are responsive to lines of specific orientation, but they, too, are not interested in the colour of the oriented line.[6] In other words, a cell in these areas responds to a line of a given orientation regardless of the colour of the line, and regardless, too, of the colour of the background against which it is presented. Because oriented lines are the components of so many forms, it seemed reasonable to suppose that these two areas are involved in the processing of signals related to the form of visual stimuli.

It is not commonly realized that this negative evidence, as far as colour is concerned, is fully as important as the positive evidence. It was to be only a matter of time before the cortical areas specialized for colour vision would be discovered. Fortunately, time could be compressed a little. To get to area V5, the electrode had to pass through V4. I commonly took the opportunity of studying the responses of cells in V4. Here, cells were more difficult to activate. But, nevertheless, the great majority of cells that I succeeded in driving were, to a greater or lesser extent, colour selective, in the sense that they responded better to lights of some wavelengths than to lights of other wavelengths[7] (Figure 14.2). Indeed, in the preliminary studies, all the cells that I managed to activate were to

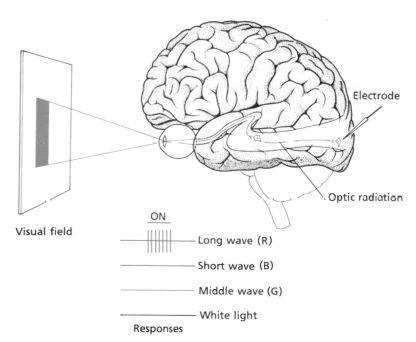

Fig. 14.2 The responses of a cell in area V4 to lights of different colours. This cell was responsive to long-wave (red) light only. For simplicity, the detailed connections linking the retina to the cortical recording site are omitted.

some degree wavelength selective. I wrote, perhaps too timidly, that though, 'It would, of course, be premature to think of this area as dealing with colour exclusively...one may suggest tentatively that this is an area in which colour is emphasised'.[7] Later studies[8] showed that there are also orientation-selective cells within V4, possibly subcompartmentalized within it,[9] but that even many of the orientation-selective cells in this area are also wavelength selective to varying degrees.[8] Here, then, was a visual area which, like V5 and V3, received its input from V1, but had properties which were remarkably different from those of V5 or V3. It seemed difficult to avoid the conclusion that there must be a division of labour among the visual areas of the prestriate cortex, with different areas undertaking different tasks in parallel.

For many years the macaque monkey stood alone, together with the dormant and imperfect clinical evidence, in speaking for a functional specialization in the visual cortex. The visual areas of the owl monkey had been charted in great detail by the early 1970s, though only in terms of the nature of the retinal maps in them. The properties of the single cells in them had not been studied. But a functional specialization in the visual areas of the owl monkey was to be confirmed about a decade after its discovery in the macaque monkey.[10] However, because of the absence of colour vision in the owl monkey, the evidence from this species was not, and perhaps continues not to be, as compelling as it is in the macaque monkey. Among the areas in the two species which show the greatest similarities are area V5 of the macaque and its homologue in the owl monkey, known as area MT. Area V5 had been identified as a separate area in 1969[11] and characterized first in a preliminary way as an area specialized for motion in 1971[12] and more extensively and definitively by 1974.[3] By contrast, its homologue in the owl monkey, area MT, was identified as a separate area in 1971[13] and was not to be studied functionally until 1980.[10] Nevertheless, area V5 is commonly referred to as MT, regardless of the species, although I prefer to use the term MT when speaking of the owl monkey alone, leaving the easier V5 for the macaque monkey and for the human brain.

By your groupings do we know you

If one were to study the physiology of these areas in greater detail, one would find that cells with common properties are grouped together in each area. This grouping gives one a fantastic insight into the precision and regularity of cortical organization. Thus, if one were to make a tangential electrode penetration through area V5 and record the directional preferences of the directionally selective cells at short intervals, for example of 50 μm, one would find a very gradual and orderly shift in the preferred directions of the successive cells, with only an occasional abrupt shift (Figure 14.3a). By contrast, if one were to make a perpendicular penetration through the cortex of area V5, one would find that most cells prefer the same direction of motion, again with occasional abrupt shifts[3,14] (Figure 14.3b). It is as if cells with common properties are grouped together in the cortex. This phenomenon of grouping was first hinted at by the studies of Vernon Mountcastle[15] and was beautifully demonstrated for the striate cortex by Hubel and Wiesel.[16] It turns out to be a general phenomenon, all areas exhibiting a grouping of cells with common properties.[17] Thus, if one were to make a long electrode penetration through area V3A, one which is parallel to the cortical surface, and record from successive cells, separated from each other by 50–100 μm, one would find that the orientational preferences of successive cells change gradually, again with some abrupt shifts. By contrast, if one were to record the activity of cells separated from each other by the same distance, but this time in a perpendicular penetration, then most cells would be found to respond to the same orientation (Figure 14.4Λ and B).

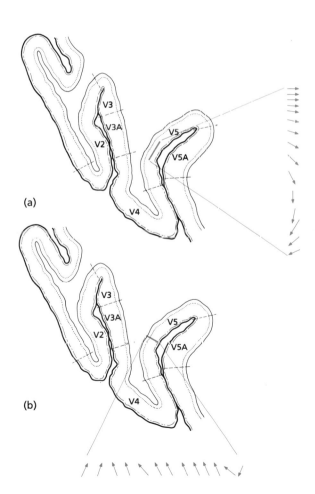

Fig. 14.3 (a) The directional preferences of successive cells, separated from each other by small distances, in area V5 encountered during a long electrode penetration made obliquely to the cortical surface of area V5. Note the orderly change in the successive directions of motion. (b) The directional preferences of successive cells in area V5, but this time encountered in a long penetration made at right angles to the cortical surface.

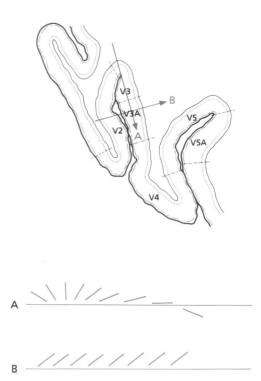

Fig. 14.4 (A) Oblique and (B) perpendicular electrode penetrations made through area V3A. The orientational preferences of the successive cells change in an orderly manner in (A) but do not vary much in (B).

In the same way, one finds that cells with common properties are grouped together in the cortex of area V4. Note that, in the area specialized for visual motion, the cells are grouped together with respect to the direction of motion, while in the area specialized for form they are grouped together with respect to orientational preferences. The grouping is more complex in V4, but is based on both wavelength and orientational preferences. In short, one can tell a great deal about an area by noting the functions which are at the basis of the groupings. Nowhere has the grouping of cells with common properties been more extensively studied than in the striate cortex, which we shall discuss in a subsequent chapter.

There remained then, and there still remains today, a great deal about these areas that we know little about. Each one of them probably has important functional subdivisions within it; each one connects with several other cortical areas as well as with subcortical stations. Above all, I have always emphasized that the functions that I have ascribed to them are not necessarily their only functions. Future studies may yet ascribe further functions to each. But, however crude and simplistic the techniques that I employed may seem in future years, the evidence was compelling enough for me to suggest a theory of functional specialization in the visual cortex.[18] This theory supposes that different attributes of the visual scene, such as form, colour and motion, are processed in separate areas of the cerebral visual cortex. It is possible that these are not the only attributes which are processed separately. Other ones, and in particular depth, may also be processed separately. But it is important for the theory that colour vision is among the attributes definitely included.

The theory of functional specialization explains a great deal that is interesting in vision. In particular, the demonstration that the 'visual association' cortex consists of several separate, and functionally specialized, visual areas overturned the ideas of hierarchy which, until then, had been considered to be the sole strategy used by the brain to 'analyze' the visual environment. They also modified the concept of association cortex as intended by Flechsig and his followers, for the specialized visual areas turned out to be in every sense visual. If they are involved in any form of association, it is that of associating the responses of cells concerned with a given submodality of vision, rather than that of associating visual signals with signals derived from other senses. Moreover, if there is a functional specialization for colour vision, then the notion that a cortical lesion may specifically involve the 'colour centre' and thus lead to a specific defect in colour vision no longer seemed as improbable as it had to generations of neurologists. This made it possible to re-examine the earlier clinical evidence on cerebral achromatopsia because the notion that a particular area in a cytoarchitectonically uniform zone of cortex might be specialized for a particular visual function no longer seemed so fantastic. The domino game was, in a sense, over. Clinicians were the first to become aware of this. Somewhat surprisingly, cases of cerebral colour blindness, which had all but disappeared from the clinical literature, began to emerge again. Meadows[19] analyzed all the frank achromatopsic patients until then and found that the lesions shared a common locus, in the lingual and fusiform gyri. And single cases, like that of Zihl and his colleagues,[20] no longer attracted the severe criticism that earlier cases had. Perhaps most significantly of all, the notion of functional specialization began to modify our view of vision as a process and of the involvement of the cerebral cortex in it. We began to ask deeper questions about colour, about motion and about why they should be separately represented in the brain. We started to conceive of vision as being the result of a series of parallel processes, undertaken more or less independently, and requiring us to understand how the results of the separate operations were then put together to give us our unitary experience of the visual world. But, even today, most of us have not realized the full implications that functional specialization has for our understanding of what the brain does.

References

1 Zeki, S.M. (1975). The functional organization of projections from striate to prestriate visual cortex in the rhesus monkey. *Cold Spring Harb. Symp. Quant. Biol.* **40**, 591–600.

2 Zeki, S.M. (1974). The mosaic organization of the visual cortex in the monkey. In *Essays on the Nervous System: A Festschrift for Professor J.Z. Young*, edited by R. Bellairs & E.G. Gray, pp. 327–343. Clarendon Press, Oxford; Zeki, S.M. (1978). Functional specialization in the visual cortex of the rhesus monkey. *Nature* **274**, 423–428.

3 Zeki, S.M. (1974). Functional organization of a visual area in the posterior bank of the superior temporal sulcus of the rhesus monkey. *J. Physiol. (Lond.)* **236**, 549–573.

4 Hubel, D.H. & Wiesel, T.N. (1969). Visual area of the lateral suprasylvian gyrus (Clare–Bishop area) of the cat. *J. Physiol. (Lond.)* **202**, 251–260.

5 Hubel, D.H. & Wiesel, T.N. (1965). Receptive fields and functional architecture in two nonstriate visual areas (18 and 19) of the cat. *J. Neurophysiol.* **28**, 229–289.

6 Zeki, S.M. (1978). The third visual complex of rhesus monkey prestriate cortex. *J. Physiol. (Lond.)* **277**, 245–272.

7 Zeki, S.M. (1973). Colour coding in rhesus monkey prestriate cortex. *Brain Res.* **53**, 422–427; Zeki, S. (1977). Colour coding in the superior temporal sulcus of rhesus monkey visual cortex. *Proc. R. Soc. Lond.* B **197**, 195–223.

8 Zeki, S.M. (1975), loc. cit. [1]; Zeki, S. (1983). The distribution of wavelength and orientation selective cells in different areas of monkey visual cortex. *Proc. R. Soc. Lond.* B **217**, 449–470; Desimone, R. & Schein, S.J. (1987). Visual properties of neurons in area V4 of the macaque: sensitivity to stimulus form. *J. Neurophysiol.* **57**, 835–868; Schein, S.J. & Desimone, R. (1990). Spectral properties of V4 neurons in the macaque. *J. Neurosci.* **10**, 3369–3389; Zeki, S.M. & Shipp, S. (1989). Modular connections between areas V2 and V4 of macaque monkey visual cortex. *Eur. J. Neurosci.* **1**, 494–506.

9 Zeki, S. (1983), Zeki, S.M. & Shipp, S. (1989), loc. cit. [8].

10 Zeki, S. (1980). The response properties of cells in the middle temporal area (area MT) of owl monkey visual cortex. *Proc. R. Soc. Lond.* B **207**, 239–248; Baker, J.P., Petersen, S.E., Newsome, W.T. & Allman, J.M. (1981). Visual response properties of neurons in four extrastriate visual areas of the owl monkey (*Aotus trivirgatus*): a quantitative comparison of medial, dorsomedial, dorsolateral, and middle temporal areas. *J. Neurophysiol.* **45**, 397–416.

11 Zeki, S.M. (1969). Representation of central visual fields in prestriate cortex of monkeys. *Brain Res.* **14**, 271–291; Cragg, B.G. (1969). The topography of the afferent projections in circumstriate visual cortex of the monkey studied by the Nauta method. *Vision Res.* **9**, 733–747.

12 Dubner, R. & Zeki, S.M. (1971). Response properties and receptive fields of cells in an anatomically defined region of the superior temporal sulcus in the monkey. *Brain Res.* **35**, 528–532.

13 Allman, J.M. & Kaas, J.H. (1971). A representation of the visual field in the caudal third of the middle temporal gyrus of the owl monkey (*Aotus trivirgatus*). *Brain Res.* **31**, 85–105.

14 Zeki, S.M. (1974), loc. cit. [3]; Albright, T.D. (1984). Direction and orientation selectivity of neurons in visual area MT of the macaque. *J. Neurophysiol.* **52**, 1106–1130.

15 Mountcastle, V.B. (1957). Modality and topographic properties of single neurons of cat's somatic sensory cortex. *J. Neurophysiol.* **20**, 408–434.

16 Hubel, D.H. & Wiesel, T.N. (1977). The Ferrier Lecture: Functional architecture of macaque monkey visual cortex. *Proc. R. Soc. Lond.* B **198**, 1–59.

17 See, for example, Goldman-Rakic, P. (1984). Modular organization of prefrontal cortex. *Trends Neurosci.* **7**, 419–429.

18 Zeki, S.M. (1974), loc. cit. [2].

19 Meadows, J.C. (1974). Disturbed perception of colours associated with localized cerebral lesions. *Brain* **97**, 615–632.

20 Zihl, J., Cramon, D. von & Mai, N. (1983). Selective disturbance of movement vision after bilateral brain damage. *Brain* **106**, 313–340.

Chapter 15: Functional specialization in human visual cortex

I had always daydreamed idly about being able to demonstrate the colour and motion areas — the two subsystems that allowed me to establish functional specialization in the macaque visual cortex — in the human brain. Daydreaming, Edwin Land kept telling me, is no bad thing provided that one sets to work to make one's daydreams come true. It frustrated me greatly that I didn't have the means of doing so unambiguously in the 1970s, when the results from the monkey were coming out. Those who work on the brain, even lowly brains, often hope that their findings will apply to the human brain. This is not surprising. To understand the brain of man is the most challenging problem in science and most neurobiologists hope that they can contribute to that understanding in some way, even if the contribution turns out to be a minor one. Indeed, the human brain was the organ of choice when neurology began as a discipline in the latter half of the last century, and many of the important observations made were based on the study of the human brain. Of these none was to have a more lasting influence than early studies of functional localization in the cerebral cortex.

The story of the discovery of functional localization in the human brain is recounted briefly in Chapter 2. One might have suspected that, given this demonstration, the idea that there may be specializations in the visual cortex should not have seemed so outrageous. But this was not so. The history of research into the visual cortex, summarized in earlier chapters, shows that the unitary nature of the visual image in the human brain — one in which all the attributes such as form, colour and motion are seen in precise registration — was to stifle any enquiry into the separation of functions within it and lead to the dismissal of any clinical evidence purporting to show such a specialization within this system. The suggestion that there may be specialized visual areas outside the striate cortex was especially odious to those who believed that the function of 'seeing' was vested in one cortical area alone — the striate area. But that was not all. Holmes and others were also intolerant of any suggestion that there may be specializations within the striate cortex itself, and asserted dogmatically that there was no dissociation of functions after lesions in the striate cortex. By 1939 Monbrun could write that, 'All authors have now rallied to the theory of a unique [visual] cortical centre'.[1]

The foundation of functional specialization in the visual system derives, therefore, from evidence in the macaque monkey, not the human brain, and is of much more recent origin. The first evidence in its favour was not behavioural, but anatomical and physiological. It lay in the demonstration that, of the several visual areas in the prestriate cortex, one (V5) is specialized for motion and another (V4) for colour.[2] It is the fact that two distinct visual submodalities are localizable to two anatomically distinct cortical areas that secured the evidence in favour of functional specialization in the visual cortex, even if the final product, vision, is unitary. This is not vastly different from the history of the cerebral cortex, where the foundations of the concept of cortical localization of function lay in the demonstration that one cortical area is critical for the production of articulate speech and another, architecturally and geographically distinct, cortical area is critical for the production of willed movement, though no one seeing a gesticulating speaker would guess that there is such a separation of function in the cortex.

Since the discovery of functional specialization in the visual cortex of the macaque brain, clinical neurologists have started to re-examine their earlier evidence and have also accumulated many new cases to show the association of different cortical fields with different visual functions. In this they have been greatly aided by new techniques of brain imaging. Through these they can localize brain damage in the living subject to a far greater extent than had ever been possible before. Unfortunately, even when their positions and extents can be determined with precision, lesions often turn out to be disappointing to those investigating the problem of functional localization. They commonly involve more than one cortical area and the white matter as well. They thus provide fertile ground, not for demonstrating the localization of function in a cortical area, but for a vivid and usually fruitless dispute among neurologists as to whether the compromised function can be localized to a distinct area. This is well demonstrated by the history of cerebral achromatopsia, recounted in earlier chapters. Another group of scientists who are now in hot pursuit of functional specialization in the human visual cortex are the psychophysicists. Armed with the most advanced technology and a conceptually far more sophisticated way of studying visual function, pioneered by Bela Julesz, they are now undertaking the most meticulous and imaginative studies of the capacities of the subsystems concerned with the different submodalities of vision. The results, which I shall return to briefly below, have been variable. Psychophysicists have been arguing among themselves as to how independent each system really is.[3] This is not surprising. Psychophysicists study the final output of the visual system, and all manner of interactions between the subdivisions of the visual system are possible before reaching the output stage. This state of affairs is clearly unsatisfactory for anyone wanting to have the satisfaction of demonstrating functional specialization in the human visual cortex directly. I wanted very much to be able to do so, but I had no idea of how to go about it.

Increases in local cerebral blood flow with local activity

Theoretically, the most obvious way of going about this task had been outlined by Broca, ever interested in problems of cerebral localization. He had applied six carefully graduated thermometers on different parts of the skulls of junior colleagues and found, in experiments which were as carefully controlled as could be under the circumstances, that there was a marked difference of temperature between the two sides of the brain, the left side being higher than the right.[4] He believed that such observations, which depended on differences in cerebral blood flow, would be useful in studies of cerebral localization in health and disease. There is little doubt that his conclusions, though derived from what might today be considered to be relatively crude experiments, carried enough conviction for others to repeat them.[5] In his usual prescient way, Broca summarized his conclusions precisely. He wrote,[6] 'The cerebral temperature is not the same at all points of the cranium: nor is it the same in all individuals and, finally, it varies in the same individual according to the state of the general circulation, *depending upon the state of rest or activity of the brain*' [my emphasis]. These observations by Broca and others must have been of sufficient interest for *The Lancet*[7] to question them in a strong editorial in 1880. It wrote, 'That there are variations in different parts of the head in individuals, and under varying conditions, is unquestionable, but it seems probable that these depend rather on the conditions of the abundant blood-supply to the scalp than on changes in the temperature of the brain. [Moreover] the summer sun acting on the head...often renders the scalp so hot that the hand can hardly bear to touch it, without any disturbance of the central functions. If changes of temperature readily permeate the skull, the cortex of the brain should be similarly heated, a supposition which is quite inconceivable'. Even in spite of the doubts voiced by the pillar of the medical establishment, the theme was taken up again towards the end of the last century by Roy and Sherrington.[8] They wrote, 'Bearing in mind that strong evidence exists of localisation of function in the brain, we are of the opinion that an automatic mechanism...is well fitted to provide for a local variation of the blood supply in accordance with local variations of the functional activity'. In other words, they hypothesized that the increase in activity in any brain area would entail an increase in the local cerebral circulation in that area. What one needed therefore was some reliable method for detecting changes in cerebral circulation and a method of localizing such changes to specific areas of the cerebral cortex. This was no easy task. Cobb and Talbot[9] stimulated rabbits with olfactory stimuli and undertook tedious post-mortem measurements of the relative areas of the capillary bed in three groups of rabbits. Two interesting facts emerged. The capillary bed was much richer in animals subjected to olfactory stimuli than in unstimulated animals and the increase was specific to olfactory cortex; the visual and motor areas showed no change. Though the results were promising, the method could not be applied to the human brain since it depended upon post-mortem measurements. But, in principle, such a method could be used to study areas of increased activity in the human brain.

It was not long before it was. In America, Fulton[10] came across a twenty-six-year-old patient with an 'angry-looking' tumour in the left occipital lobe and with a consequent right homonymous hemianopia. After operation, a bruit-producing pulsating defect remained over his left occipital lobe. Fulton was fascinated by this bruit and studied it further. It took little time '...to convince ourselves that when the patient suddenly began to use his eyes after a prolonged period of rest in a dark room, there was a prompt and noticeable increase in the intensity of the bruit. The increase was detectable within twenty to thirty seconds [and] would continue at heightened intensity for nearly a minute [after the patient had been directed to close his eyes] and then generally subside'. Nor was the increase in the bruit accompanied by changes in the blood pressure, suggesting that it was a regional affair. Fearful that no one would believe his evidence, Fulton recorded this bruit with a microphone 'placed directly on the back of his head at the point of maximum intensity of the bruit'. The results were fascinating. 'Merely shining light into his eyes when he was making no mental effort did not appear to do it. Moreover, the bruit increased very markedly when he attempted to read a paper in poor light, so that we believe that light per se had very little influence upon the results...It is also significant that auditory and olfactory stimuli did not increase the intensity of the bruit'.

It seems worth presenting these results in some detail because the thinking and principle employed is not different from the approaches used today, although the technique is. Fulton's technique of detecting a bruit depended upon the accessability of the primary visual cortex, which lies partly on the surface. The approach would have been difficult to apply to areas of the brain lying within sulci or situated on the medial side of the cerebral hemispheres. Moreover, one would probably (and hopefully) have to wait for a long time for the right patient to appear. A more accurate measuring device was needed. The opportunity arose in 1988. It was too good to miss.

The method of positron emission tomography

New advances have made it possible to look into the brain of man while he does particular things. Activity in any given circumscribed region of the brain entails a change in the local cerebral blood flow through it, much as predicted by Roy and Sherrington. This increase can be detected by the method of positron emission tomography (PET). The technique is complicated and requires the collaboration of an army of experts. In essence, it depends upon introducing some detectable substance into the blood. Knowing the amount of that substance circulating per unit volume of blood, one can calculate the amount flowing through any region and thus detect increases or decreases. In practice, a radioactive atom, say $C^{15}O_2$ is inhaled or injected. The radioactive oxygen has a very short half life of 2.1 minutes; it decays and emits positrons (positively charged electrons) which travel a short distance before hitting an electron. The result of that collision is the generation of two annihilation photons. The photons are detected by cameras installed around the head (Figure 15.1). The highest number of photons will naturally be emitted from regions where there is the highest blood flow, that is, from active regions of the brain. The picture thus obtained has subsequently to be translated, by a complex process, to produce a standard atlas of the human brain. From this one can determine the areas which showed the highest increase in blood flow, and therefore cortical activity, when the human subject was undertaking a particular task.

The spatial resolution of the brain scans obtained from such PET studies is low. Indeed, to a neurobiologist accustomed to examining individual layers of the cerebral cortex or to a physiologist spoiled enough to study the activity of single cells, the resolution, at 8 mm, is lamentable. Nevertheless, the technique has great virtues. In the first place, it is able to show active regions of the cerebral cortex and can therefore differentiate the parts of the cortex which are active in different conditions; in other words, it is a powerful tool for studying functional localization in the cerebral cortex. Indeed, one of its most successful applications has been the mapping of the extent and topographic disposition of the primary visual cortex in the human brain.[11] Next, it is able to show all the cerebral areas which are active at any given time in a single scan. Thus, if looking at a bunch of flowers entails high activity in all of four areas, all four will 'light up' in the scans. It is, in other words, a technique for studying an entire system or subsystem in the cerebral cortex. This is no mean feat, and in an important sense compensates for the low spatial resolution of PET. For if neuroanatomy and neurophysiology have taught us anything in the past two decades, it is the importance of entire systems and pathways in any given function, rather than of single areas acting in isolation. Yet it takes many years of experimentation in physiology or anatomy to determine the areas or subdivisions of areas which are involved in a particular task, say colour vision (if I may choose a task at random). PET studies, on the other hand, can show all the active areas in a single brain after a single study lasting no more than three hours. One might naturally guess that the areas which all 'light up' during a given task must be functionally related, and hence probably anatomically connected. As it turns out, one can make important inferences about the connectivity of the human cerebral cortex from PET studies.

It is this technique that my laboratory, in collaboration with that of Richard Frackowiak at the Hammersmith Hospital, used to demonstrate functional specialization directly in the human visual cortex. We could hardly have hoped for more satisfying results.[12]

Fig. 15.1 Positron emission tomography (PET) depends upon localizing the increase in regional cerebral blood flow when the brain undertakes a particular task. The increase can be detected by injecting a radioactive substance of very short half life, e.g. radioactive oxygen, into the blood stream. The radioactive atoms decay and emit positrons (positively charged electrons) which travel a short distance before colliding with electrons to produce annihilation photons (a). The photons can be detected by radiation detectors around the head (b). It is obvious that the greater the cerebral blood flow in a region of the brain, the greater the number of annihilation photons which can be traced to that region. Inset shows the part of the brain (area V5) with the greatest regional blood flow when humans look at visual motion.

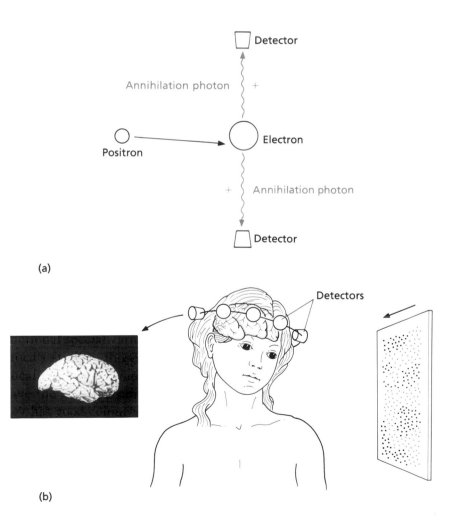

The localization of colour and motion in human visual cortex

The choice of the adequate stimulus is critical in these studies. We opted to compare the activity in the visual cortex in two experiments, one concerned with colour, the other with motion. In one set of experiments we compared the activity in the brain when subjects viewed a Land colour Mondrian, a collage of papers of variable size and colour, assembled to form an abstract scene with no recognizable objects, and when they viewed the identical scene in shades of equi-luminous grey (Plate 5, facing p. 188). The results showed that when subjects viewed the coloured Mondrian the area of heightened activity occurred in two separate regions. Posteriorly this was centred on the striate cortex and the cortex immediately surrounding it, presumably human V2. There was a second area of activation, situated more inferiorly, anteriorly and on the medial side of the brain. This was centred on the lingual and fusiform gyri, but the activity was highest in the fusiform gyrus. By contrast, when they viewed the same scene in shades of grey, the increase activity in the lingual and fusiform gyri was no more than one-third of what it had been when they had viewed the coloured display, although activity in the striate cortex was the same. Here, then, was the area which had been implicated, and then dismissed, for the better part of a century, as the colour centre in the human brain, lighting up with colour stimulation! There was only one name that it deserved to have — we called it human V4.

The fact that both the lingual and fusiform gyri were active during colour stimulation makes it difficult, from these scans, to locate V4 unequivocally in one gyrus or another. But good evidence from elsewhere suggests that V4 is located in the fusiform gyrus. There is, first, the clinical evidence[13] which shows that cerebral achromatopsia results from a lesion restricted to the fusiform gyrus. This is complemented by other clinical evidence which shows that involvement of the lingual gyrus alone does not necessarily lead to cerebral achromatopsia.[14] Next, the very anatomy of the region strongly implicates the fusiform gyrus (Figure 15.2). Human visual cortex also has an area V2, which is very similar in its cytochrome oxidase architecture to that of the monkey.[15] V2 surrounds V1. The lower part of V1 is situated in the lower lip of the calcarine sulcus and in the exposed lip of the lingual gyrus. Consequently, V2 must lie within the lingual gyrus, leaving the fusiform gyrus as the most likely site for human V4.

In the second set of experiments we compared the activity in the brains of subjects when they viewed a pattern of stationary and moving, random, black and white squares. When in motion, the pattern changed direction every six seconds, so that the subject saw all directions of motion. The resulting activity in the cortex outside

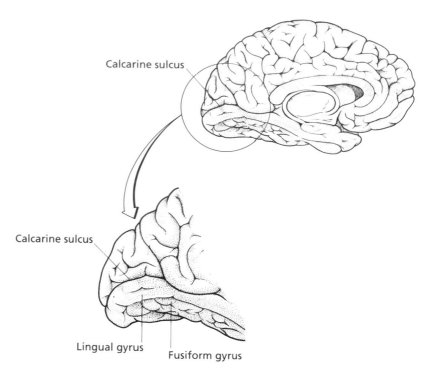

Fig. 15.2 A medial view of the brain to show the location of the lingual and fusiform gyri and their close proximity to one another and to the calcarine sulcus. It is very likely that human area V2 lies in the lingual gyrus and that human area V4 lies in the fusiform gyrus.

Calcarine sulcus

Calcarine sulcus

Lingual gyrus

Fusiform gyrus

the striate area was quite different from what we had seen with the colour experiment. Now the area of heightened blood flow (and therefore, by implication, neuronal activity) occurred in the striate cortex and in an area of the prestriate cortex located more laterally, at the junction of the occipital and temporal lobes (junction of Brodmann's areas 19 and 37). This area was far less active when subjects viewed the stationary pattern, although under this latter condition the striate cortex was as active as it had been when they viewed the moving pattern. The lesion in the unique patient of Zihl et al.,[16] which had resulted in an akinetopsic syndrome, included this area and went beyond it. We decided to call the area human V5.

The separation between the prestriate area activated by the colour stimulus and the prestriate area activated by the visual motion stimulus was impressive, and is evident at a glance (Plate 5). It provides a direct demonstration that, in addition to the striate cortex, there are other visual areas in human prestriate cortex and that there is a specialization for visual motion and for colour. But the results do more than that: they show us that the very same principle of parallelism which is so prominent a feature of the macaque visual cortex, also underlines the activity of human visual cortex.

Parallel outputs from area V1 of human visual cortex

One of the striking results obtained in this experiment is that, while different areas of the prestriate visual cortex were active in the two experiments, the same part of area V1 was active in both. In fact, the activity in what we are calling V1 was more extensive than the limits of the striate cortex, and it is almost certain that the area surrounding V1, area V2, was also active. At any rate, the results imply strongly that visual signals related to colour and to motion reach V1 first and are then distributed from V1 to these separate areas. Put more simply, the results imply that there are parallel outputs from V1 to at least two areas, V4 and V5, just as in the brain of the macaque monkey.

Perhaps a better way of demonstrating this is by the technique of co-variation. The technique is based upon choosing a pixel with high activity in the scans obtained under given conditions of stimulation and asking which other pixels in the brain co-vary consistently with the chosen pixel, either negatively or positively.[17] When, in the colour study, one selects a pixel within V4 in one hemisphere, one finds that the striate cortex, and the immediately surrounding prestriate cortex — presumably human V2 — of the same hemisphere co-vary consistently with it in a positive way. Another region which co-varies positively is V4 in the opposite hemisphere. This suggests that human V4 is connected with V1 and V2 of the same side and with its homologue in the opposite hemisphere, a pattern of connections that receives strong support from the known anatomical connections between these areas in the macaque monkey. When, in the motion study, one selects a pixel in area V5, one finds that, once again, there is a consistent positive co-variation only with the striate cortex and the immediately adjoining prestriate cortex of the same hemisphere and with V5 of the opposite hemisphere, much as one would expect from the known anatomy of these areas in the monkey brain.

It follows from all this that, not only are there parallel outputs from V1 and V2 to these areas, but that V1 (and V2) must therefore act as segregators, parcelling out different signals to different, and specialized, areas of the prestriate visual cortex for further processing.

In a sense, these PET experiments are a culmination of years of work on the functional organization of the primate brain on the one hand, and on the technology of PET on the other. The experiments described above give, however, only a first glimpse of the enormous promise that the technique holds for the future if, through adequate means of stimulation, one can demonstrate entire active systems of the cerebral cortex and infer their connectivity. Visual imagination, creativity, synaesthesias and other subjects, commonly considered more appropriate in the field of psychiatry and of art, will come firmly into the domain of scientific enquiry. The technique would be immensely enhanced if one could combine it with another one which would give a time resolution. If one could say, for example, that areas V1 and V2 were active before area V4 in the colour experiment, then there are many important features about the polarity of these connections in the human brain, and the sequence of activation of particular areas during particular tasks, that one could unravel. There is no doubt that such a sophisticated technology will be with us this decade. I have often conducted thought experiments, sometimes in public,[18] to enquire into how our subject would have developed if PET, or a technique similar to it, had been available in the 1920s and if stimulation with colour and with motion had demonstrated activity in the striate cortex as well as in separate areas of the visual association cortex. Would the resistance to the concept of specialization in the visual cortex have been quite so forceful or would we have modified our views of the cortical processes involved in vision? Would Henschen have been able to ridicule the notion of a colour centre outside the striate cortex and Holmes be able to dismiss it? Whatever the answers, the capacity to study the human brain should usher in important new concepts about the functions of the large, uncharted, parts of the cerebral cortex.

Notes and references

1 Monbrun, A. (1939). Les affections des voies optiques rétrochiasmatiques et de l'ecorce visuelle. In *Traité d'Ophtalmologie*, Vol. 6, edited by P. Baillart, C. Contela, E. Redslob & E. Velter, pp. 903–935. Société Française d'Ophtalmologie, Masson, Paris.

2 Zeki, S.M. (1978). Functional specialization in the visual cortex of the rhesus monkey. *Nature* **274**, 423–428.

3 Schiller, P.H. & Logothetis, N.K. (1990). The color-opponent and broad-band channels of the primate visual system. *Trends Neurosci.* **10**, 392–398.

4 Broca, P. (1877). Sur la thermométrie cérébrale. *Rev. Scientifique* **13**, 257.

5 Lombard, J.S. (1877). Experimental researches on the temperature of the head. *Proc. R. Soc. Lond.* **27**, 166–177; Gray, L.C. (1879). Cerebral thermometry. *J. Nerv. Ment. Dis.* **6**, 65–78; Bert, P. (1879). *C. R. Soc. Biol.* **1**(7), 28–29.

6 Broca, P. (1879). Sur les températures morbides locales. *Bull. Acad. Méd. (Paris)* **2S**, viii.

7 Editorial, (1880). Cephalic temperatures. *Lancet* **ii**, 303–304. (Note: I am much indebted to Professor Van den Berg of Groningen for drawing my attention to references [4]–[7].)

8 Roy, C.S. & Sherrington, C.S. (1890). On the regulation of the blood supply to the brain. *J. Physiol. (Lond.)* **11**, 85–108.

9 Cobb, S. & Talbot, J.H. (1927). Studies in cerebral capillaries. II. A quantitative study of cerebral capillaries. *Trans. Assoc. Am. Physicians* **45**, 255–262.

10 Fulton, J.F. (1928). Observations upon the vascularity of the human occipital lobe during visual activity. *Brain* **51**, 310–320.

11 Fox, P.T., Mintum, M.A., Raichle, M.E. *et al.* (1986). Mapping human visual cortex with positron emission tomography. *Nature* **323**, 806–809.

12 Zeki, S., Watson, J.D.G., Lueck, C.J. *et al.* (1991). A direct demonstration of functional specialization in human visual cortex. *J. Neurosci.* **11**, 641–649.

13 Lenz, G. (1921). Zwei Sektionsfälle doppelseitiger zentraler Farbenhemianopsie. *Z. Ges. Neurol. Psychiatr.* **71**, 135–186.

14 Dide, M. & Botcazo (1902). Amnésie continuel cécité verbale pure, perte du sense topographique, ramollissement double du lobe lingual. *Rev. Neurol. (Paris)* **10**, 676–680; Bogousslavsky, J.J., Miklossy, J., Deruaz, J.P., Assal, G. & Regli, F. (1987). Lingual and fusiform gyri in visual processing: a clinico-pathological study of

altitudinal hemianopia. *J. Neurol. Neurosurg. Psychiatry* **50**, 607–614; Clarke, S. & Miklossy, J. (1990). Occipital cortex in man: organization of callosal connections, related myelo- and cytoarchitecture, and putative boundaries of functional visual areas. *J. Comp. Neurol.* **298**, 188–214.

15 Burkhalter, A. & Bernardo, K.L. (1989). Organization of cortico-cortical connections in human visual cortex. *Proc. Natl. Acad. Sci. USA* **86**, 1071–1075.

16 Zihl, J., Cramon, D. von & Mai, N. (1983). Selective disturbance of movement vision after bilateral brain damage. *Brain* **106**, 313–340.

17 Friston, K. & Frackowiak, R.S.J. (1991). Imaging functional anatomy. In *Brain Work and Mental Activity*, edited by N.A. Lassen, D.H. Ingvar, M.E. Raichle & L. Freiberg, pp. 267–279. Munksgaard, Copenhagen.

18 Zeki, S. (1992). A thought experiment with PET. In *Exploring Brain Functional Anatomy with Positron Tomography*, edited by D.J. Chadwick & J. Whelan, pp. 145–154. Ciba Foundation Symposium, John Wiley, Chichester.

Chapter 16: The collapse of the old concepts

Functional specialization accounts for a great deal that is interesting in visual perception, in visual pathology and in the more detailed organization of the visual system. These are all topics which we shall return to. Here, we want to look briefly at the new concepts which the demonstration of functional specialization in the visual cortex introduced while displacing the old ones, thus ushering in new and different ideas of how the visual image is represented in the brain, and also new ideas about brain functions.

As outlined above, it was a system of beliefs, most of them fragile and vulnerable, though with a strong and usually unstated link between them, that prevented acceptance of new evidence concerning the nature of visual representation in the brain. The older concepts were not necessarily derived from the study of the visual cortex alone. Concepts such as those of strict hierarchy, of the functional uniformity of uniform cytoarchitectonic fields and of association cortex were derived as much from a study of other systems as of the visual. Yet, in the visual system they seemed to be especially well linked and to reinforce each other. Little wonder that when one collapsed, the others followed suit. The belief that a visual image is impressed upon the retina and then transmitted to be received by the primary, and sole, visual perceptive cortex was derived from the belief that objects in our visual environment are labelled or coded, requiring nothing more than an analysis. It followed from this that vision is an essentially passive process, the only active component being the requirement for interpreting the 'received' visual image and thus 'knowing' what it is. This belief gained much credibility from the clinical and experimental demonstration that, while lesions in the striate cortex led to blindness, those outside it led to mental blindness, a condition in which one could see but could not understand what was seen, or so neurologists believed. This, together with the belief in the purely analytic doctrine, in turn fed the belief in the hierarchical process, which argued for increased levels of complexity in brain function at 'higher' levels, a notion that seemed to receive powerful support not only from the physiological evidence but also from previous concepts derived from what many accepted as indisputable facts — concepts of association cortex as postulated by Flechsig and his followers. Even philosophical speculation, insofar as anyone understood it,[1] seemed to speak in favour of such a view, or was at least consistent with it. Had not

Kant, in his *Critique of Pure Reason*, proposed that the mind could be divided into two Faculties, the passive one of Sensibility concerned with the collection of raw sense data and the active one of Understanding which made sense of the raw data? Moreover, the notion that the function of the cortex outside the striate area was uniform and consisted of associating received impressions with previous impressions, seemed to receive powerful support through the demonstration of its cytoarchitectonic uniformity. And these facts seemed to speak in favour of the concept of the dual nature of visual processing in the cerebral cortex. Facts and concepts began to feed each other. All that was needed to overturn this system of beliefs was to show that one of them was fundamentally flawed.

One could choose any one of the major tenets linking this chain and show it to be false and the rest would collapse. Take the concept of a single visual 'association' cortex as the first chip in this domino game. The demonstration that this 'association' cortex consists of several separate visual areas compromised immediately not only the notion that an area of uniform cytoarchitecture corresponds to a cortical area with one and uniform function, but also the notion that the cerebral processes involved in vision are twofold. It suggested instead that the cerebral processes involved in vision must be manifold. It also immediately made plausible the clinical demonstration of specific defects in colour vision following specific lesions in cortex outside the striate area, and therefore raised the question of a functional specialization in the visual cortex which, in turn, compromised the doctrine of exclusive hierarchies. Or one could start with another chip, for example the one that supposed that vision is a strictly hierarchical process. The demonstration that the striate cortex sends separate and parallel outputs to the visual areas of the prestriate cortex called this concept into question immediately and, by showing that the separate outputs are destined for different regions of the cytoarchitectonically uniform visual 'association' cortex, suggested as well that this cortex may not be functionally uniform. It also raised the question of functional specialization in the visual cortex, for it made it plausible to suppose that the striate cortex sends different signals to the different areas of the prestriate cortex; rather, such a supposition seemed a good deal more plausible than the alternative — that it sends identical signals to these different areas. This, in turn, made the incomplete clinical evidence for a separation of functions more plausible. Either way, one would be led to ask more profound questions about the workings of the visual cortex and the functions of the brain, and these questions would ineluctably lead to the questioning of the central, but usually unspoken, doctrine that the function of the visual cortex is nothing more than an analysis of the conveniently labelled and coded visual environment. Why is colour processed separately? What kind of information does the brain need to 'analyze' colour? Why is motion processed separately? Is colour analyzed or constructed? How is it combined with form? These are all questions which have been raised by the new evidence. Just as the old system of beliefs were linked together, so are the new ones — parallelism, functional segregation, functional specialization and the multiplicity of visual areas all form part of the same chain. As surely as the old system of beliefs was rooted in the concept of a labelled image of the visual world, received and analyzed by the cortex, so the present one is rooted in the belief that an image of the visual world is actively constructed by the cerebral cortex, after discarding all the unnecessary information contained in the visual image. As surely as the old system considered that the problem of knowledge and understanding could be separated from the problem of seeing, so the present one will find it increasingly difficult to draw a dividing line between the two. It therefore involves a reappraisal of the concept of visual agnosia, which we shall undertake in a later chapter. Central to this reappraisal is the re-evaluation of the role of cortical visual areas, brought about by the demonstration of functional specialization. This evidence has shown that V1 cannot be the sole 'visual perceptive centre', as Holmes and others had supposed, since the visual image in the brain is far from constructed at the level of V1. Instead, V1 turns out to be an initial but critical cortical stage, and other cortical visual areas are also involved in a real, not an auxiliary, sense in visual perception. V1 and possibly V2 are perhaps more critical than the other stages only because all the signals are distributed to the other areas through them. Lesions in them, or at least in V1, therefore lead to almost total blindness. But lesions in the specialized areas also lead to blindness, though these are not total but submodality specific.

The important point here is that this overturning of old concepts is derived from direct experiments, rather than from merely thinking profoundly about what the brain does. It was no good fighting the established views of how the brain is organized by suggesting other ways in which it might be organized. The German Gestalt school of Wertheimer and his colleagues may well have been right in their belief that visual perception is an active process, and not the passive one that neurologists had imagined it to be. But their evidence was derived partly from relatively complex perceptual experiments and partly from thinking about the brain. The perceptual phenomena they described, for which they had no plausible physiological model, could be (and commonly were) taken to reveal higher levels of brain functioning, not the elementary processes of seeing which neurologists and neurophysiologists imagined that they were concerned with. Hence, the latter, with a few exceptions,[2] took not the slightest interest in what they considered to be idle speculations. To overturn the deeply held beliefs of the neurologists and neurobiologists direct evidence was required, evidence that could show that the cerebral visual pathways are organized differently from the way that they had supposed them to be.

The game could of course have been played differently. The scenario would then have evolved in much the same way, but the time taken could have been much shorter. The evidence for cerebral achromatopsia could have been accepted for what it was and is — a specific perceptual defect in vision arising from a specific lesion outside the striate cortex and depriving the patient of the ability to acquire a knowledge about certain properties of objects, which the brain interprets as colour. If accepted, one would have been forced to the conclusion that other attributes of vision, and hence other means of acquiring knowledge about the visual world, must be represented elsewhere, that the visual association cortex may not be a single area, that its role may therefore be different from the one ascribed to it traditionally, and that cytoarchitectonic uniformity was not a good guide to the functional identity of an area. One would then have been led ineluctably to ask the more profound question of what it is that vision actually involves. The game could have been played that way, but it was not. The prevalent concepts were too strong. Scientists like to believe that concepts are derived from facts. They like to portray themselves as deeply committed to the search for facts, unbiased and dispassionate in their collection of them, ready to renounce cherished beliefs and overthrow painstakingly constructed concepts if the new facts so dictate. Having so convinced themselves, they manage to convince others that this devotion to facts, no matter what the consequence, is the hallmark of their trade. A reading of the history of colour vision as it relates to the cerebral cortex would do little to justify this narcissistic image that scientists have of themselves.

In fairness, it is hard to believe that the bias, as well as the experience, of the scientist counts for nothing in the acceptance of certain facts, the rejection of others and in the formulation of doctrines and concepts. It is especially difficult to believe that, when studying the brain, personal experiences and beliefs do not intrude to play a powerful role in the formulation of concepts. The unitary image in the brain, a concept derived from the reality of daily visual experience of the neurologist as much as that of the common man, was at least as powerful a fact in formulating concepts of the representation of vision in the brain as were the facts derived from experimental and pathological studies.

Yet, in the long run (which, to a cynic surveying the history of cerebral colour vision, turns out to be no less than a century), the scientists' image of themselves is correct. The cynic would say, with justice, that this has more to do with the nature of the subject than with the intellect, devotion or personality of scientists. The concepts that prevented acceptance of the evidence for a separate localization of colour in the cerebral cortex, with all that it implied, were eventually overturned. The newly discovered facts would not give way. But it remains an extraordinary irony that it was the direct evidence for functional specialization that was to make the syndrome of cerebral achromatopsia credible, rather than the syndrome of cerebral achromatopsia ushering in ideas about functional specialization in the human visual cortex and raising fundamental questions about the nature of visual representation in the brain.

Notes and references

1 Healey, D. (1989). *The Time of My Life*. Michael Joseph, London. Denis Healey writes in *The Time of My Life*, his autobiography, of his struggles with Kant's description of apperception, 'surely the most difficult page of prose ever written'. He cannot have been the only one who had to struggle with the opaque writings of Kant.
2 As an example, one may cite the following two references, although it is important to realize that both consider the active process of vision only in terms of higher visual functions and of the visual agnosia which is supposedly a manifestation of the breakdown of these higher processes: Goldstein, K. & Gelb, A. (1918). Psychologische Analysen hirnpathologischer Fälle auf Grund von Untersuchungen Hirnverletzter. *Z. Ges. Neurol. Psychiatr.* **41**, 1−214; Brain, W.R. (1941). Visual object-agnosia with special reference to the gestalt theory. *Brain* **64**, 43−62.

Chapter 17: The mapping of visual functions in the brain

Why should the brain develop the strategy of functional specialization? Why could it not undertake all the necessary visual operations in a single cortical area? More broadly, why is it that the brain resorts to the strategy of assembling cells with common properties in discrete regions (areas) and in subregions of an area? This is the critical question for cortical localization of function, which itself forms the main theme of cortical studies. Cells dealing with a given modality, such as vision or audition, are assembled together to form an area. Cells dealing with a given submodality of vision, such as motion or colour, are also assembled in areas. In areas such as V1, cells dealing with submodalities of submodalities, such as the long-wave selective cells of colour vision, are assembled in discrete clusters, the blobs, with different blobs having cells of uniform wavelength selectivity (see Chapter 21). Scientists speculated on these questions, only to discover that their answers were highly speculative. Some believed that assembling cells with common properties was a more 'efficient' or 'economical' way of undertaking operations; others believed that assembling cells with common properties eliminated the need for long fibre connections between cells undertaking similar operations, as would happen if the specialized cells were widely distributed in a single area; yet others believed that to distribute cells undertaking a given operation and to connect them with long fibres might increase the number of possible errors in these connections. As commonly happens with biological speculation, evolution was usually thrown in for good measure, some scientists believing that such a system, being more efficient, has a greater survival value — a statement that explains little to the extent that it explains everything, since all biological systems are products of evolution. My own explanation has been that the requirements for constructing different attributes of the visual scene, such as colour or form, are sufficiently different for the cortex to use different algorithms, which require different anatomical machineries, and hence the need to undertake these operations in different areas,[1] a theme developed further below.

In fact, none of these arguments is at present compelling, which is not to say that they may not turn out to be true. The nervous system seems to be more than capable of connecting like with like through the use of either long of short fibres. After all, the optic nerves, or the optic tracts, consist of long fibres, and yet they are able to connect distant cells correctly and specifically, a fact made even more emphatic by the correct connections established by fibres travelling from the motor cortex to the lumbar cord. On the other hand, the cortex seems to use short fibres to connect like with like in adjacent blobs of V1[2] and slightly longer fibres to connect like with like between the blobs of V1 and the thin stripes of V2[3] (see Chapter 21). Ever since Sperry[4] demonstrated that, however hard he tried to divert retinal fibres from reaching their correct, genetically specified, destinations in the optic tectum of frogs, they outdid him and managed to reach their targets, the notion of proximity to establish specificity has seemed to be a faltering argument.

Perhaps the best way of reaching a decision is to look at the physiology of these areas. One then finds that there are similarities as well as differences in the overall organization of the different visual areas, over and above the differences in the response preferences of cells between areas described earlier. Because it has the richest architecture of all cortical areas, V1 has been studied in greater detail than any other cortical area and, because it receives the overwhelming input from the eye, area V1 will be central to the description that follows. Until relatively recently, the most detailed description of the functional architecture of area V1 came from the work of Hubel and Wiesel. They pursued ineluctably a great discovery, that of orientation selectivity, to its logical conclusion, enquiring into how orientation selectivity is represented in area V1 with respect to other features characteristic of it. The account given here and in Chapter 19, however, does not go into all the details, nor is it chronological throughout.

'Maps' in the primary areas of the brain

The most striking feature of area V1, apart from its distinctive architecture, is the precise retinal map within it that anatomists and physiologists have uncovered. In the human brain, Henschen had already reached this conclusion from his detailed pathological studies. It is indeed one of the main reasons why he called the striate cortex the 'cortical retina'. Much later, actual recording experiments revealed that area V1 in the macaque brain is similarly organized and also contains within it a highly detailed map of the retina.[5] Area V1 is not the only cortical area which contains a detailed representation of the body surface. Other sensory and motor areas also have detailed maps in them. The most famous of these is the motor cortex, which contains a 'map' in the sense that, broadly speaking, the musculature of different regions of the body is represented in different regions of the motor cortex, as if there is a 'map' of the body surface on the cortex or, worse still, as if there is a *homunculus* there, a sort of ghost in the machine, slightly deformed to give more important parts of the

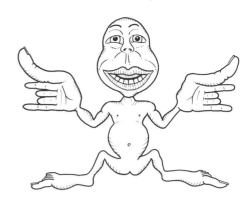

Fig. 17.1 The amount of cortex that the brain devotes to different parts of the body is in direct proportion to their relative importance. In the motor cortex, for example, relatively more space is devoted to the fingers and the lips than to the shoulder or the elbow, producing a sort of deformed map of the body. A map such as the one shown here is often called an homunculus.

body such as the hands and lips a more extensive cortical representation (Figure 17.1). Philosophers may well argue with this concept of a 'map'. But, at an operational level, there is little doubt about what the physiologist means by it. He knows that if he records the activity in a given region of a sensory surface, say V1, he will find that the cells will have receptive fields at a given position in visual space, and that they must consequently be receiving input from a given region of the retina. He knows, moreover, that whenever he records from the same region, in the same or different animals, the cells will be found to record events in the same part of visual space. There is therefore a 'map' of the retinal surface on the cortex of V1, in other words a correspondence between the two.

The overall details of the map in area V1 have been described already. Just how detailed it is can be easily gleaned from a long electrode penetration made obliquely to the cortical surface (Figure 17.2). If one were to plot the receptive fields of the successive cells, separated from each other by about 50–100 μm, encountered during the journey of the electrode, one would find that the receptive fields, being of relatively small size, are displaced from each other with a remarkable regularity. This is perhaps best seen when one connects the receptive field centres of the successive cells encountered. To be sure, there is some degree of scatter and the line connecting the centres is not straight (it is subject to a certain degree of jitter). But the overall impression is one of regularity. Moreover, the regularity is a predictable one, in the sense that if one were to make the same penetration in different brains, one would obtain very much the same results. Indeed, it is because of this precision and predictability that one is able to determine the precise part of area V1 affected by a lesion or a vascular accident, by noting the position of the scotoma in a patient, or indeed in a monkey. If the scotoma is in the upper field of view, one can predict with fair accuracy that the lesion is in the lower lip of the calcarine cortex; if it is in the far periphery, one can predict with equal accuracy that it is in the very anterior part of the

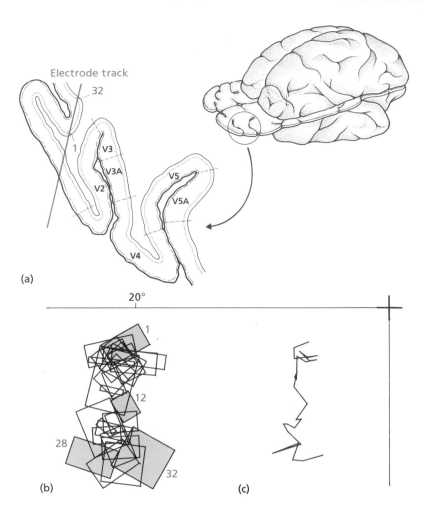

Fig. 17.2 (b) The change in the receptive field positions of successive cells (1−32, only some of which are highlighted in red), separated from each other by short distances, encountered in a long oblique penetration (a) through area V1, which has a very precise topographic map of the retina in it. (c) The displacement from the receptive field centre of one cell to that of the next. In this and the following figures, the cross marks the fovea (fixation point) projected on the screen.

calcarine sulcus. Such a map therefore gives the neurologist far more useful information than the high-sounding speculation of philosophers about what a 'map' means.

If one were to study the size of the receptive fields of cells in different parts of area V1, representing different parts of the retina, one would find that the field sizes are not uniform all over the striate cortex. They are smallest in the part of the V1 representing the central retina and increase in size as one samples from regions representing more peripheral parts. This makes sense, to the extent that finer details are observed with central vision. But an important principle of representation follows from it. The amount of cortex devoted to an organ or to its parts is not proportional to the size of the organ but to its importance or to the density of receptors in it. In the motor cortex, for example, more cortical space is devoted to the hands and to the lips than to the trunk, reflecting the relative importance of these organs. In the same way, relatively more cortical space is devoted to central than to peripheral vision. The relationship can be established quantitatively, and is known as the *magnification factor*. In the visual cortex this refers to the amount of cortex, in square millimetres, devoted to every degree of visual space.[6]

'Maps' in other visual areas

When one studies the visual areas of the prestriate cortex, one begins to find similarities between them and area V1, the most obvious similarity being that they, too, are visual areas. The next similarity is that there is an element of organization in each, in the sense that the retina appears to be mapped systematically in some and less so in others. The area surrounding V1, area V2, is topographically organized to a fair degree of precision by virtue of the point-to-point projections it receives from area V1[7] (Figure 17.3). This can be established by detailed physiological recordings which reveal the great similarities between the two areas. The overall organization of the map in V2 is different (see Chapter 12). But, as in V1, receptive fields increase in size with increasing eccentricity, although the receptive fields themselves are larger than the ones in V1. Thus, one can say that both areas contain a detailed map of the retina, though the precision of the maps is not identical, the one in V1 being the more precise.

The picture begins to differ somewhat when one records from the specialized visual areas of the prestriate cortex. The difference is not so apparent in V3, even in spite of the fact that cells have larger receptive fields here than they do in V1 or V2 (Figure 17.4). As before, there is a predictable map of the retina in V3 and the receptive field size of cells increases with increasing eccentricity,[7] i.e. with increasing distance from the centre of gaze. For both V3 and V3A, if one were to connect the receptive field centres of successive cells encountered in long, oblique, penetrations through the cortex, one would find an orderly displacement in spite of the erratic jitter from one receptive field centre to the next. But in areas V4 and V5, and especially in V6, such an order is not nearly so apparent. The receptive fields of cells in these areas tend to be larger than the ones in the previous areas, at comparable eccentricities, and the shift from field centre to field centre is not that easily predicted. To obtain an idea of the kind of differences in the overall organization of the two areas from this point of view, it is instructive to compare the picture in area V5 (shown in Figure 17.5) with the picture that one finds in V1 (shown in Figure 17.2). In the latter, if the receptive fields of the first five cells, recorded at separations of 50–100 μm, are found to be displaced in a particular direction, say downwards, the receptive fields of the successive cells will continue the trend, in spite of the jitter, until one crosses a sulcus and thus enters a part of V1 representing another part of the

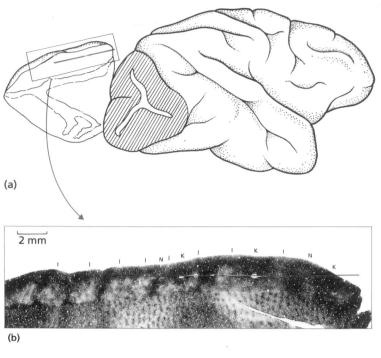

(a)

(b)

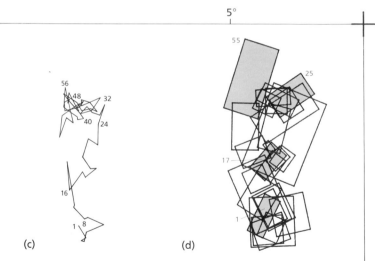

5°

Fig. 17.3 The change in the receptive field positions of successive cells encountered during a long, oblique, penetration through area V2 of the monkey (a). The penetration intersected several of the stripes which characterize the metabolic architecture of V2, as shown in (b). There was an orderly displacement of receptive fields, with the fields of cells at one end of the penetration (cell 55) being close to the fixation point and those at the other end (cell 1) further from it, as shown in (d). (c) The shifts from the receptive field centre of one cell to that of the next.

(c)

(d)

retina. In V5, however, the trend is not nearly so evident. The receptive field centres of cells in a long penetration are not displaced as regularly, the jitter is greater, and the progression is not always predictable. With V6, in which the receptive fields are larger still, the tendency to *apparent* chaos is even greater,[8] as may be seen by reference to Figure 17.6 which illustrates a long oblique penetration through it. The shift from the receptive field centre of one cell to that of the next makes little sense in retinal terms, if indeed one wishes to speak of these maps as retinal maps. The same pattern, on a smaller scale, is

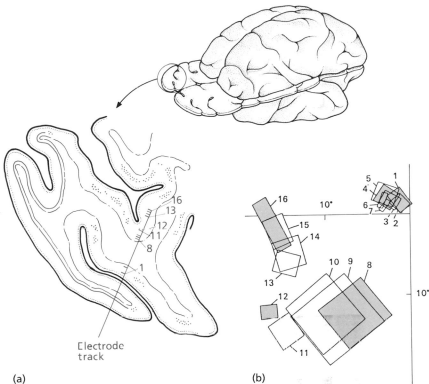

Fig. 17.4 The change in the receptive field positions (b) of successive cells (1–16) encountered in a long oblique penetration through area V3A of the monkey (a). Notice the orderly change in field position in spite of the increase in receptive field size of cells.

Electrode track

(a)   (b)

also observed in V4. This is not to say that there is a total lack of order in topographic representation in these areas. Indeed, when one records from successive cells in any given small location in them, one finds that most cells have their receptive fields in roughly the same region of visual space, though the region represented by the receptive field of even a single cell is commonly so large that to speak of these areas as containing retinal maps soon leads one to absurdities.

Scientists, like other groups, like to give difficult problems convenient labels. Having done so, they pretend that they understand the problem, which is therefore solved, at least to them. The sort of map illustrated in Figure 17.5 is commonly referred to as a 'crude' map of the retina and I take little pride in having been the first to use this silly term, though I rapidly discarded it. For such a label surely explains nothing. To repeat, maps in the brain are precise enough as they need to be to undertake their function with efficiency. Moreover, a brain that can construct a map as detailed as the one found in V1 would only construct a 'crude' map if the need for it arises, that is, if this 'retinal crudeness' is necessary for some other reason. The map shown in Figure 17.5 cannot be a map of the retina, whether crude or not, for it is a map that represents a particular type of activity only, namely motion. At the very least it is a selective map of the retina,

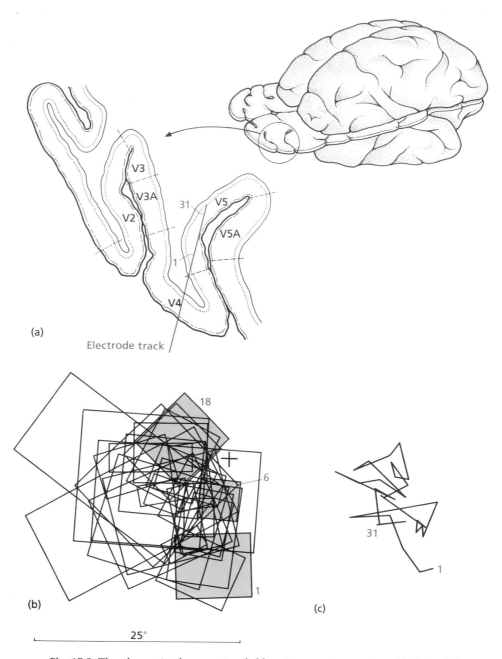

(a)

Electrode track

(b)

(c)

18

6

1

31

1

25°

Fig. 17.5 The change in the receptive field positions of successive cells (b) and their centres (c) encountered in a long oblique penetration through V5 of the monkey (a). Compare this penetration with one through V1, illustrated in Figure 17.2.

assuming it to be one at all. The real question that needs to be addressed, then, is whether these are retinal maps at all.

Imagine a thought experiment, one which can be undertaken in practice, in which one tries to plot the map of area V5 with stationary bars of light, remembering that the overwhelming majority of cells in area V5 are directionally selective. One would not be able to obtain a

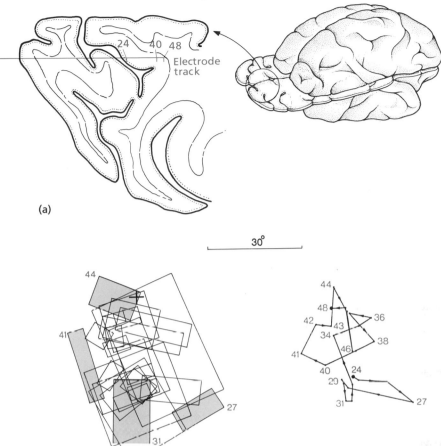

Fig. 17.6 The change in the receptive field positions of successive cells (24–48) encountered in a long oblique penetration through area V6 of the monkey. The electrode penetration is shown in (a). (b) The positions of the receptive fields of successive cells encountered during the penetration. (c) The displacement from the receptive field centre of one cell to that of the next.

map at all, since the cells will not be responsive to perfectly stationary stimuli. Or imagine trying to do the same with large stationary spots in area V3A and area V6. The cells will be unresponsive or will respond very weakly, and one wouldn't be able to learn anything at all about how the retina is mapped there. The picture becomes very different if one tries to study the way the retina is mapped in V5 by using moving spots of light. Now, many cells will become responsive, allowing one to draw their receptive fields with fair accuracy. It is obvious, therefore, that the map in V5 is in no sense a map of the retina. Rather, it is a map of a particular kind of activity, in this case motion, occurring in the field of view. Maybe we should not even call them maps; perhaps we should think of these areas as labelling a particular kind of activity in a region of visual space.

That the apparent complexity and chaos of the map in an area like V5 is only in the mind of the experimenter, not in V5 itself, can be illustrated by examples in which a single, long and continuous, penetration through it yields two patterns of receptive field displacement, one reminiscent of V1 and the other more characteristic of V5 (Figure 17.7). Moreover, one can take a long oblique penetration through V5, with its apparently irregular shift in receptive field positions, and find that otherwise the cells are organized together fairly systematically, with a fair degree of order. This can be seen by examining the directional preferences of the directionally selective cells encountered in an apparently chaotic penetration (Figure 17.7). The directional preferences

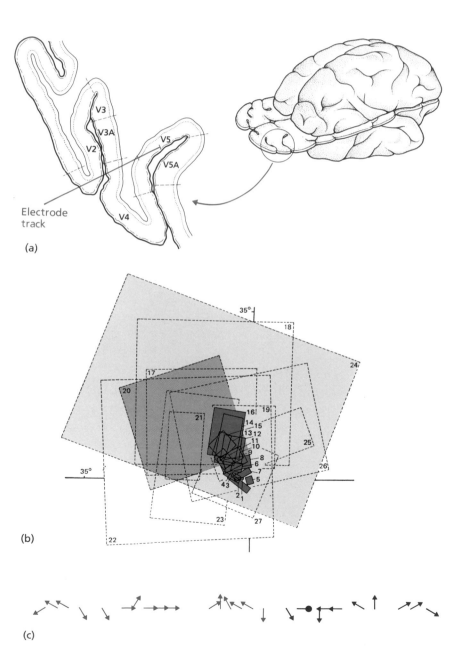

Fig. 17.7 A hint of a remarkable organization within area V5 of monkey visual cortex. Of the successive cells studied in a long oblique penetration through area V5 (a), the first sixteen (dark red) had relatively small receptive fields and their field centres were displaced from each other in an orderly way (b). By contrast the next group of cells, encountered in the same penetration, had large receptive fields and their centres were displaced from each other in an apparently chaotic way. (c) The directional preferences of all cells encountered in the penetration. The black dot indicates that the cell was motion, but not directionally, selective.

of the first ten successive cells do not show much systematic order, even in spite of the fact that the centre-to-centre shift in receptive field positions is highly orderly. By contrast, there is a systematic shift in directional preferences for the last eight cells (shown in black, Figure 17.7c), even though the centre-to-centre shift in receptive field centres seems chaotic. In the same way, one can find that the wavelength preferences of successive cells in area V4 can vary systematically while the shift of the receptive field positions of the same cells, with respect to each other, makes little sense in terms of retinal geography.[9]

There are other indications of a great deal of order in these apparently chaotic maps. If one were to look, for example, at the relationship between field size and eccentricity, one would find more or less the same relationship in each area, with field sizes increasing as a function of eccentricity. Indeed, one would hardly guess from such an orderly, and similar, relationship that the maps themselves are so very different. Again, if one were to look at the frequency of the size of shifts in the different areas, one would find a remarkable similarity. Although we still have no real clue as to the organizing principle which dictates that maps in certain areas should have a great deal of regularity and reflect fairly faithfully the retinal geography, while maps in other areas should be apparently chaotic in retinal terms, it is hard to believe that there isn't an organizing principle operating for every visual area in the cortex. It is difficult to imagine that the apparently chaotic map in area V6 is not, in fact, a highly precise map, but precise in terms of a function which demands such a chaotic map in terms of retinal geography. This would be so if the function of an area demands that the cells in it 'label' a combination of features, features which are not distributed in a precise geographic point in visual space. It may seem a little unnecessary to discuss these matters in such detail and so speculatively when nothing at all is known about the organizing principle, assuming there is one. Yet the first important element in understanding these maps is the realization that there is a problem to be solved here and that calling these maps precise or crude merely shelves the problem.

Superimposed on the similarities described above are differences. For example, it is not the same extent of the retina that is mapped in each area. In V4 it is only the central 40° of the retina that is mapped, consistent with the finding that this is an area in which colour vision and form in association with colour are emphasized, since colour perception is best with central vision and becomes increasingly weaker at more peripheral eccentricities. There is an interesting report which suggests that the lower part of the field of view is more heavily emphasized in area V5,[9] a feature which is not an obvious characteristic of the maps in V1, V2 or even V4. There are, too, differences in the way that the vertical meridian is represented in each area (discussed in the next chapter) but no one really understands what these differences relate to.

The mapping of visual functions in the visual cortex

It is results such as the ones described above that have made me wonder whether we are justified in continuing to speak of these areas as representing the retina or containing 'retinal maps', a formulation derived from our experience of the visual map in V1.[1] Perhaps a good analogy is to examine various maps of Europe. A gastronomic map of that continent would obviously have to be disproportionately weighted in favour of France, with Britain squeezed to a tiny dot, assuming that it should have any representation at all. On the other hand, a beer map would have to give greater weighting to Belgium, Denmark, Germany and Czechoslovakia and much less to Portugal and Greece. Translated to the cortex, could we not ask how a function may be mapped in the cortex? It is obvious that a 'motion map' of the cortex would give much greater weighting to V5 and would squeeze V4 to a tiny dot; by contrast, a 'colour' map of the visual cortex would give heavy weighting to V4 and none to V5. At the very least, this would lead us to ask how we would map motion or colour on the cortex, what sorts of activities would have to be magnified and what sorts of signals would have to be de-emphasized. Indeed, the maps may be dynamic ones and a good possibility is encountered in area V4. To construct a map of colour, the cells would obviously have to collate information from large parts of the field of view (see Chapter 25). But the precise extent of the field of view changes from one scene to the next, so that the importance attached to different extents will vary from moment to moment. Moreover, attention plays an important role in colour vision and it therefore becomes very interesting to note that attentional mechanisms are important in V4 and can, in fact, modify the responses of the cells and perhaps even the extent of the field of view which influences their responses.[10] In short, we may have to consider such maps in a dynamic context.

The idea that a function may be mapped in an area is not a new one. Physiologists studying the motor cortex had prolonged arguments as to whether individual muscles, groups of muscles or movements are mapped in the motor cortex, with Hughlings Jackson and Henry Head leading those who believed that the representation is that of movements. The American school, under the leadership of Clinton Woolsey, preferred to believe that it was individual muscles. It is perhaps surprising that no similar debate has occurred in the context of the maps within the visual cortex in general, and the specialized visual areas in particular. It is but one jump from asking the question of whether it is parts or functions that are mapped in the cerebral cortex to the realization that it is not adequately phrased. A better question would be to ask how colour or motion are constructed by the cortex, to consider whether the various maps in the visual cortex are influenced by the differing requirements for constructing form, colour, motion and so on. I use the term *constructional maps* to refer to this notion. We can then ask what the requirements for constructing colour or motion may be and seek to understand the extent to which the physiological architecture of the areas we study corresponds to these requirements. The answer is by no means clear and cannot become so until we recognize the problem. It is nevertheless interesting to ask what the requirements may be for constructing colours as opposed to forms and to visual motion. We shall see later that in constructing the colour of an area the brain has to collate information from large parts of the field of view simultaneously, in order to be able to compare the wavelength composition of the light coming from the area with the wavelength composition of the light coming from surrounding areas; but the exact topography of the surround is immaterial. With form, the brain again has to collate information coming simultaneously from large parts of the field of view but the exact topographic relationship of one part to another is critical, since it is the relationship of adjacent parts to one another that determines the form of an object. Finally, for motion, it is contiguity in time and space, and not simultaneity, that is critical. Such differences suggest that if the maps are indeed constructional maps, then they should vary. Although the relationship cannot be drawn directly, it is therefore perhaps suggestive in this context that, outside areas V1 and V2 (the two segregator areas), the most topographic maps are those of areas V3 and V3A, the very ones which contain the highest concentration of orientation-selective cells, the ones presumed to be of importance in the perception of forms. By contrast, the map in area V4 is much less so and perhaps reflects the underlying requirement that the precise topographic relationship of surfaces to one another is, to a large extent, immaterial in determining the colour of a surface.

The functional architecture of area V1

The most detailed map of the retina is found in area V1. This detail goes hand in hand with a very rich functional architecture, uncovered by Hubel and Wiesel in their physiological studies.[11] They proposed on the basis of their experiments that V1 was made up of a set of orientation columns and a set of ocular dominance columns. Perhaps the best way to understand this is to see how cells encountered in a penetration made perpendicular to the cortical surface of V1 respond (Figure 17.8). It is usual to plot the receptive field for each eye one at a time, by keeping one eye open and the other shut. This establishes

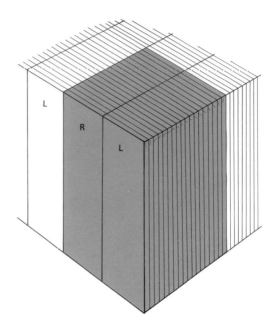

Fig. 17.8 A model of the orientation columns and ocular dominance columns in area V1 of monkey cortex. All cells in one perpendicular penetration (from above down) will respond to the same orientation and prefer the same eye. By contrast, both orientation and eye preferences will change in a penetration parallel to the cortical surface. For details, see text. (Redrawn from Hubel, D.H. & Wiesel, T.N. (1977). *Proc. R. Soc. Lond.* B **198**, 1–59.

whether the cell can be driven by stimulation of one eye, the other eye or both and, if the latter, which eye is more potent in activating the cell. As well, one tests the preferred stimulus for a cell by flashing different visual stimuli in its receptive field. It was found that in a perpendicular penetration, all the cells encountered responded to the same orientation and all cells were activated by one eye only or dominated by that eye, in the sense that their reaction to stimulation of that eye was much more powerful than to stimulation of the other eye (the cells of layer 4C, which receives the predominant input from the lateral geniculate nucleus, are driven exclusively by one eye). Hence cells seemed to be arranged in columns, all the cells in one column having a common orientation preference or a common eye preference (Figure 17.8). These columns of cells were referred to as the orientation columns and the ocular dominance columns. By contrast, in an oblique penetration, the orientation preferences of successive cells, removed from each other by small distances, of the order of 50–100 μm, varied with great regularity. As the orientation preference of successive cells changed systematically, the eye preference would remain the same and then suddenly change to the other eye, though without a break in the orientation sequence. The electrode had to travel a minimum distance of about 0.8 mm for the cells to respond to the right eye plus the left eye, and then start the sequence again, a distance comprising the ocular dominance hypercolumn. Equally, an electrode had to travel about 1 mm for all 18 orientations to be covered, a distance comprising the orientation hypercolumn. It so happens that in travelling tangentially for at least 2 mm through the cortex of V1, one moves from the representation of one small region of the field of view to the representation of an adjacent region. This detailed and repetitive map in V1 gives, therefore, a clue as to why V1 is so extensive an area. Each small part of the field of view is screened for one eye and then for the other eye, and each small part is simultaneously screened for different orientations, the entire process being repeated again in the adjacent millimetre for an adjacent small part of the field of view. As we shall see in the next chapter, there is in fact a great deal more that area V1 does in terms of screening the field of view.

Thus, to all intents and purposes, area V1 was found to possess a highly modular architecture. It was very exciting that this modularity, or at least the modularity of the eye dominance system, could be actually demonstrated anatomically[11] (Figure 17.9). If one eye of the monkey is injected with a suitable marker, such as labelled amino acids, the marker is taken up by the cells of the retina, is incorporated into proteins and travels up the axons to the lateral geniculate nucleus where it crosses the synaptic separation between the optic nerve terminals and the geniculate cells and continues its journey to the cortex. When the cortex is subsequently sectioned and suitably treated, the distribution of the label can be easily visualized. In the experiment described above, when one eye only is injected, the label is found to fall into small compartments in layer 4 (the layer which receives the

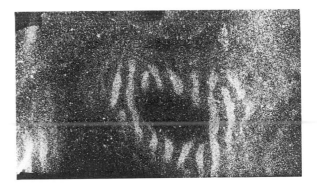

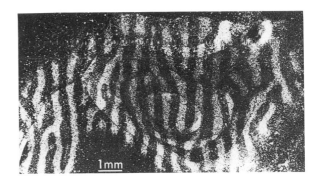

Fig. 17.9 The ocular dominance columns demonstrated anatomically. Injection of labelled amino-acids into one eye of a monkey resulted in the label being transported to the primary visual cortex. Sections taken parallel to the cortical surface and treated to show the label (above and below) demonstrate the alternation of the labelled zones (light) with the unlabelled zones in between. (Reproduced by permission from Hubel, D.H. & Wiesel, T.N. (1977). *Proc. R. Soc. Lond.* B **198**, 1−59.)

geniculate axons); the labelled compartments are separated from each other by unlabelled compartments which belong, consequently, to the other, uninjected eye. It is interesting to note that this is one of the relatively rare examples in which functional groupings have been found physiologically and then confirmed anatomically without any hint of an architectonic difference that might differentiate the regions of the cortex of V1 belonging to one eye from those belonging to the other.

The areas of the prestriate visual cortex have not been studied in anything like the same detail, at least partly because they were discovered much more recently. It is, however, obvious that there is a basic similarity in organization which is common to all visual areas, to the extent that cells with common properties are also grouped together in the prestriate areas, as indeed they appear to be in all cortical areas (see Chapter 14). One very obvious difference between V1 and the visual areas of the prestriate cortex is the eye preferences of cells.[12] The overwhelming majority of cells in all prestriate areas are binocularly driven (Figure 17.10), and this may be of some consequence in trying to learn about depth perception and its neurological basis, to understand how the sensation of two different images vanishes to yield single or cyclopean vision. But it means essentially that the

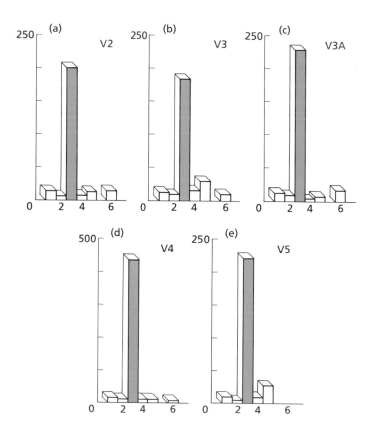

Fig. 17.10 The eye preferences of cells in areas of the prestriate visual cortex. 1 = cells driven by the ipsilateral eye only; 2 = cells dominated by the ipsilateral eye; 3 = binocularly driven cells; 4 = cells dominated by the contralateral eye only; 5 = cells driven by the contralateral eye only; 6 = cells driven only by simultaneous binocular stimulation. (Redrawn from Zeki, S. (1979). *Proc. R. Soc. Lond.* B **204**, 379–397.)

visual areas of the prestriate cortex cannot be divided into ocular dominance columns. This does not mean to say that they cannot be divided into groupings according to, for example, the strength of the interocular interactions, the degree to which the stimulation of the two eyes simultaneously potentiates or inhibits the response of the cells; nor does it exclude other possible ways in which these areas can be subdivided. As we shall see in Chapter 19, one of the prestriate visual areas has in fact been subdivided in a fairly elaborate way and there is no reason to suppose that a similar elaborate subdivision will not be discovered for other visual areas.

The extraordinary regularity and precision of the retinal map in V1 may have misled us into thinking that it must be the retina that is mapped in all visual areas. But the results from studies of the prestriate cortex suggest that we may need a new concept of what a map in the cortex means. We are perhaps a little too inclined to think of these maps as static maps of the retina. It may in fact be useful to think of them as dynamic maps and even constructional maps. We may try to think of the kind of map that might be necessary to construct the colours of surfaces, and study the map in V4 within that framework. This is not to suggest that colour, with all that it entails, is constructed uniquely in area V4, although the latter is critical to it. In fact, as we shall see later, the back connections between area V4 and the visual areas that feed it (areas V1 and V2) may also be necessary for the conscious experience of colour. The dynamic component in constructing colour then becomes much more extensive; it involves several areas. This, in turn, entails an extension of what we mean by a map in the cerebral cortex.

References

1 Zeki, S. (1981) The mapping of visual functions in the cerebral cortex. In *Brain Mechanisms of Sensation*, edited by Y. Katsuki, R. Norgren & M. Sato, pp. 105–128. John Wiley, New York.

2 Ts'o, D.Y. & Gilbert, C.D. (1988). The organization of chromatic and spatial interactions in primate striate cortex. *J. Neurosci.* **8**, 1712–1727.

3 Livingstone, M.S. & Hubel, D.H. (1984). Anatomy and physiology of a color system in the primate visual cortex. *J. Neurosci.* **4**, 309–356.

4 Sperry, R.W. (1963). Chemoaffinity in the orderly growth of nerve fiber patterns and connections. *Proc. Natl. Acad. Sci. USA* **50**, 703–710.

5 Daniel, P.M. & Whitteridge, D. (1961). The representation of the visual field on the cerebral cortex in monkeys. *J. Physiol.* **159**, 203–221; Hubel, D.H. & Wiesel, T.N. (1974). Uniformity of monkey striate cortex: A parallel relationship between field size, scatter, and magnification factor. *J. Comp. Neurol.* **158**, 267–294.

6 Daniel, P.M. & Whitteridge, D. (1961), loc. cit. [5].

7 Zeki, S.M. (1969). Representation of central visual fields in prestriate cortex of monkeys. *Brain Res.* **14**, 271–291; Cragg, B.G. (1969). The topography of the afferent projections in circumstriate visual cortex of the monkey studied by the Nauta method. *Vision Res.* **9**, 733–747; Van Essen, D.C. & Zeki, S.M. (1978). The

topographic organization of rhesus monkey prestriate cortex. *J. Physiol.* **277**, 193–226.

8 Unpublished results from this laboratory.

9 Maunsell, J.H.R. & Van Essen, D.C. (1987). Topographic organization of the middle temporal visual area in the macaque monkey: representational biases and the relationship to callosal connections and myeloarchitectonic boundaries. *J. Comp. Neurol.* **266**, 535–555.

10 Moran, J. & Desimone, R. (1985). Selective attention gates visual processing in the extrastriate cortex. *Science* **229**, 782–784.

11 Hubel, D.H. & Wiesel, T.N. (1977). The Ferrier Lecture: Functional architecture of macaque monkey visual cortex. *Proc. R. Soc. Lond.* B **198**, 1–59.

12 Zeki, S. (1979). Functional specialization and binocular interaction in the visual areas of rhesus monkey prestriate cortex. *Proc. R. Soc. Lond.* B **204**, 379–397.

Chapter 18: The corpus callosum as a guide to functional specialization in the visual cortex

Making inferences from clues is always fun in science, especially if the inferences turn out to be correct. I therefore digress here slightly to look at the sort of inferences about functional specialization that one can make by observing nothing more grand than the manner in which the two hemispheres of the brain are connected with one another.

There have been many speculations as to why there are two halves of the brain. In man, there are cerebral dominances for language, handedness and many other functions. In lower animals, including primates, cerebral dominance is less obvious, which is not to say that it is not there, at least for some functions. But, whether in animals or in man, it is obvious that there is no marked dominance for the most primordial functions. There is no hint, for example, that the striate cortex of one hemisphere is dominant. Equally, no one has yet produced convincing evidence to show that the specialized visual areas in the prestriate cortex of one hemisphere are dominant, although recent positron emission tomography (PET) evidence from the human brain suggests that some may be so. One remarkable feature about these areas is that they are all interconnected with their counterparts in the opposite hemisphere by means of a massive cerebral commissure known as the corpus callosum (Figure 18.1). The corpus callosum was a mysterious organ for many years; indeed, mysterious enough for Lashley to suggest once, perhaps jocularly, that its only function was to hold the two halves of the brain together. With further study it became obvious that it has many functions. One of these is to link the representation of the midline in the two hemispheres.

The input from the periphery to the brain is organized in such a way that it is the contralateral half of the body that is mapped in each cerebral hemisphere. For example, the right hand and arm and the right side of the trunk are represented in the motor cortex of the left cerebral hemisphere. Equally, it is the contralateral field of view that is mapped in each primary visual cortex, or V1 (see Figure 18.2). But our view of the world is not interrupted at the midline. Hence, somehow, the visual cortex of one side must communicate with that of the other. This communication is brought about by the corpus callosum.

If one were to study the manner in which the two hemispheres are connected with each other through the corpus callosum, one will find

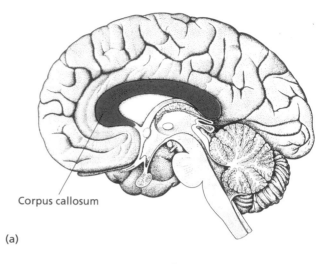

Corpus callosum

(a)

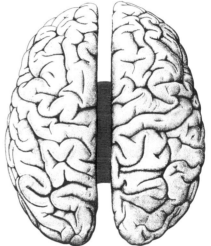

Fig. 18.1 The corpus callosum, linking the two halves of the brain, seen from the inside of the brain in (a) and from above (b).

(b)

that it is only strips of cortex in which the midline is represented that are so connected.[1] For example, it is only the parts of V1 in which the vertical meridian is represented that are connected with their counterparts in the opposite hemisphere; parts of V1 in which other regions of the retina or the field of view are mapped are not connected with their counterparts in the striate cortex of the opposite side. This is generally true of all primary areas. For example, in the somatosensory cortex, it is only the representation of the midline of the trunk in one hemisphere that is connected with its counterpart in the other; the representations of the distal extremities, the fingers and so on, are not interhemispherically connected.[2]

When one examines the prestriate visual cortex, one finds that the callosum distributes its fibres there irregularly, some parts of the prestriate cortex being heavily connected with the opposite hemisphere, others not. To show the regions in which callosal fibres

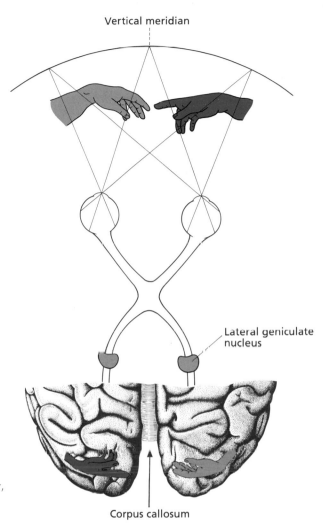

Vertical meridian

Lateral geniculate nucleus

Corpus callosum

Fig. 18.2 The projections from the eyes to the brain are so arranged that it is the contralateral field of view, right up to the midline, that is represented in each hemisphere.

terminate is easy. One cuts the corpus callosum and waits for about a week for the callosal fibres to degenerate. The brain can then be sectioned and stained to reveal the degenerated fibres. The striking fact about the distribution of callosal fibres in the prestriate cortex is that they always occur at the borders, or within the territory, of the visual areas there (Figure 18.3). So far, no visual area of the cerebral cortex without its own set of connections with the opposite hemisphere has been identified. Callosal connections are thus a guide to the presence, and sometimes to the borders, of the separate visual areas; indeed, I used this distribution when trying to define the visual areas of the prestriate cortex.[3] But is it still the case that, even outside V1, areas of midline representation are connected interhemispherically through the corpus callosum?

The answer to this question is easy to obtain. All one needs to do is to cut the corpus callosum and, after a few days, record from the

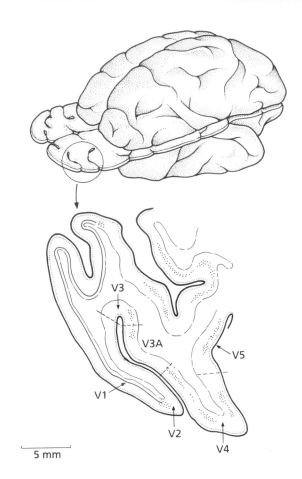

Fig. 18.3 The distribution of the fibres of the corpus callosum (shown as dots in a horizontal section taken through the brain) within areas of the visual cortex. Note that the fibres distribute to certain regions of each area only. These are the regions at which the vertical meridian of vision is represented.

prestriate cortex, noting the receptive field positions of cells in the penetrations and, after the brain is sectioned and stained, noting the position of the electrode tracks with respect to the bands of callosal degeneration in the prestriate cortex.[4] The result is that, yes, each area has a separate map which includes the vertical meridian. Moreover, the vertical meridian representation in each area is connected with its counterpart in the opposite hemisphere through the corpus callosum, since it is only within zones of callosal fibre degeneration that one finds cells whose receptive fields include, or extend to, the midline. This is surprising. One might have thought that uniting the representation of the two hemispheres once would be enough; instead, the cortex prefers to do it repeatedly, once for each area. Why? And what else does the callosal connectivity of the visual areas tell us?

If one looks more closely at the pattern of callosal distribution within each cortical area, one finds a good deal of variation. Both areas V1 and V2 have a precise retinal map in them and the callosal connections of both areas reflects this precision. The strip of V1 cortex which is connected with the opposite hemisphere is narrow and restricted to the very borders of V1 at which the vertical meridian is represented. The same is true of V2 (Figure 18.3). The callosally connected strip here is broader than the one in V1, though still narrow and restricted to the region at which the vertical meridian is represented. When one examines V3, the callosal strip is found to be broader; in V4 it is quite broad and diffuse, as it is in V5 (Figure 18.3). The retinal map in V4 and V5 is nothing as orderly as the one in V1 or V2; correspondingly, the callosal connections of both former areas are not as neatly arranged as those of the latter. The callosal strips mirror, therefore, the topographic organization of the visual areas. Where the topography, *in retinal terms*, is very precise, so is the callosally connected zone within that area; where the topography, *in retinal terms*, is crude, the callosal strip is diffuse. From which one can derive a simple rule: *The pattern of the distribution of the callosal fibres within an area is a good guide to the topographic precision with which the retina is mapped in that area.*

Let us suppose that each area of the prestriate visual cortex is undertaking a separate operation, in parallel but more or less independently from the other areas. Let us also suppose, moreover, that each one of these areas is dealing with a different attribute of the visual scene, such as motion or colour. To be able to construct motion or colour, the visual system has to compare signals coming from large parts of the field of view, a problem that we shall examine in greater detail in Chapter 23. Here, it is sufficient to emphasize that, whatever that operation, it must involve signals coming from both halves of the field of view. Hence, each area needs to be connected with its other half, representing the other half of the field of view. We suppose that the operations themselves are kept separate in the separate visual areas of the two hemispheres because the machineries required to undertake the different operations are themselves different, and in this machinery we include the anatomical wiring. *It is not surprising to find, then, that each area is connected separately with its counterpart in the opposite hemisphere, precisely because the two halves of the area (one in each hemisphere) have machineries which are different from those of other areas and thus require to be separately connected.* This way the machineries are not mixed. Indeed, we shall see (p. 254) that the corpus callosum is critical for generating colour when the brain has to compare signals coming from the two hemi-fields. But the generation of colour requires a distinct machinery, different from that involved in constructing dynamic forms. The machinery in V3, important for dynamic forms, requires that the area be more or less topographically organized — less than V1 or V2 but more so than V4 or V5. This machinery is reflected in its callosal connectivity which, in turn, is less precise than that of V1 or V2 but more so than that of V4 and V5. More significantly, the callosal connections of V3 are kept distinct from those of V4. Had the exclusive cortical strategy for vision been the hierarchical one, in which each area would be involved in 'analyzing' all the same attributes as the previous area but at a higher level of sophistication, then there would probably have been more reason for the representation of the two visual hemi-fields to be united once only. At any rate, it would have been more difficult to account for the repetitive linkage across the hemispheres. Thus, the repetitive callosal connections between the visual areas is itself indicative of the importance of parallelism as a general strategy for visual processing.

In summary, the pattern of callosal connectivity between the visual areas of the prestriate cortex is a good guide to the number of distinct visual areas and to the precision with which the retina is mapped in each area. Moreover, the fact that each area must have its separate connections with its counterpart in the opposite hemisphere argues for the fact that each area undertakes its operation with a certain level of autonomy. It is only a matter of time before the technology to study callosal connections non-invasively in the human brain will be sufficiently developed to give important insights into the number and organization of the visual areas in human cerebral cortex. It is an approach which we are already exploiting.

References

1 Whitteridge, D. (1965). Area 18 and the vertical meridian of the visual field. In *Functions of the Corpus Callosum*, edited by E.G. Ettlinger, pp. 115–120. Churchill, London.
2 Jones, E.G., Coulter, J.D. & Wise, S.P. (1979). Commissural columns in the sensory motor cortex of monkeys. *J. Comp. Neurol.* **188**, 113–137.
3 Zeki, S.M. (1975). The functional organization of projections from striate to prestriate visual cortex in the rhesus monkey. *Cold Spring Harb. Symp. Quant. Biol.* **40**, 591–600; Zeki, S.M. (1977). Colour coding in the superior temporal sulcus of rhesus monkey visual cortex. *Proc. R. Soc. Lond.* B **197**, 195–223; Zeki, S.M. (1978). Functional specialization in the visual cortex of the rhesus monkey. *Nature* **274**, 423–428; Van Essen, D.C. & Zeki, S.M. (1978). The topographic organization of rhesus monkey prestriate cortex. *J. Physiol. (Lond.)* **277**, 193–226.
4 Zeki, S.M. & Sandeman, D.R. (1976). Combined anatomical and electrophysiological studies on the boundary between the second and third visual areas of rhesus monkey cortex. *Proc. R. Soc. Lond.* B **194**, 555–562.

Chapter 19: Functional segregation in cortical areas feeding the specialized visual areas

Functional segregation in area V1

Perhaps the major reason why functional specialization in the visual cortex gained only a grudging acceptance initially is because it faced a formidable obstacle in the form of V1, the primary visual cortex. The specialized areas of the prestriate visual cortex receive most of their visual input from V1 and an area adjacent to it, area V2. It seemed natural to expect some degree of functional specialization within V1 itself, as indeed a theory of functional specialization had predicted.[1] One might expect, for example, that cells in V1 dealing with colour would be segregated from cells dealing with, say, motion or orientation. Indeed, such a segregation had even been posited by some of the early neurologists who had imagined, on the basis of altogether indifferent clinical evidence, that the segregation might occur in different layers of V1.[2] Yet the most detailed physiological studies of V1 — those of Hubel and Wiesel — contained no hint of such functional groupings. Instead, their 1977 Ferrier Lecture, which summarizes their work to that date, showed that all the cells outside the layer which receives the predominant input from the lateral geniculate nucleus (LGN) were orientation selective[3] (see Chapter 17). In their schema, whether one recorded from cells in an electrode penetration made perpendicular to the cortical surface or one which was parallel to it, all cells were orientation selective, without any breaks in the sequence that one might have expected had functional specialization also been a feature of V1. In brief, there was no hint of any kind of functional specialization or segregation within V1. If there was no functional segregation in the visual area that fed the other visual areas, the idea that the latter might be functionally specialized did not seem compelling, at least to many neurobiologists.

This created a puzzle, though a muted one. Today, many might wish to point to other papers, more or less contemporaneous with those of Hubel and Wiesel, which spoke otherwise and testified to the presence of large numbers of unoriented wavelength-selective cells in V1,[4] thus suggesting a separation between form and colour. Michael[5] especially had made a point of emphasizing that colour cells are grouped together in V1 and are separated from the orientation-selective cells, though he considered the former to be orientation selective as well, with wavelength selectivity added on, so to speak. While it would therefore be true to say that there had been substantial hints from other studies of a segregation of function within V1, the fact also remains that such reports made little impression on most, and made no impression at all on Hubel and Wiesel. And theirs had been the dominating position ever since the discovery of orientation-selective cells in the visual cortex.

The kind of uniform functional architecture proposed by Hubel and Wiesel for V1 correlated very well with the apparently uniform anatomical architecture of V1 revealed by the cytoarchitectonic method, a coincidence that was to play a cruel trick on Hubel and Wiesel, as it had on so many others before. For, like others, they had assumed that any functional inhomogeneity would be revealed by the architectural inhomogeneity and, likewise, that architectural uniformity implied functional uniformity. Understandably, and like others before them, they seem to have ignored the fact that the cytoarchitectural picture may not be a good index of an area's architecture. To this must be added the fact that they had focused on a great discovery, in particular, that of orientation selectivity. It soon became obvious, however, that the picture of V1 obtained by Hubel and Wiesel ignored all non-oriented cells, including wavelength-selective cells, in the striate cortex, even though the latter constitute an important percentage of the total. It also became obvious that the uniform architectural picture of V1, revealed by the cytoarchitectonic method, concealed another and far richer architecture, one which correlated well with the functional segregation within it.

In the late 1970s, Margaret Wong-Riley[6] applied the technique of cytochrome oxidase histochemistry to the cerebral cortex. When applied to the striate cortex, the method reveals the features that are revealed by the cytoarchitectonic method, but reveals much else besides. Chief among these is the characteristic blobs, which have been described before, and a much more distinctive layer 4B (Figure 19.1). If the axiom that architectural differences mean functional differences is true, then these inhomogeneities in structure must reflect an inhomogeneity in function, not hinted at by Hubel and Wiesel's earlier studies. Livingstone and Hubel[7] began recording from V1 all over again, to learn whether cells in the blobs were indeed functionally different from surrounding zones. They 'found to our amazement that cells in the blobs are not orientation specific'.[8] About half were wavelength selective, with a special arrangement of their receptive field, for which they are known as the double opponent cell. This type of cell, described in greater detail below, is not found in the retina or the LGN. The remaining cells in the blobs were broad band, i.e. responsive to light of all wavelengths, though without being orientation selective. By contrast, the majority of the cells between the blobs (the interblob cells) were orientation selective, without

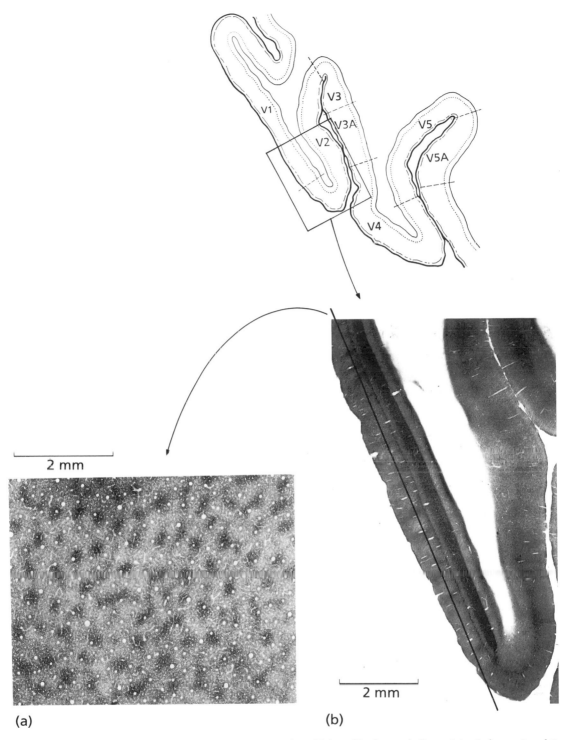

(a)   (b)

Fig. 19.1 (a) The cytochrome oxidase 'blobs' of high metabolic activity in layers 2 and 3 of area V1 viewed when the cortex is cut parallel to the surface, as in (b).

being especially concerned with the colour of the stimulus. In sum, these new studies showed that there was indeed a segregation of function within V1, at least between form and colour. Hubel and Livingstone said, 'At any rate, the apparent tendency of the visual cortex to process form and colour separately would seem to vindicate those who in recent years have argued for a processing of different kinds of perceptual information along separate parallel channels'.[8]

This segregation entailed a revision of the model for the functional architecture of V1 proposed earlier by Hubel and Wiesel (Figure 19.2). It turned out that the blobs occupied the centres of the ocular dominance columns and thus interrupted the orientation sequence. It thus turned out, too, that the manner in which the retina is mapped in V1 is even more complex than earlier results had suggested. V1 not only screens every given small region of visual space for one eye and then for the other eye and for all possible orientations, but for wavelengths as well. Nor was this all. Many years before, it had been discovered that the direction- (and orientation-) selective cells of V1 are located in layer 4B[9] and project to area V5,[10] the motion area of the prestriate cortex. When the distribution of the V5 projecting cells in layer 4B was studied,[11] it was found that they also occurred in discrete clusters, separated from each other by cells of layer 4B projecting elsewhere (Figure 19.3). These 'motion-selective patches' bear no

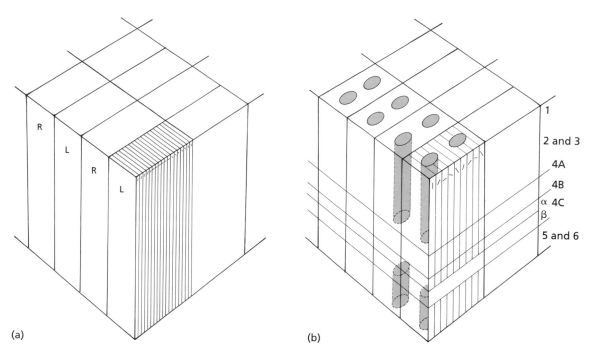

(a)   (b)

Fig. 19.2 (a) The model of the organization of area V1 proposed by Hubel and Wiesel and (b) its later modification by Livingstone and Hubel. (Redrawn from Hubel, D.H. & Wiesel, T.N. (1977). *Proc. R. Soc. Lond.* B **198**, 1−59 and Livingstone, M.S. & Hubel, D.H. (1984). *J. Neurosci.* **4**, 309−356.)

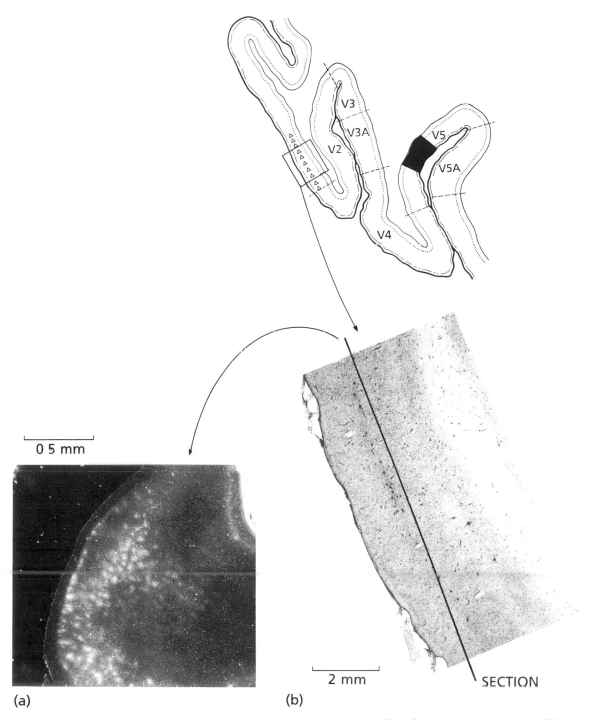

Fig. 19.3 The patches of 'motion selective' cells in layer 4B projecting to area V5, seen in a section cut parallel to the cortical surface (a) and a section cut perpendicular to the cortical surface (b).

relation to the cytochrome oxidase blobs and must be considered to be a separate functional system incorporated into V1. Thus, in addition to everything else that it does, V1 also screens every small region of the field of view for visual motion. It is as if V1 contains a set of anatomically identifiable 'pigeon-holes' into which it assembles different kinds of visual signals. And this does not exhaust all the possibilities, for there are other functions of V1, for example its involvement in depth perception,[12] which are not nearly so well studied. In brief, the vast extent of V1 is due in large measure to its role as an area which scans the field of view for all visual activities, and all sub-modalities of vision are repetitively represented in it. Indeed, it could be said that there are multiple maps in V1, each registering a different kind of activity in the visual field.

Imagine a thought experiment again, one in which you are to undertake a mapping experiment in V1 by making one or more long tangential electrode penetrations through it, a thought experiment which is technically feasible. Suppose, moreover, that you intend to concentrate only on wavelength-selective cells, that is, to discard all cells which are not wavelength selective, and record the position of the receptive fields of the wavelength-selective cells only at intervals of about $500\,\mu m$. You would end up obtaining a very precise map of V1, indeed as precise as the one you would obtain by recording the receptive field positions of the orientation-selective cells only. Moreover, the overall map would be very similar to the one obtained by recording unselectively from all cells in V1. Or imagine that you were to make a long tangential penetration through layer 4B and record only the receptive fields of cells which show orientation plus direction selectivity. You would again end up with a map which is very similar to the one obtained by recording from the wavelength-selective cells. In brief, one might legitimately consider that there are several maps, each devoted to a different visual attribute, that co-exist within V1.

What factor is it that made Hubel and Wiesel miss out on these non-oriented cells for so long, and thus miss out on one of the most fundamental aspects of the organization of the visual system, namely the subdivision of labour within it? It is difficult to imagine that they were unaware of the possibility that non-oriented cells may exist in the cortex. Indeed, for much of the 1970s, they were involved in a controversy as to whether orientation-selective cells are present in the newborn animal, at birth, or are environmentally determined and thus appear later in life. In a paper published in 1974,[13] they described the properties of cells in V1 of the newborn monkey. They had encountered cells 'that could only be driven with difficulty, or whose orientation seemed less critical than usual'. Upon checking the experiment they found that the level of CO_2 in the air expired from their artificially respirated animals was excessive. 'Within a few moments of correcting this the cells were responding with an orientation precision seen in normal adult cells'. A much more likely answer would therefore seem to be that Hubel and Wiesel, like others before them, came under the spell of cytoarchitecture. For, by way of an explanation for the earlier omission, Livingstone and Hubel[7] write that, 'without any anatomical hints of inhomogeneity in the upper cortical layers, it would have been easy to dismiss occasional, apparently sporadic groups of unoriented cells', although there is nothing occasional about the distribution of the blobs nor sporadic about the organization of the unoriented cells. It was, in brief, a repeat of history. They thus acknowledged the critical role that the uniform cytoarchitecture played in misleading them into ignoring non-oriented cells. But it is worth noting here that, as before with the prestriate cortex, it was colour vision that was to suffer most under the spell of cytoarchitecture. For there were no anatomical or cytoarchitectonic hints to the ocular dominance columns either, and yet Hubel and Wiesel found them, and their findings in this regard remain without blemish even over a quarter of a century later.

At any rate, with the discovery of functional segregation within V1, the last obstacle to an acceptance of functional specialization in the cortex was removed. And, since then, evidence has accumulated to show that functional specialization is a general feature which can be traced back to the retina itself and forwards to the area interposed between V1 and the specialized visual areas of the prestriate cortex, area V2.

Functional segregation in area V2

V1 is not the only area which contains a representation of all sub-modalities of vision. Area V2, which surrounds V1,[14] also contains all functional groupings of cells[15] and projects to the same specialized visual areas of the prestriate cortex as does V1, i.e. to areas V3, V4 and V5.[16] In other words, it is subject to the same law of parallelism as V1 and, indeed, as all other cortical areas. The existence of V2 as a separate entity was not suspected for a long time because, cytoarchitecturally, it is similar to the rest of the cortex known as Brodmann's area 18, a cortical field which was considered by most eminent neurologists to constitute a single functional area. In fact, V2 constitutes less than half of area 18, one that receives a topographically organized, that is to say point-to-point, input from V1.[14] Moreover, the physiology of V2 shows that it contains a functionally heterogeneous population of cells, i.e. that orientation-selective, direction-selective and wavelength-selective cells are all found within it.[15] It can therefore be easily inferred that V2, like V1, will send signals related to different attributes of the visual scene to different specialized areas of the prestriate visual cortex. In other words, it acts as a segregator, just like V1. Given the picture obtained for V1, it would not be too idle to hope that V2 will also have a distinctive architecture, one which reflects the functional subgroupings within it, that it too contains anatomically identifiable 'pigeon-holes' into which signals can be assembled. Moreover, since the submodalities of vision represented in V1 are also represented in V2, it would not be surprising to find that the connections between V1 and V2 obey the 'like with like' principle, i.e. the pigeon-holes of V1 assembling particular kinds of signals will connect specifically with their counterparts in V2. Thus, the wavelength-selective cells of the two might be expected to be specifically connected with each other, and the orientation-selective cells might also be expected to be specifically connected with each other but not with other groups of cells, and so on. Finally, given that V2 has all the submodalities of vision represented in it, we would not be wrong in suspecting that it, too, must contain multiple maps, each map being devoted to a different attribute and all the maps contained within the overall map of V2.

If sections through V2 are stained for the metabolic enzyme cytochrome oxidase, it can, like V1, be characterized by zones which are rich in cytochrome oxidase activity. This architecture has been described before. In brief, zones which are rich in cytochrome oxidase come in stripes of two types, thick ones and thin ones, the two sets of stripes being separated from each other by interstripe zones which are much poorer in metabolic activity and therefore do not stain so densely (Figure 19.4). The tracing of the more intimate details of the connections between V1 and V2 has shown that the connections are highly specific, that is, they obey the 'like with like' principle. Thus,

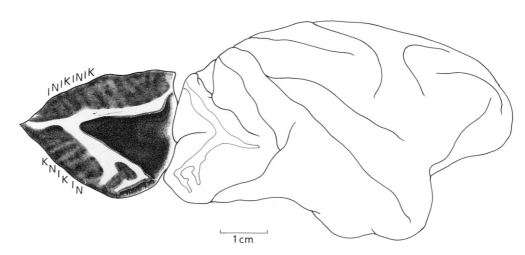

Fig. 19.4 The cytochrome oxidase architecture of area V2, showing the thin (N) and thick (K) stripes separated from each other by the interstripes (I).

the blobs in layers 2 and 3 of V1 connect with the thin stripes of V2 and the interblobs connect with interstripes[7] while layer 4B connects with the thick stripes.[17] Now, the details of the connections between V2 and the specialized visual areas reveal that the thick stripes of V2 connect with areas V3 and V5 and the thin stripes and interstripes connect with area V4.[18] These connections are of great significance and we shall return to them later.

Given that the thin stripes of V2 receive their input from the blobs of V1, where the majority of cells are not orientation selective and about half are wavelength selective, and given that the thin stripes project to area V4, one might expect to find that the physiology of the thin stripes is also concerned with colour, which is indeed the case.[19] Given, next, that the interstripes of V2 receive their input from the interblobs of V1, and given that the majority of the cells in the latter are orientation selective but not wavelength selective, one might also expect most cells in the interstripes to be orientation selective but not wavelength selective, which is also the case.[19] The interstripes project to V4, and may actually overlap with the projection there from the thin stripes, since most orientation-selective cells in V4 are also wavelength selective to variable degrees. Finally, given that the thick stripes of V2 receive their inputs from layer 4B, where orientation-selective and orientation- plus direction-selective cells are predominant, and given that they project to areas V3 and V5, one might expect that cells in the thick stripes will also be orientation selective and that the directionally selective cells of V2 will be concentrated in the thick stripes, which again has been observed physiologically.[19] It follows that area V2, like V1, has multiple compartments in it, different compartments being dedicated to different visual attributes. Thus the cytochrome oxidase architecture of V2, like the patchy connections linking it to V1 on the one hand and to the specialized visual areas on the other, is a good guide to its functional architecture.

The functional diversity of these two areas is therefore reflected in their architecture. This correspondence between function and architecture takes the axiomatic belief of neurologists, formalized by the Vogts in 1919[20] — that areas which differ in their architecture will be found to differ in their functions — to the more intimate organization of single cortical areas. Not all cortical areas, even visual areas, have been studied in as much detail as V1 and V2, in terms of both anatomical and functional architecture. Yet the evidence from these two areas is sufficiently compelling for us to be able to derive a general rule about cortical architecture. *If physiological studies reveal repetitive differences in the functional groupings of cells, then it is almost certain that a corresponding architectural pattern will be found, even if that pattern is not revealable by one of the known techniques, for example that of cyto- or myeloarchitecture. By the same token, if any of the anatomical methods reveals a specific and well-defined architecture, in which adjacent cortical subregions within an area differ obviously and repetitively from each other, it is certain that sooner or later a functional difference corresponding to the architectural heterogeneity will be found.*

From the observations described above, and by analogy with area V1, it follows that, if one makes a long tangential penetration through area V2, one should be able to detect multiple topographic maps, all contained within the overall topographic map of V2. Once again, this appears to be the case.[21] A tangential penetration through V2 would intersect the stripes more or less at right angles. One can then record the response properties and the receptive field positions of cells separated from each other by small intervals of, say, 50–100 μm. Such penetrations show that the receptive field positions of cells in adjacent stripes overlap to a great extent. For example, there is a good deal of overlap between the receptive field positions of cells in a thick stripe and an adjacent interstripe. However, when one plots the receptive field positions of cells belonging to different stripes of the same set, e.g. two thin stripes separated from each other by a thick stripe and two interstripes, one finds that the overlap is minimal. One can thus get a continuous topographic map of the retina by plotting the receptive fields of cells in one set of stripes only. This is really the thought experiment suggested above for V1, applied to V2 and found to be true. It shows that there are at least three independent maps in V2, each devoted to a different attribute of vision.

Tracing functional specialization back to the LGN...

Functional specialization in the visual system was first found in the higher visual areas, and then traced back to the much more minutely studied primary visual cortex. If it could be traced back to V1, could one find any trace of it at even earlier levels, say that of the even more minutely studied LGN or the retina itself?

The predominant input to V1 comes from the LGN. This nucleus has six layers, of which the upper four have small cells and are known as the parvocellular or P layers and the lower two have large cells and are known as the magnocellular or M layers (Figure 19.5). The two sets of cells have different destinations in V1 (see below). Early physiological recordings from the LGN[22] showed that most cells in the P layers have some degree of wavelength specificity, whereas those in the M layers do not. This was done before the discovery of functional specialization in the visual cortex in the early 1970s, and its real significance was missed by all. This is surprising. When trying to dismiss the evidence for a cortical specialization for colour vision

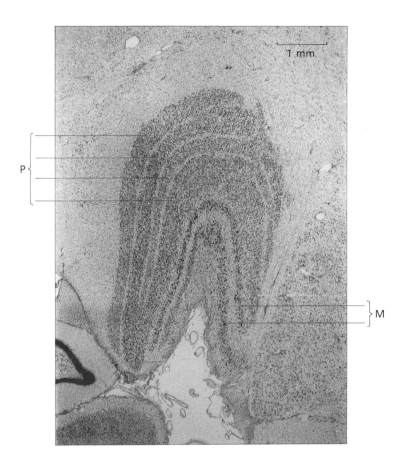

Fig. 19.5 A section through the lateral geniculate nucleus (LGN) of the macaque monkey, stained to show its six layers. The upper four layers, marked P, have small cell bodies and are therefore known as the parvocellular layers. The lower two, marked M, have large cell bodies and are known as the magnocellular layers.

within V1 (the calcarine cortex), Magitot and Hartmann had, in 1926, relied on the fact that no one had shown any neurons specialized for colour in the optic pathways. They had asked menacingly, 'in admitting a chromatic functional specialization for the calcarine cells, should we admit equally the presence of specialized neurons in the optic pathways?'.[23] Now that such specialized neurons were discovered, no one knew what to make of them, in terms of functional specialization at any rate. No one speculated the reverse, that this segregation along the optic pathways, in the LGN, might imply a segregation in V1, at least for colour. It was only after the specializations within the prestriate cortex and the subdivisions within V1 itself were demonstrated, and after the detailed connections between the subdivisions of the LGN and those of V1 became evident, that the subdivision of the LGN began to be seen in the broader context of functional specialization within the visual system.

The connections between the LGN and area V1 have been studied in very considerable detail.[24] One can summarize these connections by saying that the output from the P layers of the LGN is relayed to layers 2 and 3, where it divides to constitute two pathways. One of these feeds the blob cells and is therefore concerned with colour, while the other feeds the interblob cells and is therefore concerned with form. By contrast, the output from the M layers is relayed to layer 4B of area V1, and also divides into two components. One component feeds the orientation- plus direction-selective cells of layer 4B and is therefore concerned with motion, while the other feeds the orientation-selective cells of the same layer and is therefore concerned with form.

...and then on to the retina

The story as it relates to the retina is even more interesting. The retina is a layer-rich structure and its first layer, that of the photoreceptors, consists of two types of cell, the rods and the cones. It was Max Schulze who first suggested, in the latter half of the nineteenth century, that the rods are responsible for night vision and the cones for daylight vision, and hence that there is a functional differentiation at the very first layer of the retina. This idea was later developed into what has become generally known as the duplicity theory of vision. Physiologists have since found many categories of cells in the other layers of the retina. In the present context, the layer that interests us most is the ganglion cell layer, the one whose axons form the optic nerve which feeds the layers of the LGN.

One of the earliest subdivisions was found in the ganglion cell layer of the cat by Robson and Enroth-Cugell.[25] The initial subdivision was between what were called X and Y cells. The former had sustained responses to visual stimuli, remaining active as long as the stimulus was in the cell's receptive field. The latter had transient responses, the cells firing transiently when the stimulus was switched on or off only. Colour was not an important variable, presumably because the cat has only a very rudimentary colour vision, if it has one at all. This work had, early on, suggested that the pathways from the retina to the cortex must be parallel ones. But when the attempt was made to translate these findings to the monkey retina, the result was not as neat. Presumably because of this, physiologists did not even try to translate the findings to monkey cortex. It was only several years after the discovery of functional specialization in the prestriate visual cortex that physiologists began to find that, in the monkey, the layer of the retina that feeds the LGN, the ganglion layer, also has two types of cells, though the presence of colour vision in the monkey aided the classification considerably.[26] One type, the M cells, is sensitive to low contrasts, responds transiently, and has axons which conduct very rapidly. It is not selective for the wavelength of the stimulus. It projects to the M layers of the LGN. The other type, the P cells, responds to high contrasts, has a sustained response and many of its constituent cells are wavelength selective. It projects to the P layers of the LGN. This subdivision, made in the early 1980s, is now commonly considered to be the basis of the specializations observed in the prestriate cortex, since the outputs from the M and P layers of the LGN themselves have different cortical destinations. To many, it may seem surprising that such a discovery in the retina should have been made so many years after the discovery of functional specialization in the prestriate cortex, since the number of studies on the former outnumber by far those on the latter. The chronology serves merely to emphasize the futility of the 'systematic' approach as a research policy.

A motion pathway, a colour pathway and two form pathways

We can now try to spin all these results together and talk of the four pathways in the visual cortex (Plate 6, facing p. 188). The simplest of these is the motion pathway. It has its origin in M ganglion cells of the retina, which relay to the M layers of the LGN. From the LGN the output is relayed to layer 4B and from there to area V5, both directly and through the thick stripes of area V2. The pathway can be referred to as an M pathway insofar as it is derived principally from the M layers of the LGN. Another M pathway, again derived from the M ganglion cells of the retina, is also relayed to layer 4B. This is the M dynamic form pathway, since it relays to the orientation-selective cells of layer 4B and from there to area V3, both directly and through the thick stripes of V2.

The P pathway has its origin in the P ganglion cells of the retina and ultimately divides to form a colour pathway and a form pathway linked to colour. From the P layers of the LGN, the signals are relayed to layers 2 and 3 where they feed the blobs (colour) and the interblobs (form), these two subdivisions eventually relay to area V4 through the thick stripes and interstripes of area V2 and also directly.

We can therefore speak of two form pathways, one derived principally from the M system, and much more concerned with dynamic form, and the other derived principally from the P pathway and much more concerned with form in association with colour. In addition to these, there is a principally M-derived motion pathway and a principally P-derived colour pathway. There is ample opportunity for the P and the M signals to mix in the cortex, so that the input to the specialized visual areas may consist of signals from either source. We shall later see that these pathways and the areas associated with them can be selectively compromised, leading to strange visual syndromes.

This almost minute subdivision of the visual cortex into small modules perpetuates the ineluctable tendency of cortical studies to identify histologically distinct parts of the cerebral cortex and assign specific functions to each. Those who were vilified earlier this century for the modest subdivisions of the cortex which they proposed would be surprised at how much further the process of subdivision has been taken. They should not feel too vindicated. The present subdivisions are compelling because one can attach specific functions to them. Earlier subdivisions were bewildering because no one could attach functions to any but a few of them. Although the tendency in cortical studies has remained the same, the quality of the evidence has improved beyond recognition.

References

1 Zeki, S.M. (1975). The functional organization of projections from striate to prestriate visual cortex in the rhesus monkey. *Cold Spring Harb. Symp. Quant. Biol.* **40**, 591–600.

2 Wilbrand, H. (1884). *Ophthalmiatrische Beiträge zur Diagnostik der Gehirn-krankheiten.* J.F. Bergmann, Wiesbaden; Poppelreuter, W. (1923). Zur Psychologie und Pathologie der optischen Wahrnehmung. *Z. Ges. Neurol. Psychiatr.* **83**, 26–152; Halpern, F. & Hoff, H. (1929). Kasuistische Beiträge zur Frage der cerebralen Farbenblindheit. *Z. Ges. Neurol. Psychiatr.* **122**, 575–586.

3 Hubel, D.H. & Wiesel, T.N. (1977). The Ferrier Lecture: Functional architecture of macaque monkey visual cortex. *Proc. R. Soc. Lond.* B **198**, 1–59.

4 Dow, B.M. (1974). Functional classes of cells and their laminar distribution in monkey visual cortex. *J. Neurophysiol.* **37**, 927–946; Poggio, G.F., Baker, F.H., Mansfield, R.J.W., Sillito, A. & Grigg, P. (1975). Spatial and chromatic properties of neurons subserving foveal and parafoveal vision in rhesus monkey. *Brain Res.* **100**, 25–59.

5 Michael, C.R. (1981). Columnar organization of color cells in monkey's striate cortex. *J. Neurophysiol.* **46**, 587–604.

6 Wong-Riley, M. (1979). Changes in the visual system of monocularly sutured or enucleated cats demonstrable with cytochrome oxidase histochemistry. *Brain Res.* **171**, 11–28.

7 Livingstone, M.S. & Hubel, D.H. (1984). Anatomy and physiology of a color system in the primate visual cortex. *J. Neurosci.* **4**, 309–356.

8 Kolata, G. (1982). Color vision cells found in visual cortex. *Science* **218**, 457–458.

9 Dow, B.M. (1974) loc. cit. [4].

10 Lund, J.S., Lund, R.D., Hendrickson, A.E., Bunt, A.H. & Fuchs, A.F. (1975). The origin of efferent pathways from the primary visual cortex (area 17) of the macaque monkey as shown by retrograde transport of horseradish peroxidase. *J. Comp. Neurol.* **164**, 287–304.

11 Shipp, S. & Zeki, S. (1989). The organization of connections between areas V5 and V1 in macaque monkey visual cortex. *Eur. J. Neurosci.* **1**, 309–332.

12 Poggio, G.F. & Fischer, B. (1977). Binocular interaction and depth sensitivity in striate and prestriate cortical neurons of behaving rhesus monkey. *J. Neurophysiol.* **40**, 1392–1405.

13 Wiesel, T.N. & Hubel, D.H. (1974). Ordered arrangement of orientation columns in monkeys lacking visual experience. *J. Comp. Neurol.* **158**, 307–318.

14 Zeki, S.M. (1969). Representation of central visual fields in prestriate cortex of monkey. *Brain Res.* **14**, 271–291; Cragg, B.G. (1969). The topography of the afferent projections in the circumstriate visual cortex of the monkey studied by the Nauta method. *Vision Res.* **9**, 733–747.

15 Baizer, J.S., Robinson, D.L. & Dow, B.M. (1977). Visual responses of area 18 neurons

in awake, behaving monkey. *J. Neurophysiol.* **40**, 1024–1037; Zeki, S.M. (1978). Uniformity and diversity of structure and function in rhesus monkey prestriate cortex. *J. Physiol. (Lond.)* **277**, 273–290.

16 Zeki, S.M. (1971). Cortical projections from two prestriate areas in the monkey. *Brain Res.* **34**, 19–35.

17 Livingstone, M.S. & Hubel, D.H. (1987). Connections between layer 4B of area 17 and the thick cytochrome oxidase stripes of area 18 in the squirrel monkey. *J. Neurosci.* **7**, 3371–3377.

18 Shipp, S. & Zeki, S. (1989), loc. cit. [11]; Shipp, S. & Zeki, S. (1989). The organization of connections between areas V5 and V2 in macaque monkey visual cortex. *Eur. J. Neurosci.* **1**, 333–354; Zeki, S. & Shipp, S. (1989). Modular connections between areas V2 and V4 of macaque monkey visual cortex. *Eur. J. Neurosci.* **1**, 494–506.

19 Shipp, S. & Zeki, S. (1985). Segregation of pathways leading from area V2 to areas V4 and V5 of macaque monkey visual cortex. *Nature* **315**, 322–325; De Yoe, E.A. & Van Essen, D.C. (1985). Segregation of efferent connections and receptive field properties in visual area V2 of the macaque. *Nature* **317**, 58–61; Hubel, D.H. & Livingstone, M.S. (1987). Segregation of form, color and stereopsis in primate area 18. *J. Neurosci.* **7**, 3378–3415.

20 Vogt, C. & Vogt, O. (1919). Allgemeinere Ergebnisse unserer Hirnforschung. Vierte Mitteilung. Die physiologische Bedeutung der architektonische Rindenfelderung auf Grund neuer Rindenreizungen. *J. Psychol. Neurol. Lpz.* **25**, 399–462.

21 Zeki, S. & Shipp, S. (1990). Functional segregation within area V2 of macaque monkey visual cortex. In *Seeing Contour and Colour*, edited by J.J. Kullikowski, C.M. Dickinson & I.J. Murray, pp. 120–124. Pergamon Press, Oxford.

22 Wiesel, T.N. & Hubel, D.H. (1966). Spatial and chromatic interactions in the lateral geniculate body of the rhesus monkey. *J. Neurophysiol.* **29**, 1115–1156.

23 Magitot, A. & Hartmann, E. (1926). La cécité corticale. *Bull. Soc. Ophtalmol. (Paris)* **38**, 427–546.

24 Fitzpatrick, D., Itoh, K. & Diamond, I.T. (1983). The laminar organization of the lateral geniculate body and the striate cortex in the squirrel monkey (*Saimiri sciureus*). *J. Neurosci.* **3**, 673–702; Lund, J.S. (1988). Anatomical organization of macaque monkey striate visual cortex. *Ann. Rev. Neurosci.* **11**, 253–288.

25 Enroth-Cugell, C. & Robson, J.G. (1966). The contrast sensitivity of retinal ganglion cells of the cat. *J. Physiol. (Lond.)* **187**, 517–552.

26 Leventhal, A.G. (1979). Retinal ganglion cells in the old-world monkey: morphology and central connections. *Science* **213**, 1139–1142; Perry, V.H., Oehler, R. & Cowey, A. (1984). Retinal ganglion cells that project to the dorsal lateral geniculate nucleus in the macaque monkey. *Neurosci.* **12**, 1101–1123.

Chapter 20: The P and M pathways and the 'what and where' doctrine

Just over one century ago, Lissauer speculated that the cortical processes involved in vision were twofold. His speculations were derived from clinical observations but were influenced by a strong philosophical view of the role of the brain in general and of its role in vision in particular. Distorted and simplified by the neurologists, his doctrine proved to be seductively and deceptively simple. Through its very simplicity it was to have a powerful hold over neurologists for almost a century. Experience had taught them that they could account for visual perception in these terms, or so they believed. So clear did the entire process become to them that they were able to localize each of Lissauer's two processes, apperception and association, to separate parts of the cerebral cortex, with the visual perceptive centre being located in V1 and the associational centre in the surrounding prestriate cortex. In time, neurologists gained sufficient confidence to account for all manner of visual disturbances by references to these two processes, or to dismiss them if they couldn't.

Today, we are faced with another doctrine,[1] also derived from clinical observations, and equally seductive in its simplicity. This one also tries to oversimplify the cerebral machinery involved in vision. Like the earlier doctrine, this one also supposes that vision is a dual process and tries to attach each process to a separate visual pathway. But the two postulated processes are very different from the ones proposed by Lissauer. This new doctrine supposes that there are two, and only two, visual pathways emanating from area V1 (Figure 20.1). They are conceived as being mutually exclusive and hierarchically

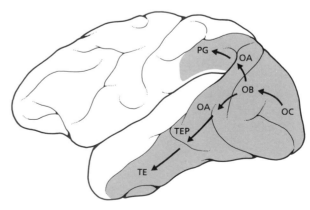

Fig. 20.1 The postulated 'two pathway organization of the visual cortex'. (Redrawn from Mishkin, M., Ungerleider, L.C. & Macko, K.A. (1983). *Trends Neurosci.* **6**, 414–417.)

organized. One pathway, known as the ventral pathway because it is thought to lie more ventrally and to terminate in the temporal lobe, is considered to subserve exclusively form vision, including colour vision, in all its varieties. It supposes that the 'analysis of the physical properties of a visual object…may even be completed within this tissue'.[1] The other pathway, known as the dorsal pathway because it is considered to lie dorsally and to terminate in the parietal cortex, is thought to be specialized exclusively for spatial vision. Because of this dichotomy the doctrine is referred to as the 'what and where' doctrine, a doctrine which does not address the question of how and where the knowledge of 'what' an object is may be integrated with the knowledge of 'where' it is. This dual pathway hypothesis derives from the perfectly correct observation that lesions in the parietal cortex and in the inferior temporal cortex have very different effects.[2] The consequence of lesions in the parietal cortex is complex, but among its major features is a spatial disorientation, hemi-neglect of space and of body and other disabilities where the relations between objects in the field of view are difficult to perceive correctly. By contrast, lesions in the posterior and inferior temporal cortex lead to pronounced defects in object recognition. As with Lissauer's doctrine before, attempts have been made in recent years to tie this doctrine into a neat anatomical system and to account for much in vision in terms of these two cortical pathways. It was not long before attempts were made to see these pathways as cortical prolongations of pathways that start in the retina itself and are known as the parvocellular or P and magnocellular or M pathways.[3] It is the validity of this doctrine that we shall examine here. Because in the last few years the doctrine has become enmeshed with this doctrine of separate P and M pathways, discussed in the last chapter, we will examine both simultaneously.

The P and M pathways

As described before, the different visual cortical pathways have their origins in two different types of retinal ganglion cells. One type (the P type)[4] terminates in the P layers of the lateral geniculate nucleus (LGN) and has general characteristics which make it more suitable for form and colour vision, while the other (the M type) terminates in the M layers and has characteristics which make it more suitable for detecting dynamic form and motion. Different signals from the retina are relayed to area V1 through the P and M layers of the LGN, and the cortical termination sites (in V1) derived from the two sets of LGN layers themselves have very specific, and different, further connections with different visual cortical areas (see Chapter 19). Because of this, it has been supposed that the entire visual pathways in the cerebral cortex can be referred to as the P or the M pathways. In the cortex, the M pathways are thought to consist of layer 4B of V1, the output from layer 4B to area V5, directly and through V2, and then the further output from area V5 to the parietal cortex. This is the pathway that is thought to be concerned with spatial relations and with 'where' an object is. By contrast, the P pathway in the cortex is thought to consist of layers 2 and 3 of V1, the output from these two layers to V4, both directly and through V2, and from V4 to the inferior temporal cortex, 'the highest-order area for the visual perception of objects'.[1] Hence, the fate of the two systems, the P and M on the one hand and the 'what and where' on the other, have become inextricably linked. Any demonstration of substantial interconnections between the P and M pathways in the cortex would compromise the 'what and where' doctrine. Here it is important to understand that, from the point of view of functional specialization in the visual areas of the prestriate cortex, it is immaterial whether an area receives input from one or other of the pathways, or from both. Thus, when I suggested that V5 is specialized for motion, I did so in reference to its physiology alone, not to the input to it from one or the other pathway, which indeed had not been traced in such detail at the time. There is no a priori reason to suppose that V5 does not receive any input from the P pathways, any more than there is to suppose that V5 cells will not be able to detect the motion of an object which differs from its background in colour alone, although this may well turn out to be so. Equally, when I charted the physiology of V3 and V3A and showed that most cells there are interested in the orientation of the visual stimulus, and hence that these areas may be concerned with form, I did not do so with reference to the input, which was also not at the time traceable to the M pathway, but by reference to the physiology alone.

The initial mistake is to suppose that there are only two pathways emanating from V1. Whichever way one looks at this proposition, it turns out to be wrong. If one were to accept it literally, one would be driven to the conclusion that it is false because V1 has direct as well as indirect outputs to areas V3, V4 and V5, as well as an output to area V3A and possibly also to area V6 (see Chapter 12). Thus, to speak of two pathways only as emanating from V1 is obviously wrong. On the other hand, one may want to look at it in another way, and speak of two functionally different pathways with different derivations, each one of which may contain several subpathways. But here again, the proposition turns out to be false. In the 'what and where' formulation, the output to area V3 is combined with the output to area V4, and is considered to relay to the temporal sulcus. But areas V3 and V4 are not in any sense functionally equivalent, nor can they be equated with the P system alone or the M system alone. Area V3, a cortical region in which most cells are orientation selective, derives its input from layer 4B and from the thick stripes of V2, and therefore mainly

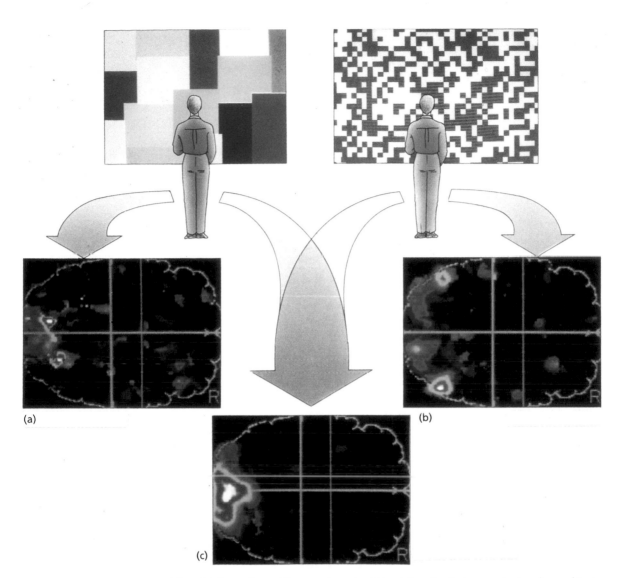

Plate 6 The regions of increased cerebral blood flow in the human brain when subjects view (a) a multi-coloured Mondrian display and (b) a pattern of moving squares. Highest increases are shown in white, red and yellow. The regions of high cerebral blood flow are indicated in horizontal slices through the cerebral cortex. Note the difference in location between the area activated by the colour stimulus (human V4) and the one activated by the motion stimulus (human V5). Note that area V1 and the adjoining area V2 were active with both stimuli, suggesting that both colour and motion signals reach V1 and are distributed from it to the specialized visual areas V4 and V5. (Reproduced by permission from Zeki, S. (1990). *La Recherche* **21**, 712–721.)

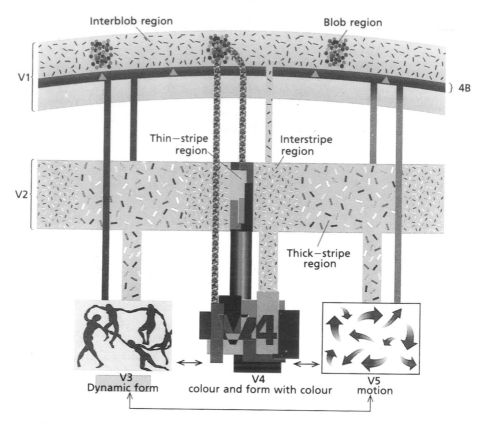

Plate 6 Summary diagram of the four perceptual visual pathways and their anatomical connections, from V1 to the specialized visual areas of the prestriate cortex. (Reproduced by permission from *The Visual Image in Mind and Brain* by S. Zeki. Copyright © 1992 by Scientific American, Inc. All rights reserved.)

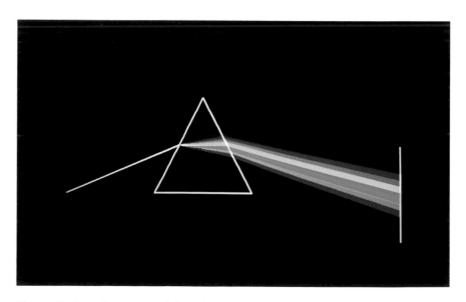

Plate 7 Sir Isaac Newton's celebrated experiment, perhaps the most influential one in colour vision. In this, he passed white light through a prism and observed that it could be broken down into many different wavelengths, each having a different colour to a human observer.

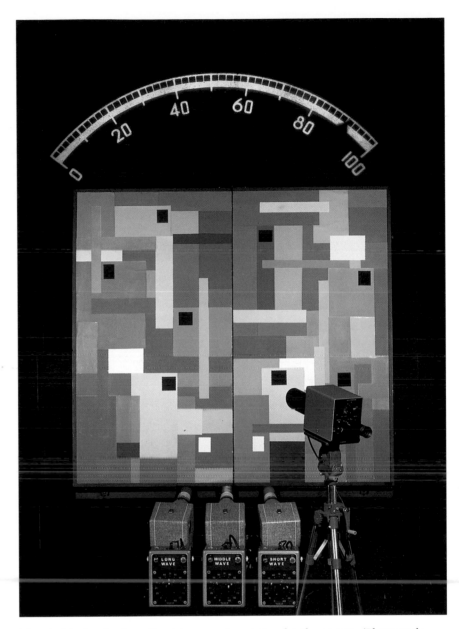

Plate 8 The Land colour Mondrian experiment. For details see text. (Photograph courtesy of Mr J. Scarpetti, Rowland Institute, Cambridge, MA.)

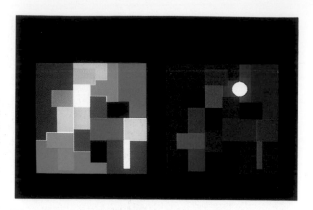

Plate 9 (*right*) The Land Mondrian experiment repeated on a single patch of the display (void viewing mode). The rest of the patch is obscured and the green patch is made to reflect the standard triplet of energies. Its colour, when thus viewed, is a very light grey but reverts to green at once when, without changing the energies coming from it, the surround is brought into view (natural viewing mode) (left).

Plate 10 The lightness record of a simple scene for a given wavelength of light is generated by comparing the reflectance of the two surfaces for light of the same waveband. In this example, the two contiguous areas, one red and one green (c), are illuminated with long-wave light (a). The red area looks light because it reflects a great deal of long-wave light while the green area looks dark because, in comparison, it reflects very little long wave light. When the same scene is illuminated with middle-wave light alone (b), the green area (which reflects a great deal of middle-wave light) looks light while the red area becomes dark in comparison.

(a)

(b)

(c)

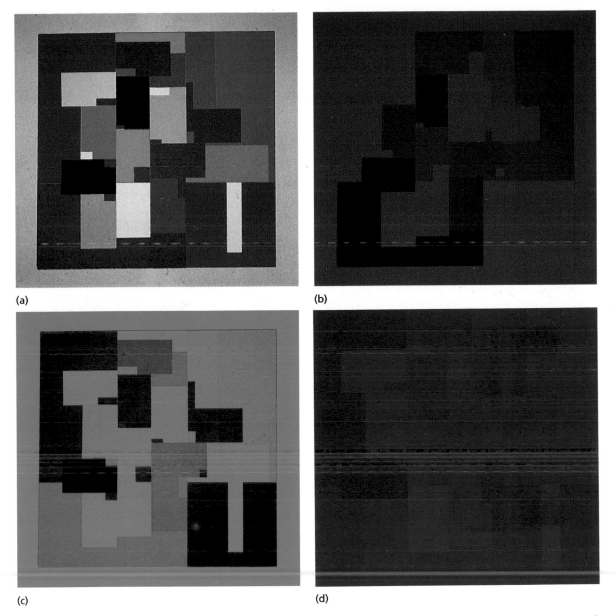

Plate 11 The lightness record of a complex, multicoloured scene (a) when it is viewed in long-wave (red) light alone (b), in middle-wave (green) light alone (c) and in short-wave (blue) light alone (d).

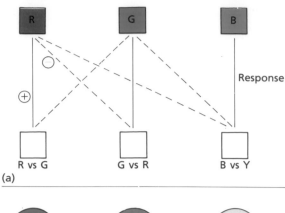

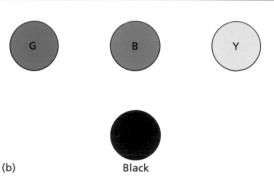

(a)

Plate 12 (a) The opponent inputs from the three cone types to the ganglion cells of the retina. Long-wave (R) cones are opposed by middle-wave (G) cones in the so-called red-green channel. Short-wave (B) cones are opposed by the long- plus middle-wave cones in the so-called blue-yellow channel. These are the colour pairings that have been described as the ones that cannot live with each other and cannot live without each other. If you stare at any one of the spots and then look at a neutral white or grey patch, the opponent colour will appear.

(b)

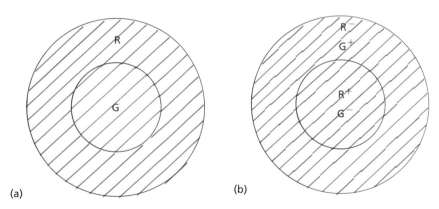

(a)　(b)

Plate 13 (a) The receptive field organization of a wavelength selective opponent cell in the lateral geniculate nucleus. The cell is excited by long-wave (red) light in the centre and by middle-wave (green) light in the surround. (b) The receptive field organization of a double opponent cell. The cell is excited by long-wave (red) light and inhibited by middle-wave (green) light in the centre and is excited by middle-wave and inhibited by long-wave light in the surround. Other double-opponent cells have the reverse arrangement.

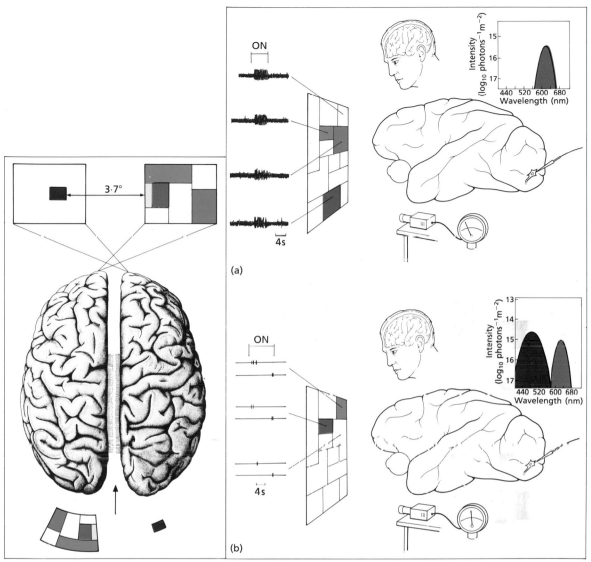

Plate 14 (*left*) An experiment to show that the corpus callosum (arrow), linking the two hemispheres, is essential for assigning the correct colour to a surface, when the surface is presented to one hemi-field and the rest of the multicoloured display to the other hemi-field. If the two are separated by 3.7°, the normal human brain can use the information coming from one hemi-field to generate the colour of the patch presented to the other hemi-field. If the corpus callosum is cut or absent, the colour generating interactions cannot occur. Since V4 is the first visual area which has wavelength selective cells and callosal connections extending beyond the representation of the 1° strip of the vertical meridian, it follows that V4 is the first possible area in which such colour generating interactions can occur. (Redrawn from Land, E. *et al.* (1983). *Nature* **303**, 616–618.)

Plate 15 (*right*) (a) The responses of a narrow-band, wavelength selective cell (inset shows its wavelength sensitivity profile) in area V1 to different areas of a Mondrian. When each area was put in the cell's receptive field, it was made to reflect the same amount of long-, middle- and short-wave light. Clearly, the cell is not interested in the colour of the area in its receptive field but only in the wavelength composition of the light reflected from it. (b) The responses of a short-wave (blue) ON, long-wave (red) OFF cell in area V1 to different areas of a Mondrian. Inset shows the wavelength selectivity profile of the cell. The cell could be made to give an ON or an OFF response to an area of any colour, by simply changing the wavelength composition of the light reflected from it, without changing the colour.

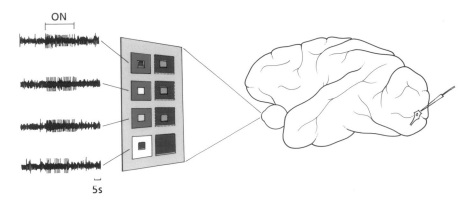

Plate 16 The responses of a double-opponent cell in V1 to rectangles of different colour in a display. The cell was excited by long-wave light and inhibited by middle-wave light in the centre of its receptive fields and had a reverse sensitivity in the surround. It responded well to a red, white or yellow square against a green background (left-hand column). The common feature is that, when illuminated with long-wave light, the centre in each case appears very light compared with the surround (right-hand column). On the other hand, the cell was less responsive to a red patch against a white background (bottom record), because both areas have a high lightness for long-wave light and the entire display therefore looks very light when illuminated with long-wave light alone. Such cells may be the first ones to undertake the wavelength-differencing which is critical for generating colours.

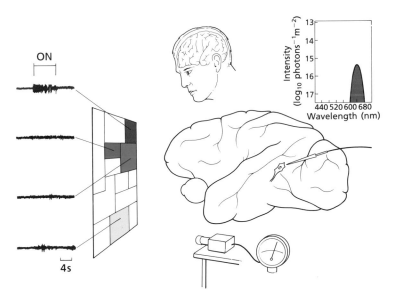

Plate 17 The responses of a true colour-sensitive cell in area V4. The cell had a wavelength sensitivity profile similar to the cell of V1 illustrated in Figure 26.2 but, unlike that cell, this one only responded to the red area, even when all the areas were made to reflect the same triplet of energies when put in the cell's receptive field.

from the M system. By contrast, area V4 derives its input from the blobs and interblobs of V1 and from the thin stripes and interstripes of area V2, and therefore belongs more properly to the P system. It follows therefore that area V3 does not share a common derivation with area V4. Instead, it shares a common derivation with area V5, the motion area, though it is distinct in function (see Chapters 12 and 20).

Nor is it true to suppose that area V3 has a direct and heavy output to the temporal cortex. In fact, much of its output is to the parietal cortex.[5] Area V4, by contrast, sends a heavy output to the inferior temporal cortex.[6] Thus, while both areas V3 and V4 deal with form, their involvement is different. In keeping with its derivation, area V3 is more involved with dynamic form, whereas V4 is more involved in form in association with colour, since it is derived from the P system. It follows, moreover, that form perception is not the exclusive province of the inferior temporal cortex, but is a more widely distributed activity. This accounts for why there has never been a description in the clinical literature of a total and specific loss of form vision alone (see Chapter 27). Whichever way one looks at it, the premise that there are two, and only two, exclusive pathways would therefore not appear to be sustained by the experimental evidence, which also speaks against equating the P system exclusively with form vision and the M system exclusively with spatial, but not form, vision. Moreover, experimental evidence also speaks against a total isolation of the M system from the P system.

Equiluminance experiments

In general, visual stimuli can be discriminated because of a difference in luminance or in colour, or both. Consequently, if one could arrange things in such a way that a stimulus has the same subjective intensity (luminance) as the background and differs from it in colour alone, one should be able to force the individual to discriminate stimuli on the basis of colour alone. Such stimuli are called *equiluminous* (or isoluminant). This approach of studying psychophysical function was pioneered in the 1970s[7] and has been used on an almost industrial scale since. One might expect, then, that the visual motion system, consisting of the M pathway and its prolongation in the cortex, would be inactive under equiluminous conditions since, not having any wavelength selectivity, it might be considered to be 'colour blind'. Thus, if the motion system is indeed 'colour blind', then one should not be able to detect motion when a moving stimulus is equiluminous with the background against which it is presented. The colour pathway, on the other hand, should be very active under these conditions. One can try, in other words, to isolate the two systems perceptually.

The most dramatic perceptual equiluminous experiment uses the same two submodalities that were used to demonstrate functional specialization in the visual cortex, namely colour and motion. Take a system consisting of red dots against a green background, with the dots and the background differing in both colour and luminance. The dots can be made to move coherently in such a way that one perceives a rotating globe. If, on the other hand, the luminance difference between the dots and the background is eliminated, the same motion of the dots is no longer seen as coherent and a globe can no longer be perceived, though the motion of the individual dots can still be perceived. The experiment is convincing and can be repeated easily with a good-quality TV monitor. This does not mean that there is no interaction between colour and motion. It only means that at some level of the visual pathways the processing of colour and of motion is sufficiently separate for the effect to be demonstrable. On the other hand, the fact that dots equiluminous with the background can still be seen in motion suggests that the motion system can use wavelength information. An equally dramatic experiment concerns the perception of depth using red and green anaglyphs.[7] Here, a depth figure is perceived if the red and green dots forming the figure differ in both colour and luminance. If the two are made to be equiluminant, depth perception is severely compromised. One might conclude from this that the depth system is also colour blind.

One might conclude from such results that isoluminance experiments are an ideal way of demonstrating the autonomy of the two systems and that such experiments could be extended to the study of single cells in the two pathways of the visual cortex.[8] Thus, a cell in the M layers of the LGN or in layer 4B or in V5 might be expected to be unresponsive when the stimulus in its receptive field is equiluminous with the background, whereas a cell in the P layers or in area V4 should respond with undiminished vigour to such stimuli, provided of course that the colour is right. If only things could be that simple.

The very fact that motion can still be perceived, even if incoherently, when stimuli are made isoluminant with their background suggests that the motion system is able to use wavelength information to undertake its task, a fact confirmed by subtle psychophysical experiments.[9] These have shown that there is a certain level of interaction between the colour and the motion systems, leading one group to the conclusion that '. . . color information can, to some extent at least, be used for processing the information required by these tasks'.[10] If luminance contrast is held at some constant value, while colour contrast is varied between 0 and 100%, performance is improved with increased colour contrast. 'Thus color cues, although less effective than are luminance cues, can indeed be used for the perception of texture, motion and stereoscopic depth perception',[10] a statement which is entirely unexceptionable as far as functional specialization in the visual cortex is concerned. These findings have led to the view that '...impairment of visual capacities at isoluminance cannot be uniquely attributed to either of these two systems and that isoluminant stimuli are inappropriate for the psychophysical isolation of these pathways',[10] once again a perfectly reasonable conclusion as far as functional specialization is concerned.

The reaction of single cells to isoluminant stimuli

If the picture that one obtains from such perceptual studies implies that there must be some connections between the P and the M pathways and that the two are therefore not as isolated as one might have supposed, the study of the reaction of single cells to isoluminant stimuli suggests much the same picture. The responses of the cells in the M layers of the LGN are indeed diminished when such stimuli are used, but not to any greater extent than those of the P layers according to some authors,[11] while others believe that the responses of such cells are diminished at points of equiluminance to a much greater extent than those of the P cells,[12] although the responses of the latter too are diminished somewhat. In summary, both agree at least that M cells, or at least some of them, can respond to equiluminous stimuli. Again, many cells in layers 2 and 3 of V1 behave in a way to suggest that they receive both P and M contributions.[13] This observation is interesting and important in trying to interpret some of the characteristics of syndromes resulting from brain lesions (see Chapter 27). It has been shown, for example, that an orientation-selective but not wavelength-selective cell in layers 2 and 3 of area V1 can respond to the border between two isoluminant stimuli, provided that the border is held at the right orientation for the cell, which is otherwise indifferent to the colour of the two isoluminant stimuli.[8] Therefore, substituting one set of isoluminant colour stimuli for another makes little impact on the responses of the cell, which is interested in the orientation of the stimulus alone. Recordings in area V5 have shown that only about 50% of cells become unresponsive at isoluminance. The remaining half continue to do so, though commonly with a diminished vigour, suggesting that substantial numbers receive some input which is more characteristic of the P system.[14] Results such as these suggest that there must be some interactions between the M and the P systems and speak against a total isolation of the two systems.

The anatomical basis of interactions between the P and the M systems

Such an interaction should not be surprising, given the anatomical opportunities that exist for the two systems to 'talk' to each other. First, there are modest connections between layer 4B (which receives its input from the M system) and layers 2 and 3 (which receive their inputs from the P system).[15] Next, there is a system of horizontally coursing fibres within layer 3 of area V2.[16] These are roughly about 4 mm in extent and thus are sufficiently long to allow interactions between all three sets of stripes within V2, keeping in mind that the dimensions of one cycle of a thick stripe, thin stripe and two interstripes is roughly about 4.5 mm.[17] Moreover, there are direct connections between areas V3, V4 and V5.[18] Finally, there is an important system of back projections (re-entrant projections), discussed in detail in Chapter 31, from the specialized visual areas to areas V1 and V2. These could serve to unite signals derived from the M and the P pathways.[18] Anatomically, there is therefore no total isolation of the two systems in the cortex. Rather, the organization seems to be such that the specialized areas of the visual cortex will draw on signals from any source, be it the P or the M system, to undertake their specialized functions. Moreover, the fact that there are massive connections linking the cortex of the superior temporal sulcus to the parietal cortex would suggest that the two systems are not isolated from each other.

This last conclusion is made even more emphatic by observing the projections of two areas, V4 and V5, which are known to have different principal derivations and different functions, to the temporal and parietal cortex.[18] One observes here that both V4 and V5 project to the parietal cortex, from which it follows that both P and M signals find their way to the parietal cortex. There is no suggestion that the input from V5 is stronger than that from V4. The projections are to contiguous regions of the intraparietal sulcus, with only partial overlap. This finding is sometimes dismissed by saying that only peripheral parts of V4 project to the parietal cortex. But the terms peripheral and central as applied to V4 do not have the same significance as when applied to the retina. In the retina, anything outside of the central 2° is concerned with peripheral vision. But in V4, the receptive fields of cells are relatively large, and a cell with a receptive field of 5° could well include the fovea. Moreover, cells have strong and silent surrounds which can extend to or include the fovea. While it is probably true that the most central representation in V4 does not project to the parietal cortex, this should not be taken to imply that signals relating to colour or to form in association with colour do not reach the parietal cortex. At any rate, the observation of a projection from V4 to the parietal cortex shows that the input to the parietal cortex cannot be conceived of as consisting of one system only.

The same is true to a lesser extent of the anterior end of the superior temporal cortex, since area V5 has been consistently found to project there, though not nearly as massively as area V4. The projection of the M-dominated V5 to the temporal cortex is interesting in view of the fact that complex forms can be generated from moving patterns, as Johanssen strongly emphasized in his pioneering work.[19] This projection shows that the temporal cortex is not the exclusive preserve of the P system but receives a contribution from the M pathways as well. Indeed, recent physiological evidence suggests that there are cells in the superior temporal sulcus of the monkey which are able to respond specifically to patterns of motion characteristic of biological motion.[20]

The fact that both the parietal and temporal cortex receive inputs from the same specialized areas indicates that the latter perform functions which are of interest to both these widely separated zones of the cortex. Moreover, the fact that more 'peripheral' regions of areas V3 and V4 project to the parietal cortex might imply that the parietal cortex is less involved with fine detail than is the infero-temporal cortex, which is a very different statement from saying that the parietal cortex is not involved with form vision. In fact, the temporal cortex interconnects with the parietal cortex, thus giving the lie to the isolation of the two systems.

Incapacitating the M and the P layers of the LGN

At what level do the two systems interact? Obviously a good way of answering this question would be to go to the source of the separation, and ask what happens when the layers of the LGN that give the two systems their names are selectively damaged. There are two ways of doing this, both dependent on injecting neurotoxins.[21] In one, systemic injections of acrylamide, a toxin that selectively destroys small cells with fine axons and therefore destroys the parvocellular system, are made. In the other, ibotenic acid is injected at determined sites of the LGN, either into the P or the M layers. The results show that destruction of the P layers of the LGN does indeed result in a severe deficit in colour discrimination. But the deficit is not limited to colour. It also includes defects in shape perception, including texture and pattern perception, though coarse shape perception is only mildly affected. By contrast, injections which destroy the M layers of the LGN do not have any effect on these discriminations. Instead, the defect is now restricted to motion perception. The above experiments have not tested the possibility that dynamic form may be compromised after M layer lesions, so the question remains open. But, on the whole, these experiments provide good evidence that the P and the M pathways are concerned with different attributes of the visual scene. The picture becomes a good deal more complicated, however, when one examines the cortex and, in general, cortical studies have been less satisfactory in design and outcome than the LGN studies, at least in the monkey. In theory at least one might expect that lesions of a specific visual area, such as V4 or V5, might lead to very specific visual defects, such as a defect in colour vision and in motion perception, irrespective of whether they derive their inputs from the P or the M system. This does happen in man, as the review in earlier chapters and in Chapter 27 shows. We shall therefore defer considering the effects of experimental cortical lesions until we consider the effects of such lesions in man in greater detail.

'What' and 'where' in a single area

Recent experiments have shown that, to reach the conclusion that an area is involved in form vision only because the cells in it are orientation selective may be a great oversimplification. In particular, it has been shown that the orientation-selective cells of area V3 and area V3A are commonly gaze-locked, in that they will only respond to the appropriate orientation if the monkey gazes in a particular direction.[22] What does this make of these areas, one of which (V3) has been included in the 'what' system and the other of which is still unclassified? If one considers them to be part of the 'what' system, as the proponents of the 'what and where' doctrine do, then one is forced to the conclusion that the 'what' system may also undertake a 'where' task. If, on the other hand, one considers that they are part of the 'where' system because of the derivation of their input from the M layers and because of the presence of gaze-locked cells in them, then one will be forced to the conclusion that the 'where' system must also be concerned with the 'what' system. Whichever way one turns, the evidence speaks against the kind of segregation into two separate, isolated and hierarchically organized systems, dealing with object and spatial vision respectively, that the proponents of the doctrine seek to establish.

Perhaps a far better way to look at this system is to accept that each area will draw on any source to undertake its specialized task. Examples of one source of information providing material for another are common. Shape can be derived from shading; depth can be derived from motion. The precise position of an object and its relationship to other objects (spatial vision) can give the vital clue to the identity of the object, and the precise shape of an object can give the vital clue to its position.

There are, in brief, far too many facts militating against the 'what and where' doctrine for it to be retained as a serious indicator of how the visual cortex is organized.

Notes and references

1 Mishkin, M., Ungerleider, L.G. & Macko, K.A. (1983). Object vision and spatial vision: two cortical pathways. *Trends Neurosci.* **6**, 414–417.

2 Pohl, W. (1973). Dissociation of spatial discrimination deficits following frontal and parietal lesions in monkeys. *J. Comp. Physiol. Psychol.* **82**, 227–239.

3 Livingstone, M.S. & Hubel, D.H. (1987). Psychophysical evidence for separate channels for the perception of form, color, movement, and depth. *J. Neurosci.* **7**, 3416–3468.

4 The terminology used here is simplified. In fact the P ganglion cells are known technically as the P_b cells and the M ganglion cells are known as the P_a cells.

5 Unpublished results from this laboratory.

6 Desimone, R., Fleming, J. & Gross, C.G. (1980). Prestriate afferents to inferior temporal cortex: An HRP study. *Brain Res.* **184**, 41–55.

7 Lu, C. & Fender, D.H. (1972). The interaction of color and luminance in stereoscopic vision. *Invest Ophthalmol.* **11**, 482–490; Ramachandran, V.S. & Gregory, R.L. (1978). Does colour provide an input to human motion perception. *Nature* **275**, 55–56.

8 Gouras, P. & Kruger, J. (1979). Responses of cells in foveal visual cortex of the monkey to pure color contrast. *J. Neurophysiol.* **42**, 850–860; Thorell, L.G., De Valois, R.L. & Albrecht, D.G. (1984). Spatial mapping of monkey V1 cells with pure color and luminance stimuli. *Vision Res.* **24**, 751–769.

9 Cavanagh, P., Boeglin, J. & Favreau, O.E. (1985). Perception of motion in equiluminous kinematograms. *Perception* **14**, 151–162.

10 Logothetis, N.K., Schiller, P.H., Charles, E.R. & Hurlbert, A.C. (1990). Perceptual deficits and the activity of the color opponent and broad-band pathways at isoluminance. *Science* **247**, 214–217.

11 Schiller, P.H. & Colby, C. (1983). The responses of single cells in the lateral geniculate nucleus of the rhesus monkey to color and luminance contrast. *Vision Res.* **23**, 1631–1641; Logothetis, N.K., Schiller, P.H., Charles, E.R. & Hurlbert, A.C. (1990), loc. cit. [10].

12 Derrington, A.M. & Lennie, P. (1984). Spatial and temporal contrast sensitivities of neurones in lateral geniculate nucleus of macaque. *J. Physiol. (Lond.)* **357**, 219–240; Hubel, D.H. & Livingstone, M.S. (1990). Color and contrast sensitivity in the lateral geniculate body and primary visual cortex of the macaque monkey. *J. Neurosci.* **10**, 2223–2237.

13 Hubel, D.H. & Livingstone, M.S. (1990), loc. cit. [12].

14 Saito, H., Tanaka, K., Isono, H., Yasuda, M. & Mikami, A. (1989). Directionally selective response of cells in the middle temporal area (MT) of the macaque monkey to the movement of equiluminous opponent color stimuli. *Exp. Brain Res.* **75**, 1–14.

15 Blasdel, G.G., Lund, J.S. & Fitzpatrick, D. (1985). Intrinsic connections of macaque striate cortex: axonal projections of cells outside lamina 4C. *J. Neurosci.* **5**, 3350–3369.

16 Rockland, K.S. (1985). A reticular pattern of intrinsic connections in primate area V2 (area 18). *J. Comp. Neurol.* **235**, 467–478.

17 Shipp, S. & Zeki, S. (1989). The organization of connections between areas V5 and V1 in macaque monkey visual cortex. *Eur. J. Neurosci.* **1**, 309–332; Shipp, S. & Zeki, S. (1989). The organization of connections between areas V5 and V2 in macaque monkey visual cortex. *Eur. J. Neurosci.* **1**, 333–354.

18 For a general review see, Zeki, S. & Shipp, S. (1988). The functional logic of cortical connections. *Nature* **335**, 311–317.

19 Johnassen, G. (1973). Visual perception of biological motion and a model for its analysis. *Perception Psychophys.* **14**, 201–211.

20 Perret, D.I., Smith, A.J., Mistlin, A.J. *et al.* (1985). Visual analysis of body movements by neurones in the temporal cortex of the macaque monkey: a preliminary report. *Behav. Brain Res.* **16**, 153−170.
21 Schiller, P. & Logothetis, N. (1990). The color-opponent and broad-band channels of the primate visual system. *Trends Neurosci.* **13**, 392−398.
22 Galletti, C. & Battaglini, P.P. (1989). Gaze-dependent visual neurons in area V3A of monkey prestriate cortex. *J. Neurosci.* **9**, 1112−1125.

Chapter 21: The modularity of the brain

There is a common thread that runs through the history of cerebral studies, from its earliest days to the present time. That thread may be broadly, but accurately, defined as the thread of functional subdivisions. The history of cerebral physiology can then be summarized as having consisted largely of an attempt to chart histologically distinct parts of the cerebral cortex and to assign specific functions to each. In spite of many difficulties and setbacks, cortical physiology has been remarkably successful in this endeavour. At one level, the result of these researches allows us today to subdivide the cortex into a number of areas dealing with different activities. The specializations of some of these areas, such as V1, are relatively well understood, though there remains much to discover about them. The specializations of other areas, such as the auditory cortex or the motor areas, are less well understood and the specializations of yet other areas, such as those in the temporal or frontal cortex, are only very vaguely understood or not understood at all. At the next level, individual cortical areas have now been found to possess anatomical subdivisions within them, corresponding to various functional subdivisions. Nowhere is this more apparent than in V1 and V2, although it is likely to prove an elegant feature of other cortical areas as well. Whether one looks at the callosal or intrinsic connections of these uncharted areas, or whether one studies them physiologically, a periodicity becomes evident, which is an almost certain guide to their mosaic organization (Figure 21.1).

In the visual cortex, and to a certain extent in other cortical areas such as the auditory and the somatosensory, the process of subdivision can be taken further. For example, it is becoming clear that the functions of the blobs in the upper layers of V1 are uniform only to the extent that they deal with low spatial frequencies and with colour. But not the same region of the spectrum is represented in every blob, some blobs having predominantly short-wave-selective cells, others middle-wave-selective cells and yet others long-wave-selective cells[1] (Figure 21.2). Equally, there are strong hints that any given set of stripes in V2 is not necessarily uniform. For example, the thick stripes project to V3 and V5,[2] two areas with different specializations. It is possible that the same cells project to both areas by bifurcating axons, but no one has yet demonstrated such dual projections and there are good grounds for believing that different groups of cells project to V3 and to V5. After injecting a tracer into V5 to label the

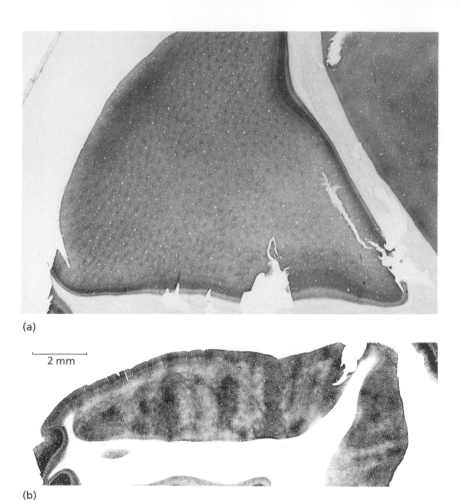

(a)

2 mm

(b)

Fig. 21.1 The mosaic organization of area V1 (a) and of area V2 (b), revealed by the cytochrome oxidase method.

cells in the thick stripes of V2 projecting to it, one finds that the label occurs in the form of small clusters or islands within the thick stripes, with the rest of the thick stripe remaining unlabelled[2] (Figure 21.3). This is almost certainly an indication of the fact that not all cells in a given thick stripe project to V5 — other cells project elsewhere — a sure sign that there is a functional specialization even at the level of the thick stripes. Wherever one looks in the cortex, if one notices that only a small proportion of cells in a certain area, or one of its subzones, connect with another area, one must suspect that other cells in that area will connect elsewhere — one must suspect, in brief, a functional specialization.

The module, though present, is difficult to define

This capacity to subdivide the cerebral cortex into areas, subareas, and then into a seemingly endless set of subregions, has prompted

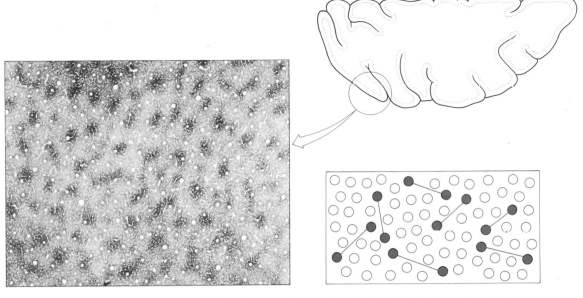

Fig. 21.2 Blobs with a certain wavelength selectivity in layers 2 and 3 of V1 (left) connect with other blobs of the same wavelength selectivity (right).

talk of the modular organization of the cortex. But the term module is not used in the same sense by all scientists, a good sign that no one has yet discovered a definite cortical entity with the same properties everywhere in the cortex, and which everyone can agree on. Some like to think of the column as a module. As defined for V1, the column is a set of cells stacked upon one another, all sharing the same property (for example, that of orientation selectivity) and extending from surface to white matter (Figure 21.4). Columns with such a definition are likely to exist in V2 and probably also in V5, where cells registering the same directional preference have been found to be stacked upon each other as in a column.[3] But is this a feature of V4, or of the higher visual areas in the parietal and temporal lobes? No one knows. Others may think of a grouping of columns as constituting a module. They might think, for example, that a hypercolumn in V1, whether of orientation or ocular dominance, might constitute a module. But since it was proposed,[4] the orientation hypercolumn has had to be modified because of the presence of the non-oriented cells in the metabolically active blobs.[5] These blobs occur in the centre of an ocular dominance hypercolumn, thus possibly justifying its further subdivision (Figure 21.5). Some may like to think of the blob as a module, since it has a definite (cytochrome oxidase) architecture and cells in it share the common property of preferring low spatial frequencies. If the blobs are thought of as modules, then the obvious temptation would be to consider the metabolically active

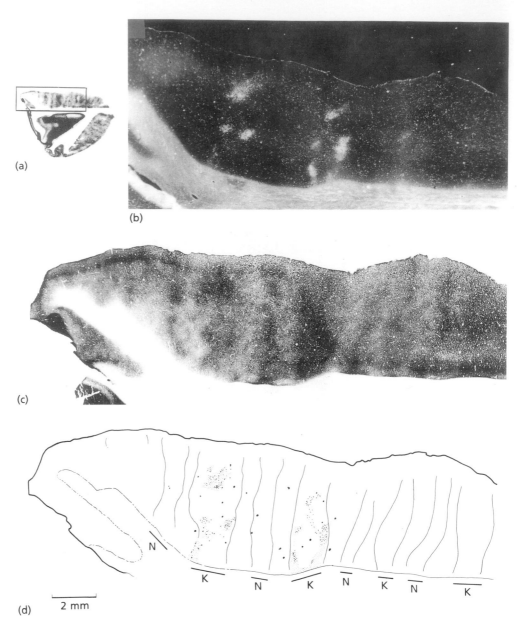

Fig. 21.3 Cells within V2 which project to V5 are concentrated in the thick stripes. (b) and (c) are contiguous sections taken through the part of V2 boxed in (a) in a brain in which V5 was injected with the retrograde tracer, horseradish peroxidase (HRP). Comparison of (b) and (c) shows that the islands of labelled cells in (b) fall within the territory of the thick stripes of V2 (see (d), where N = thin stripes and K = thick stripes). (Reproduced by permission from Shipp, S. & Zeki, S. (1989). *Eur. J. Neurosci.* **1**, 309−332.)

thin stripes of V2, in which cells also prefer low spatial frequencies, as modules. But since the two differ in their dimensions, one cannot make an argument in favour of a ubiquitous module of uniform dimensions. Others might consider that a cycle of thin stripe, thick

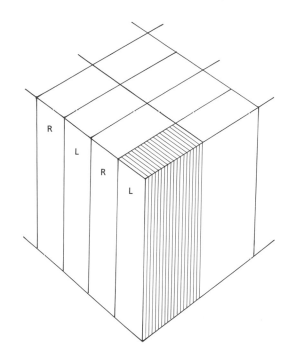

Fig. 21.4 The orientation columns of area V1 in an earlier model. (Redrawn from Hubel, D.H. & Wiesel, T.N. (1977). *Proc. R. Soc. Lond.* B **198**, 1–59.)

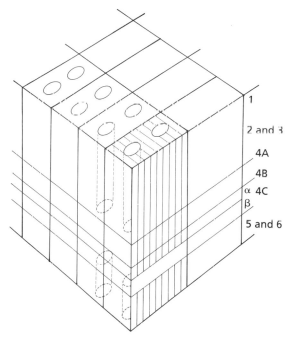

Fig. 21.5 The blobs situated in the centre of the orientation columns form another modular system. (Redrawn from Livingstone, M.S. & Hubel, D.H. (1984). *J. Neurosci.* **4**, 309–356.)

stripe and two interstripes, in which a given retinal position is represented for all the visual submodalities, a better candidate for a module. But, if so, what is the module in V5? Others have written of the specialized visual areas themselves as modules,[6] and some might even be tempted to include an entire specialized pathway — for example, P layers of the lateral geniculate nucleus to blobs to thin stripes to V4 — in their definition of the term module. Finally, some usually use the term in quotes, a certain sign that, for good reason, they do not understand what it really means and cannot therefore communicate it to others. Thus, while there is no doubt that the cerebral cortex is modular in its organization in the sense that, even for a given modality, it assigns geographically separate cortical areas and subregions of areas to different specializations, we still have no agreement as to whether there is a unit of organization which is repetitive, and the same everywhere in the cortex, and which we can think of as the cortical module.

The basic unit of cortical organization is difficult to define

The cytoarchitecture of many cortical areas is remarkably similar. This homogeneity is even more striking up to 110 days of gestation.[7] It is only then that the extrinsic connections of the cortex develop, endowing different cortical areas with greater differences. Scientists, especially the atomistic ones amongst them, have therefore been encouraged to ask whether there is a basic unit of organization in the cortex, reflected in its largely uniform cytoarchitecture, much as the atom is the basic unit of all matter. They have wanted to learn whether this basic unit, if it exists, might be undertaking the same operation everywhere in the cortex. Such an operation would be in addition to the other, and more specialized, operations of the cortex. But what could this basic unit be? A column of cells extending from surface to white matter? Or a cluster of cells restricted to the input layer, layer 4? Some believed, though without much conviction, that it was 200–300 μm in diameter, while others thought that 400 μm was a more likely figure.[8] And what would the basic operation consist of? An input–output relationship, a facilitation, an excitation, an inhibition? Or the detection of co-variation? In the late 1970s and early 1980s, the great neurobiologists debated the issue and came out as confused as ever, or at any rate not any more enlightened than they had been before.[8] And for very good reason. Wherever they looked they saw marked differences. Soon they realized that this was not the most fruitful occupation for scientists with a claim to eminence. The subject ceased to occupy their attention.

The uniformity of cortical operations

Yet it remains an interesting problem. Perhaps a better approach is not to confine oneself to a region of cortex of hypothetical dimensions, since such a region has eluded definition, but to concentrate instead on the cortex as a whole, considering it as a homogeneous sheet with no boundaries. Could each zone of this cortex, defined as a region with a dimension of 1 mm diameter or more, be said to perform broadly a similar operation?

No terminal station in the cerebral cortex

Wherever one looks in the cerebral cortex, one finds certain anatomical rules which are ubiquitous. The first of these rules is that there is no cortical region which is only recipient — all cortical areas have outputs as well as inputs. The anatomical connections of V2, discussed above, illustrate this well. But the principle could be equally well illustrated by studying the anatomical connections of V3 or of any other cortical area, visual or non-visual. Moreover, both recipient and output zones are located within the same 1-mm-diameter zone, though in different layers. This first rule, derived from anatomical studies, may seem obvious and even trivial. Yet it is also profound for it implies that there is no cortical terminus, no final destination where the soul or consciousness, for example, may reside.

Each cortical area or zone undertakes multiple operations

In general, a zone of cortex has multiple cortical connections, as is well exemplified by the parallel projections from area V1, or indeed from the thick stripes of V2, which project to both V3 and V5. But the principle can equally well be exemplified by reference to any other cortical region or subregion. From this second rule, two conclusions which are not mutually exclusive, follow. The first is that each cortical zone in each of the separate cortical areas is probably undertaking more than one operation and relaying the results of these operations to further, distinct, cortical areas. The second is that the results of the same operation are of interest to more than one other cortical area, which explains the need for multiple projections. That both principles are valid and may operate simultaneously is shown by V1 (Figure 21.6). We may take as an example a small region of V1 extending from surface to white matter, with a diameter of about 350 μm, and centred on a blob. The cells within the blobs, being wavelength selective, would be performing an operation relevant to colour vision and relaying their signals to the thin stripes of V2. The cells just beneath the blobs, in layer 4B, would be performing an operation relevant to the perception of motion and relaying their signals to V5. These two operations could well be supplemented by others. If we look yet deeper beneath the cortical surface, we find that the Meynert cells of upper layer 6 project to both the superior colliculus and to V5, implying that the results of the same operation are relayed to the two distinct visual centres.

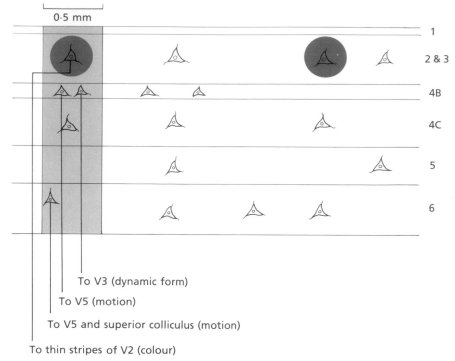

Fig. 21.6 The separate but simultaneous operations performed by a small region of area V1, roughly 0.5 mm in diameter and centred on a blob (red). The cells in the blobs are concerned with colour, those in layer 4B with motion and with dynamic form and those in layer 6 with cortical and subcortical motion mechanisms. All these subdivisions are contained within the same small part of area V1 in which a given part of the field of view is represented.

To V3 (dynamic form)

To V5 (motion)

To V5 and superior colliculus (motion)

To thin stripes of V2 (colour)

This leads us to consider the operational connection,[9] one which with variations may be present everywhere in the cerebral cortex (Figure 21.7). If one were to study the connections between areas V1 and V2 by injecting the latter with horseradish peroxidase (HRP) label, one would find that every given small region of V1, though not necessarily every layer, projects to V2. Indeed, a characteristic of the connections between V1 and V2 is that they are 'point-to-point' or

Fig. 21.7 The topographic connection and the operational connection. (a) Every part of area A, defined as a region of a given diameter (say 1 mm) connects in a systematic and topographic way with area B, thus constituting a topographic connection. (b) A large part of the cortex of area A is involved in undertaking an operation which is of interest to area B, with which area A connects. But not every part of area A needs to connect with B. Instead, the results of all the operations undertaken by A are reported to zone X of A, which alone needs to communicate with B. This constitutes an operational connection.

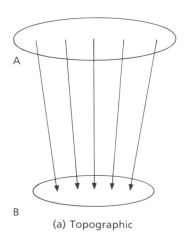

(a) Topographic

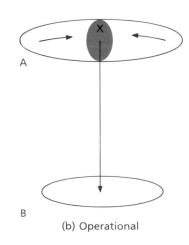

(b) Operational

topographic. By contrast, if one were to inject HRP label into a large portion of area V5, one would find that only a small zone of V4 is labelled; the connections between the two do not appear to be of the point-to-point variety. I have therefore sought for a more general rule to describe these connections.

By an operational connection I mean one in which not every part of a given area X connects with area Y. Rather, we suppose that, although the integrity of the whole of area X is necessary for X to perform its function, not all the activity in X needs to be communicated to area Y. Instead, the results of activity in area X may be communicated to one small region of it and it is this small region of X alone that needs to communicate with Y, thus forming an operational rather than a topographic connection. In a general sense, we know that something like this does happen in the cortex. For example, we know that it is predominantly the cells of the upper layers in the cerebral cortex that project to other cortical areas. But it is at least plausible that these cells are signalling the results of an operation whose execution depends upon the integrity of other cells, in lower layers, and ones which do not themselves project out of the cortical area.

Each cortical zone undertakes operations which are of interest to the cortex and to the subcortex

This introduces the third rule, which is derived from the observation that there is no cortical area which does not have a subcortical projection, predominantly from the lower layers. It follows from this that each region of the cortex must be undertaking an operation which is relevant to both the cortex and the subcortex. Whether it is the result of the same operation that is relayed to other cortical areas and to the subcortex is not clear. The fact that it is usually different cells that project to the cortex and the subcortex would suggest that the results of different operations are relayed to the two destinations.

These anatomical observations lead us to the conclusion that each cortical zone must be undertaking at least two operations and possibly more, given that each cortical zone has multiple cortical and subcortical projections. The operations themselves may differ from one zone to another, but the rules enumerated above suggest that there is a common theme in cortical activity which one can glimpse by studying the anatomical connections. I do not wish to imply that, over and above these rules, there is not a common physiological operation, repeated everywhere in the cortex. But if there is, it has proven remarkably difficult to define. One can only hope that our ever-increasing knowledge of the anatomy and physiology of the cerebral cortex will allow us to formulate more general rules about the operations of the cerebral cortex.

References

1 Dow, B.M. & Vautin, R.G. (1987). Horizontal segregation of color information in the middle layers of foveal striate cortex. *J. Neurophysiol.* **57**, 712–739; Ts'o, D.Y. & Gilbert, C.D. (1988). The organization of chromatic and spatial interactions in the primate striate cortex. *J. Neurosci.* **8**, 1712–1727.

2 Shipp, S. & Zeki, S. (1985). Segregation of pathways leading from area V2 to areas V4 and V5 of macaque monkey visual cortex. *Nature* **315**, 322–325.

3 Zeki, S.M. (1974). Functional organization of a visual area in the posterior bank of the superior temporal sulcus of the rhesus monkey. *J. Physiol. (Lond.)* **236**, 549–573; Albright, T.D. (1984). Direction and orientation selectivity of neurons in visual area MT of the macaque. *J. Neurophysiol.* **52**, 1106–1130.

4 Hubel, D.H. & Wiesel, T.N. (1977). The Ferrier Lecture: Functional architecture of macaque monkey visual cortex. *Proc. R. Soc. Lond.* B **198**, 1–59.

5 Livingstone, M.S. & Hubel, D.H. (1984). Anatomy and physiology of a color system in the primate visual cortex. *J. Neurosci.* **4**, 309–356.

6 Julesz, B. (1984). Toward an axiomatic theory of preattentive vision. In *Dynamic Aspects of Neocortical Function*, edited by G.M. Edelman, W.E. Gall & W.M. Cowan, pp. 585–612. John Wiley, New York.

7 Rockel, A.J., Hiorns, R.W. & Powell, T.P.S. (1980). The basic uniformity in structure of the neocortex. *Brain* **103**, 221–244.

8 Phillips, C.G., Barlow, H.B. & Zeki, S. (1984). Localization of function in the cerebral cortex: past, present and future. *Brain* **107**, 327–361.

9 Zeki, S. (1990). The motion pathways of the cerebral cortex. In *Vision: Coding and Efficiency*, edited by C. Blakemore, pp. 321–345. Cambridge University Press, Cambridge.

Chapter 22: The plasticity of the brain

The connections between the visual areas and their subdivisions are not only highly intricate but also highly specific. It would be surprising if such specific connections were not genetically determined at least in part, but biology is full of surprises and experiments are needed to settle the question. In fact, it would be equally surprising if the visual pathways were completely genetically determined and hard-wired, and therefore unable to undergo any modification. *A totally hard-wired nervous system might make sense in a rigidly coded world, where everything can be identified by a unique label, where nothing changes and where every condition that an organism is likely to encounter, and every possible reaction to it, is predetermined and known beforehand.* This, of course, is far from true. One of the chief features of our environment is that it is in a state of continual change. A hard-wired system in an environment of continual change would run counter to the great biological principles enshrined in the Darwinian doctrine of survival, which implies adaptability to change; of adaptability, which implies plasticity; and of plasticity, which implies variability. One should expect to see, therefore, a certain amount of plasticity or modifiability in cortical connections. As we shall see, this is the case. And the answer which the physiological and anatomical experiments in this area hint at is in fact one which will assist us in understanding the construction of the visual image by the brain.

But the problem of the extent to which the wiring of the nervous system is predetermined and the extent to which it is plastic and modifiable is not merely a problem of visual neurobiology, though it can perhaps best be studied in the visual cortex. It is a more general problem that has fascinated thinkers for ages, namely the problem of nature versus nurture, the extent to which the cortex is a tabula rasa upon which the environment can act, and the extent to which it is predetermined, selecting certain features of the environment through its genetically endowed apparatus, modifying them through its own rules, and then imposing those rules on the environment. It may seem far-fetched to begin studying this problem by studying complex behaviour — of sexuality, of maternal love and of group behaviour. But, apparently, the rules governing the working of the visual system are, in this context, remarkably similar to the ones that govern such complex activities, which is why the study of the visual system gives us so breathtaking a vision of the brain.

Ordinary people with common sense have long recognized the importance of different stages during the development of an organism, at any rate long before physiologists began profaning the secrets of the cerebral cortex with their electrodes. Chief among them have been those interested in education, and who have long known that there are certain periods in the life of an individual when the brain is maximally receptive to certain kinds of training and that a similar training outside these periods is comparatively ineffectual. Everyone knows that mathematical or musical training is best achieved during the early years. This is not to say that there isn't a special kind of neural organization which predisposes its possessor towards music and mathematics. It only implies that, if that special neural organization, whatever it may be, is not adequately nurtured during a critical time, it will wither. Wilder Penfield, the Canadian neurosurgeon, spoke of a 'biological time-table of learning language', emphasizing the importance of acquiring linguistic skills by the age of nine.[1] Western society has inherited an aphorism, commonly, but wrongly, attributed to the Society of Jesus. This states, 'Give us a child until the age of seven and you can have him for life'. Whatever its source, it goes a step further, beyond specific aptitudes and abilities, to supposing that a whole system of complex behaviour, and indeed of morals, is dependent upon early training. If there is cynicism in this aphorism, there is also a profound physiological truth. It implies that the thinking, behaviour and even morality of a human individual can be modified during these tender years in a way that cannot be done later in life, which is not to say that people are immune to influences later in life. It also implies that the desired effects, as well as the undesirable ones, can be more or less permanent. No wonder that Sigmund Freud considered that, psychologically, the child is the father of the man.

The importance of the early years of life, and in particular the relationship to the father and the mother, in developing the later character and profile of individuals is a theme which Freud was very influential in establishing more firmly in the popular mind and in Western thinking. He had been trying to account for the psychoses and neuroses and, 'In my search for the pathogenic situations...I was carried further and further back into the patient's life and ended by reaching the first years of his childhood. What poets and students of human nature had always asserted turned out to be true: the impressions of that remote period of life, though they were for the most part buried in amnesia, left ineradicable traces upon the individual's growth...'.[2] Freud was not only concerned with trying to account for aberrant behaviour and for the psychoses and neuroses; he went beyond and tried to explain much in apparently normal behaviour, and even in artistic achievement, by reference to the formative influences during the early years of life. A remarkable, and charming, example is his attempt to account for the art of Leonardo da Vinci by the experiences of the great master's early life, the emphasis on his early relationship with his simple peasant mother, Catarina, and his early sexual development. Some may find fault with many of the details in Freud's psychobiography of Leonardo. Neurobiologists may well raise an eyebrow at the quality of Freud's evidence; they may be appalled by his retrospective approach. But none can deny the seriousness with which he approached the subject or, in the context of what we have since learned, the physiological basis of his conclusions. A critical passage in his book[3] on the illegitimate Leonardo, who had been discarded by his father at birth, reads as follows: 'In the same year that Leonardo was born...his father...married a lady of good birth; it was to the childlessness of this marriage that the boy owed his reception into his father's...house — an event which had taken place by the time he was five years old...*And by then it was too late. In the first three or four years of life certain impressions become fixed and ways of reacting to the outside world are established which can never be deprived of their importance by later experiences*' [my emphasis].

Love created, love destroyed, love (partly) regained

Freud sought to dissect out the various influences that may operate in early childhood in establishing the later personality of the individual. To most neurobiologists this is too daunting a task, because it deals with so many unknowns and so many variables. Factors that are of importance in shaping the personality and conduct of individuals are complex, as indeed are the personalities themselves. Those who study the brain directly feel a lot more comfortable if they can isolate a given nervous pathway and study its development and maturation. Untold numbers of nervous pathways must be involved in complex behaviour. Yet Freud's approach has been refined in stages, from specific kinds of complex behaviour right down to the development of specific pathways and the responses of single cells in the cortex. And in general terms the conclusions that Freud reached from studying complex behaviour have been found to be mirrored at the single cell level.

One of the major workers in this field has been the American neuropsychologist, Harry Harlow. The system that he studied, the affectional system in monkeys, is still very complex in terms of neural pathways and organization. It is part of the system that determines adult behaviour. Yet it is more limited than the system that determines entire personalities, favoured by Freud in his largely retrospective psychoanalytic approach. To Harlow, Freud's studies had an inherent defect: '...they start with the disorder and work backward in time, retracing the experiences of the individual as he and his relatives and associates recall them...Plainly there is a need to study the development of personality forward in time from infancy'.[4] To do this, Harlow and his colleagues studied complex behaviour in the macaque monkey. The origin of their studies was almost accidental. They had isolated monkeys at birth in order to breed a colony of infection-free monkeys, only to find that they had bred a colony of neurotic monkeys. This led Harlow and his colleagues to a more systematic study of the consequences of isolating monkeys.

How would newborn monkeys, who are totally isolated by being housed in cubicles with solid walls and deprived of the chance of seeing another living being, respond to being introduced into monkey society, to being liberated from their prisons? 'They responded to their liberation by the crouching position with which monkeys typic-ally react to extreme threat...they froze or fled when approached and made no effort to defend themselves from aggressive assaults'. Their abnormal behaviour had not been greatly modified after two years spent in the company of other, normal, monkeys.[4]

Enquiring next into the details, Harlow and his colleagues separated infant monkeys from their mothers a few hours after birth and reared them in individual cages in monkey rooms, so that they could see and hear other monkeys but had no physical contact with them. Physical contact was therefore the only missing feature of their lives. Animals raised in this way and then studied at various ages thereafter showed severe abnormalities. They '...sit in their cages and stare fixedly into space, circle their cages in a repetitive stereotyped manner and clasp their heads in their hands...for long periods of time. They often develop compulsive habits such as pinching precisely the same patch of skin...hundreds of times a day; occasionally such behaviour may become punitive and the animal may chew and tear at its body until it bleeds'. By contrast, animals born in the wild, brought to the laboratory as adolescents or preadolescents and then housed in identical cages and conditions as the laboratory-bred monkeys did not develop such neurotic behaviour. This led Harlow to two conclusions. The first was that normal sensory experience, excluding physical contact, was not enough for normal development; physical contact was also neces-sary. The second was that, 'In line with the "paramount importance" that Freud assigned to experience in the first years of life, our experi-ments indicate that *there is a critical period somewhere between the third and sixth months of life during which social deprivation, par-ticularly deprivation of the company of its peers, irreversibly blights the animals' capacity for social adjustment'*[4] [my emphasis]. The experimental approach, the ability to study the 'development of per-sonality forward in time' enabled Harlow to be more precise about the critical period than Freud had been able to from his retrospective approach, but the conclusions were the same.

The next step was to study the relationship of the newborn monkey to its mother, since 'The first love of the human infant is for his mother. The tender intimacy of this attachment is such that it is sometimes regarded as a sacred or mystical force, an instinct incapable of analysis'.[5] Comparing groups of monkeys reared with and without their mothers, he found that '...the mothered infants entered into more lively and consistent relations with one another than did the four motherless ones'. Moreover, when the 'motherless' mothers delivered their own infants after successful mating, their own behaviour towards their offspring was abnormal, and was characterized by abuse and indifference. Unlike normal monkeys, who fiercely fight any attempt to remove their infants from them, the motherless mothers paid no attention when their infants were removed from them. This inadequacy could be compensated for by infant–infant interactions, which he judged to be at least as important, if not more so, than the mother–infant relationship. The desire and love of the infant monkey for its mother was obviously instinctual, genetically programmed. When real mothers were replaced by inanimate surrogate mothers, some made of wire, others clothed, and all provided with the 'nipple' of the feeding bottle protruding from the 'breast', the infant monkeys became much attached to the clothed mothers and rejected the 'wire' mothers. Making the mothers in some way aversive did little to diminish the love of the infant. Thus developing an 'air-blast' mother, which provided a noxious stimulus in the form of compressed air released under high pressure whenever the monkey approached, did not break this genetically programmed bond. 'The blasted baby never left the mother, but in its moments of agony and duress, clung more and more tightly to the unworthy mother. Where else can a baby get protection?...love conquered all'.[6] But obviously these surrogate mothers never replaced the real mothers because, '...the behaviour of these monkeys...is indistinguishable from that of monkeys raised in bare wire cages with no source of contact comfort'. Nor could later exposure to other monkeys alter their fundamentally abnormal behaviour. 'Apparently their early social deprivation permanently impairs their ability to form effective relations with other monkeys, *whether the opportunity was offered to them in the second six months of life or in the second to the fifth year of life*'[4] [my emphasis]. Moreover, even '...a brief separation experience, involving removal of the mother but no exposure to a strange environment, can produce effects lasting for months or years in rhesus monkeys'.[7]

Thus the affectional system studied by Harlow was a 'love created, love destroyed, love regained' system.[8] Love was created by a genetic programme which was the basis of the bond between mother and infant and between infant and infant, it was destroyed by isolation and separation, and regained, though partially and depending upon the extent of deprivation, by interaction with other, mainly younger, monkeys.

Feral man

Naturally such experiments are impossible to undertake in humans, but everyone who reads newspapers knows about the trail of tragedy that a deprived childhood leaves behind. We do, however, have a set of almost natural experiments, conducted in feral man, in which the development of the deprived human infant forward in time can be studied.[9] The term feral, introduced by Linnaeus, refers to human infants who, for one reason or another, have been deprived of all other human contact and have grown up in the wild, either on their own or in the company of animals. Such 'natural' experiments are difficult to control because many variables are unknown, and some authorities have disagreed on whether the behaviour of feral man should be attributed to the circumstances of their development or to their inferior cerebral capacity. There are about forty recorded cases of feral man, of which the two most famous and best documented are Victor, '*Le sauvage de l'Aveyron*' (the wild boy of the Aveyron) and Amala and Kamala, the wolf children of Midnapore in India. Certain characteristics that they share with other examples of feral man provide a consistent account of the effects of early deprivation of human contact, one that is also consistent with the results of Harlow's experiments on monkeys. There is little reason to doubt their veracity and little reason to doubt that they provide us with profound insights into the developing brain.

The wild boy of the Aveyron was eleven or twelve years old when found totally naked in a forest in the Tarn, southwest France, in 1797.[10] He excited much interest because men, among them Champigny, a minister who was also a protector of science in revolutionary France, believed that the study of Victor could provide some insights into the moral condition of man and test the ideas of John Locke and his French disciple Condillac. John Locke had written, 'But alas, amongst *Children, Ideots, Savages*, and the grossly *Illiterate*, what general Maxims are to be found? What universal Principles of Knowledge? Their Notions are few and narrow, borrowed only from those Objects, they have had most to do with, and which have made upon their Senses the frequentest and strongest Impressions...But he that from a Child untaught, or a wild Inhabitant of the Woods, will expect these abstract Maxims, and reputed Principles of Science, will I fear, find himself mistaken' [original emphasis]. Here then was Victor, a wild inhabitant of the woods. How much would he know?

Very little, it turned out. His entire behaviour was asocial. Perhaps the most surprising feature was that, although given the most extensive care, when Victor died at the age of forty, he could not speak more than a few words as if, having missed the opportunity of learning a language during the critical years, he was forever blighted, like Harlow's monkeys. This feature is in fact not unique to Victor. Inability to talk after prolonged training in feral humans who do not appear to have been otherwise imbeciles, is common. Indeed, one of the characteristics assigned to feral man by Linnaeus is that of *mutus*. Amala and Kamala were found by the Reverend Singh, director of an orphanage at Midnapore, in 1920 in a cave in the company of wolves. Amala was about one and a half years old while Kamala was about eight years old. Their conduct was very much like that of wolves. Soon after their transfer to the orphanage, Amala died. But Kamala lived on for another nine years and her behaviour and development were chronicled by the Reverend Singh and his wife. Of great interest is the fact that the best that Kamala was able to achieve linguistically during these nine years was fifty words, an observation that is consistent with the experience of Victor and other wild children. It is perhaps significant that in a summary of thirty-one cases of feral man,[11] only one was able to talk fluently after training and there is reason to suppose that he was exposed to language at some time after birth.

Perhaps not too much should be made of these cases of feral man. Indeed, because of the uncontrolled nature of these 'experiments', most respectable biologists would not even want to consider this evidence. But whatever the nature of the 'experiments', the final outcome is consistent with what we know from more controlled experiments in development. There are many other, far better, examples which show the importance of the critical period in shaping the nervous system. Imprinting in chicks has been much written about. I have chosen these examples of complex behaviour, of language and of love and affection, to contrast them with the much more extensively studied developing visual system and to show that, in fundamentals, the strategy employed to shape the adult brain is much the same for all these diverse systems. In neurological terms, the affectional system in primates and the linguistic system in man are highly complex. They involve a multitude of cortical systems — auditory, gustatory, visual, as well as other systems such as the autonomic and hormonal ones. On the other hand, the locomotor system is a good deal simpler. But one does not need to know all the details of either the more complex or the simpler system. *From the experiments of Harlow and his colleagues and from observations made on feral man one can derive some quite simple rules which apply to all systems: (1) a genetically programmed system which attaches infant to mother and attracts infants to other infants, and which allows infants to walk and to talk; (2) a critical period of development during which such attachment, in the form of actual physical contact, is mandatory if the individual is to develop normally;*

the development of language and locomotor skills is also subject to a critical period; and (3) the consolidation of the neural mechanisms responsible for normal adult behaviour during this critical period, so that deprivation later in life is without effect, or has less severe consequences. These simple rules can be observed in the visual system.

Vision created, vision destroyed

It is not surprising that in considering human knowledge John Locke should have thought about the visual system, through which so much knowledge of the external world is acquired. If the notions of children, idiots, savages and the illiterate are 'few and narrow, borrowed only from those Objects...which have made upon their Senses the frequentest and strongest Impressions', what knowledge would a visually 'illiterate' person have? In a passage approvingly quoted by Bishop Berkeley in his book *An Essay Towards a New Theory of Vision*, John Locke wrote, '...I shall here insert a Problem of that very Ingenious and Studious promotor of real Knowledge, the Learned and Worthy Mr. Molineux...and it is this: *Suppose a Man born blind, and now adult, and taught by his touch to distinguish between a Cube, and a Sphere of the same metal, and nighly of the same bigness, so as to tell, when he felt one and t'other, which is the Cube, which the Sphere. Suppose then the Cube and the Sphere placed on a Table, and the Blind Man to be made to see. Quare, Whether by his sight, before he touch'd them, he could now distinguish, and tell, which is the Globe, which the Cube.* To which the acute and judicious Proposer answers: *Not. For though he has obtain'd the experience of how a Globe, how a Cube affects his touch; yet he has not yet attained the Experience, that what affects his touch so or so, must affect his sight so or so; or that a protruberant angle in the Cube, that pressed his hand unequally, shall appear to his eye, as it does in the Cube.* I agree with this thinking Gent. whom I am proud to call my Friend...and am of the opinion, that the Blind Man, at first sight, would not be able with certainty to say, which was the Globe, which the Cube, whilst he only saw them'. Obviously this was not what Locke's contemporaries believed for he continues that, '...this observing Gent. farther adds that *having upon the occasion of my Book, proposed this to divers very ingenious Men, he hardly ever met with one, that at first gave the answer to it, which he thinks true, till by learning his reasons they were convinced*' [original emphasis].

The thought experiment that Locke had in mind, one in which a man born blind is made to 'see' in adulthood, is similar to the experiments of Harlow, except of course that it is confined to the visual system. In fact such an 'experiment' has been conducted many times since, through an unfortunate accident of nature. When a human infant is born, it is equipped with an intact visual apparatus, consisting of the retina and the visual pathways leading from it to the cortex. Some unfortunate individuals are born with a congenital cataract, a condition in which the lenses in the eye, which focus the light rays on the retina, are opaque and thus incapable of transmitting light. A cataract develops commonly in adults and, if correctly treated, leaves no lasting visual impairment. But the story is very different with patients who are born blind because of congenital cataract. There are many descriptions of cataractous patients, all but blind at birth, who had undergone operations to remedy the condition, and thus render the optic apparatus clear and healthy at some period or another of their life. Some of these are more reliable than others because the precise age and state of the patient before the onset of the cataract is not always adequately documented.[12] But the common theme that runs through these descriptions is the difficulty that patients have in learning to see, like the difficulty that Harlow's monkeys experienced when liberated from their prolonged isolation. Von Senden writes that '...the process of learning to see in these cases is an enterprise fraught with innumerable difficulties, and that the common idea that the patient must necessarily be delighted with the gifts of light and colour bequeathed to him by the operation is wholly remote from the facts'.[12] This is not something which those who have been blessed with sight at birth can easily understand.

How does a blind patient react to 'liberation'? An example is given in an early description of a fourteen-year-old female patient in Vienna.[13] After her 'sight' had been 'restored' to her, she complained, 'How come that I now find myself less happy than before? Everything that I see causes me a disagreeable emotion. Oh, I was much more at ease in my blindness', adding that, '...if I were always to feel such uneasiness as I do at present at the sight of new things, I would sooner return on the spot to my former blindness'. The very question asked by Locke was studied by Uhthoff in a congenitally blind boy whose vision had been restored to him. Through training undertaken before the operation, the boy had been acquainted with objects by touch, but after the operation, '...he showed no visual recognition of any of the objects presented though they were perfectly familiar to him by touch'. These difficulties are well summarized in a long and moving article by Moreau.[14] After operating on his eight-year-old cataractous patient, he had anticipated the return of vision with pride and enthusiasm. 'But the deception was great'. It took many months of patient training to teach him to recognize objects by sight, and two years after the operation much of what was learnt visually was forgotten. Moreau concluded that, 'It would be an error to suppose that a patient whose sight has been restored to him by surgical intervention can thereafter see the external world. The eyes have certainly obtained the power to see, but the employment of this power...still has to be acquired from the very beginning. The operation itself has no more value than that of preparing the eye to see; education is the most important factor. The occipital lobes can only register and preserve the visual impressions after a process of learning...To give back his sight to a congenitally blind patient is more the work of an educationalist than that of a surgeon'. Seemingly, vision, like the affectional system, is genetically predetermined, and like it has to be nourished or 'educated' during an early period of life. It was to be many years before detailed anatomical and physiological studies were to show what an insurmountable difficulty the educationalist faced.

The critical period for vision

In the late 1960s and early 1970s, Hubel and Wiesel, impressed by the remarkable order in the organization of the visual system of the adult animal, wanted to learn whether this organization is genetically determined.[15] The chances that this was so were high, since it is difficult to believe that such a degree of order can be established by chance encounters with the visual environment. Moreover, it was known that the consequences of depriving monkeys of vision at birth were as severe as those described in the human. Nevertheless, it was not clear whether the properties of cells in the newborn animal are as specific in their behaviour as those of the adult animal. They consequently undertook a study in which they deprived animals (first the cat and then the monkey) of vision in one or both eyes for varying periods of time, at varying periods after birth, and studied the anatomical and physiological consequences of this deprivation. Note that the general question that they were asking — what would the effect of deprivation be — was the same as that asked previously by Harlow. The system chosen and the techniques employed were vastly different. Hubel and Wiesel wanted to study the properties of single cells in the primary visual cortex, area V1, and learn whether these cells could be activated in the same way as those of an adult animal. There are two features of area V1 which lend themselves particularly well to such a study: one is the binocularity, the other orientation selectivity.

The general organization of V1 has been described before (see Chapter 17). Here we need only emphasize that the cells in layer 4 of area V1, which receive the predominant input from the lateral geniculate nucleus (LGN), are exclusively monocular, i.e. responsive to the stimulation of one eye only, and the territory occupied by each eye within this layer is the same. This can be readily ascertained if one were to make an electrode penetration through layer 4C, parallel to the cortical surface, and determine eye preferences for cells separated from each other by about 50 μm. In the other layers cells are binocularly driven, but show preferences for one eye or the other. Eye preferences are usually established by determining the strength of the response to the optimal visual stimulus through each eye in turn. One can then classify cells in a more or less arbitrary way into seven groups (Figure 22.1), with group 1 representing cells driven only by the contralateral eye (i.e. opposite to the hemisphere being recorded from) and group 7 representing cells driven only by the ipsilateral eye. In a normal adult monkey only a relatively small proportion of cells is driven equally well by both eyes and most of these are situated outside layer 4C; most prefer one eye or are driven exclusively by one eye.

The other feature of cells studied developmentally was the property of orientation selectivity. Recall that most cells in the cortex outside layer 4C are orientation selective and that in a long oblique penetration through the cortex of V1, the orientation preferences of successive cells separated from each other by small distances (ca. 50−100 μm) change gradually and in an orderly manner (Figure 22.2). How do these two properties, binocularity and orientation selectivity, develop?

When born, monkeys come with what appears to be an intact visual apparatus from retina to cortex, at least as judged macroscopically. Recordings from the visual cortex of newborn monkeys show that some cells at least are orientation selective and that in monkeys which are only a few weeks old the ocular dominance columns are remarkably similar to those found in the adult monkey, suggesting that these properties are to a large extent genetically determined.[16] But this work also showed that this genetically determined

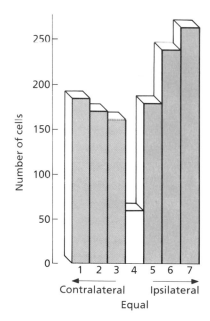

Fig. 22.1 The ocular dominance histogram, obtained by determining which eye best activates the cell. Cells in group 1 are activated exclusively by the contralateral eye (the eye opposite to the hemisphere in question) while those in group 7 are activated exclusively by the ipsilateral eye. (Redrawn from Hubel, D.H. (1979). *American Scientist* **67**, 532−543.)

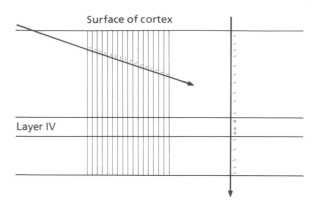

Surface of cortex

Layer IV

Fig. 22.2 The gradual change in the orientation selectivity of successive cells encountered during a long, oblique, penetration through area V1. (Redrawn from Hubel, D.H. & Wiesel, T.N. (1977). *Proc. R. Soc. Lond.* B **198**, 1–59.)

apparatus is not rigid but is subject to modification. Such a finding confirms, at a microscopic level, the earlier findings of Harlow at a complex behavioural level.

When an animal was deprived of vision in one eye during the first three months after birth, by suturing the eyelids together, the effects were catastrophic. Many cells responded in 'a vague and unpredictable manner', making them difficult to study. The cells that could be driven were the ones that were activated through the eye that had remained open during the first three months of life and they displayed the normal orientation selectivity. Stimulation through the eye that had been closed during the critical period was completely ineffective in driving the cells. The ocular dominance histogram of such animals was therefore very different from that of normal monkeys (Figure 22.3). These results show, then, that the connections of each eye to cells in the visual cortex are sufficiently labile for them to be disrupted or become ineffective if the relevant eye is disused. The eye is disused if it is not properly stimulated with patterned light. The presence of light, as such, was not in itself sufficient. Thus, fitting the eyes with translucent lenses, allowing light to pass through but depriving the animals of the ability to see forms, had equally severe consequences, the cells again being unresponsive to visual stimulation and certainly lacking the orientation selectivity that is so prominent a feature in adult primary visual cortex. Such catastrophic effects were only obtained if the monkeys were deprived of vision during the first three months of life. If monkeys were deprived completely of vision during adulthood, the effects were not noticeable, the cells being apparently as normal as they are in a monkey without a history of deprivation. In a sense, this is similar to Harlow's earlier experiment, in which a normal environment without physical contact was insufficient to rear normal monkeys. In sum, this set of experiments showed that, *at the cellular level, there is a critical period, during which adequate visual stimulation is mandatory if the animal is to be able to see at all,*

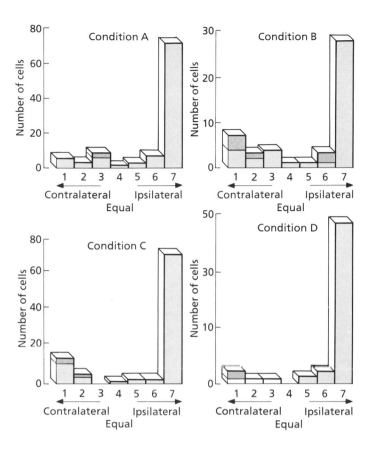

Fig. 22.3 The ocular dominance histogram obtained by recording from the left striate cortex of animals deprived of vision in the right eye, from birth or during the critical period. Whether the animal is deprived of vision for the first two weeks of life (A), for five days only during the critical period (B), for nine days only from birth, and then left open for four years (C), the result is the same — the great majority of cells are driven by the eye which was open during the critical period only. (D) When the right eye was closed seven days after birth and left closed for one year, at which time it was opened and the open eye closed for a year, most cells are again driven by the eye which was open during the critical period only. (Redrawn from Hubel, D.H. (1979). *American Scientist* **67**, 532–543.)

even if to all appearances the visual pathways and cortex appeared to be intact. Thus, 'The effects of monocular deprivation for the first 3 months of life tend to be permanent, with very limited morphological, physiological, or behavioural recovery'.[17] This conclusion is remarkably similar to that of Harlow, that, 'there is a critical period somewhere between the third and sixth months of life during which social deprivation . . . irreversibly blights the animals' capacity for social adjustment'.

With a more accurate and sensitive measure of the consequences of deprivation, physiologists were able to narrow down the critical period in the visual system of the cat to the first three months of life. But within this three month span there were periods when the cortex was more susceptible to deprivation than during other periods since ' . . . the susceptibility to the effects of deprivation, which appears rather suddenly near the beginning of the fourth week and is very great during that week, begins to fall some time between the sixth and eighth week, continues to decline during the third month, and has disappeared by the end of that month'.[18] In other words, there is a period of high susceptibility, in the fourth and fifth weeks, during this critical period. During this time of high susceptibility, eye closure 'for as little as

3–4 days' leads to a sharp decline in the number of cortical cells that can be driven through that eye and 'A six day closure is enough to give a reduction in the number of cells that can be driven by the closed eye to a fraction of the normal'.[17] Once again, one is impressed by the similarity between this statement and that derived from behavioural studies.[7] '...that such a brief separation experience, involving removal of the mother but no exposure to a strange environment, can produce effects lasting for months or even years'. The systems and the techniques are different, the principles much the same.

The plasticity of the brain

In the infant monkey deprivation of contact with the mother or with other infant monkeys blights the affectional system irreversibly but can be partially compensated for by infant–infant interactions; deprivation in adolescent life has no effect. With vision, deprivation early in life blights forever the visual capacities, but deprivation in adult life has no measurable effect. A lesion sustained in adulthood and affecting the speech areas of the brain impairs speech permanently, but an individual who sustains a similar lesion in early childhood can nevertheless learn to speak. What does all this tell us about the brain? Speaking in terms of language, Penfield believed that it reveals something about the plasticity of the brain. He wrote, 'The brain of the child is plastic. The brain of the adult, however effective it may be in other directions, is usually inferior to that of the child as far as language is concerned'.[1] The consequences of early and late destruction of the speech areas in humans was one reason which led Penfield to his conclusion. He wrote, 'This [plasticity] is borne out still further by the remarkable re-learning of a child after injury or disease destroys the speech areas in the dominant left hemisphere. Child and adult, alike, become speechless after such an injury, but the child will speak again, and does so, normally, after a period of months. The adult may or may not do so, depending upon the severity of the injury'.[1] But what, in terms of hard currency, that is, the physiological properties of cells and their connections, does plasticity mean? Does it entail a change in properties of cells? Do they establish new connections? The best evidence comes from the visual system.

Recall again that in a normal adult monkey the territory occupied by each eye in layer 4 is roughly about the same. There is an anatomical way of demonstrating this and it consists of injecting one eye of a normal adult monkey with labelled amino acids. These are taken up by the retinal cells and incorporated into proteins, which then travel down the optic nerves to the LGN, cross the synaptic clefts there and then travel in the optic radiations to the primary visual cortex. When

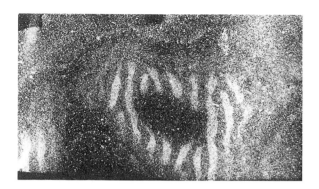

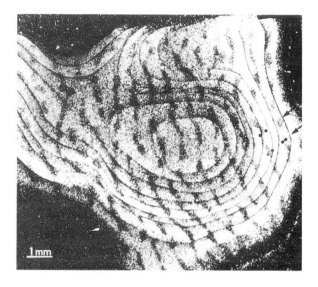

Fig. 22.4 The labelling of cortical zones receiving input from one eye (label is shown as white). (Above) When the label is injected into one eye of a normal animal and sections through layer 4 of V1 are taken parallel to the cortex, labelled zones are found to alternate with unlabelled zones, each occupying roughly the same space. (Below) What happens when an animal is deprived of vision in one eye during the critical period and the eye which was open during that time is subsequently injected with label. The labelled zones are much larger, showing that the open eye had expanded its cortical territory and taken over cortical space which, by genetic right, had belonged to the other (closed) eye. (Reproduced by permission from Hubel, D.H. & Wiesel, T.N. (1977). *Proc. R. Soc. Lond.* B **198**, 1–59.)

sections taken through the primary visual cortex are appropriately treated, the label is found to be distributed in bands, separated from each other by unlabelled bands (Figure 22.4, above). The labelled bands belong to the injected eye and the unlabelled bands to the other eye. But this is not the picture that is found in the newborn monkey. When an experiment similar to the one described above is repeated in a one-day-old monkey, this separation into bands is not found. Instead, the label resulting from the injection of one eye is continuously distributed in the primary visual cortex.[15,18] This result was confirmed by physiological recordings from monkeys only a few days old, which showed that most cells in layer 4C of V1 are binocularly driven, whereas by six weeks the adult pattern of segregation into left eye and right eye bands is already complete. These results suggest, then, that the segregation of the input from the two eyes in the cortex occurs later. In fact, it occurs during the critical period. A direct anatomical way of demonstrating this is to close one eye of a monkey during the critical period and, following this, to inject the eye that was maintained open during that period with labelled amino acids. What one finds in the cortex is now very different. Instead of the labelled bands occupying the same amount of cortical space as the unlabelled ones, the territory now occupied by the labelled bands (coming from the eye that was open and thus functioning normally during the critical period) has expanded very substantially, at the expense of the territory occupied by the unlabelled bands (belonging to the eye that was closed during the critical period) (Figure 22.4, below). The open eye has apparently taken over territory which, by genetic right, belonged to the closed eye. This result is confirmed by physiological recordings which show that in such animals most cells are driven by the eye that was open during the critical period, that few are driven by the eye that was closed and that those few are abnormal in their responses. Here we begin to obtain some insight into plasticity. The connections established between eye and brain are not rigid. They are labile. They can expand to take over territory not belonging to them genetically, but their ability to do so declines with time. Moreover, reverse suture experiments, in which one eye is sutured for a few days, followed by closure of the other eye, during the critical period, have shown that this process of encroachment, of the taking over of territory belonging to the 'bad' eye, is not an irreversible one, especially during the critical period.[19]

The importance of these anatomical observations is perhaps better appreciated by studying the results of physiological experiments which, in fact, were undertaken earlier and revealed some oddities. The first of these was that the effects of binocular closure could not be predicted from that of monocular closure, and instead gave a counter-intuitive result, always the most interesting in science. If a cat is deprived of vision in one eye during the critical period, cells in the cortex cannot be driven by that eye. One might have expected from this that binocular closure during the critical period will render all cortical cells abnormal and that one would end up with a visually unresponsive cortex. Not so. 'Contrary to what had been expected, responsive cells were found throughout the greater part of all penetrations, and over half of these cells seemed perfectly normal. The cortex was nevertheless not normal in that many cells responded abnormally, and many were completely unresponsive'.[20] It thus seemed that when the input to the cortex was equalized (in this case no visual input from either eye), the effects of deprivation were less drastic. How can this be accounted for?

Plasticity as a competition for cortical cells

When one eye alone is shut during the critical period, it is placed at a severe disadvantage with respect to the other eye, since it receives no input to transmit to the cortex. When both eyes are shut, the cortex is at a severe disadvantage, in that it receives no visual input at all. But one eye is no longer at a disadvantage with respect to the other. One can suppose that the input from each eye, via the LGN, competes for space on cortical cells. Put more anatomically, one can suppose that the axons from the two sets of layers of the LGN, each set belonging to one eye, compete for space on the cortical cells upon which they terminate. If the axons belonging to one eye do not transmit signals to the cortex, they would be at a competitive disadvantage compared with the axons belonging to the other eye, which will consequently monopolize more cortical cells and eventually more cortical space. This was tested in an ingenious anatomical experiment[21] (Figure 22.5).

Cells in different layers of the LGN project to the striate cortex, cells representing a given point in space in a layer belonging to, say, the right eye projecting to a given part of layer 4 and cells representing the identical point in visual space in a layer belonging to the left eye projecting to the adjacent part. If the animal is deprived of vision in one eye, the LGN cells belonging to that eye will atrophy and shrink in size, while the cells in a corresponding part of the adjacent layer, which belongs to the normal, open, eye, will retain a normal size. In the cortex, the territory occupied by the normal eye increases in extent, at the expense of territory belonging to the closed eye, suggesting that the closed eye had 'lost out' in the competition for cortical space. But what would happen if one were to contrive a situation where there is a monocular closure and no competition? Such a situation is there, waiting only to be exploited. There is a segment of the LGN, known as the monocular crescent, which represents a part of the extreme periphery of the nasal retina for which there is no corresponding temporal retina (Figure 22.5). The cells here project to the corresponding monocular crescent of the cortex and there cannot be any competition for space between the two eyes. If the shrinkage and atrophy of cells in the LGN and the loss of cortical territory are to be explained by competition, then it follows that the cells of the monocular crescent should not atrophy when the eye is closed during the critical period, for the simple reason that they have no competition even though they are not able to transmit signals to the striate cortex. By contrast, the cells in the remaining part of the same layer, those which have to compete for cortical space with the input from the normal eye, will shrink and atrophy. This is precisely the result that was obtained.[21] Plasticity, then, is the manifestation of the ability of cells to compete for space on a third, common, cell.

How late into adult life is the nervous system plastic and can the connections established postnatally during the critical developmental periods be modified later in life, through rules of competition which evidently operate during the critical period? Interesting experiments

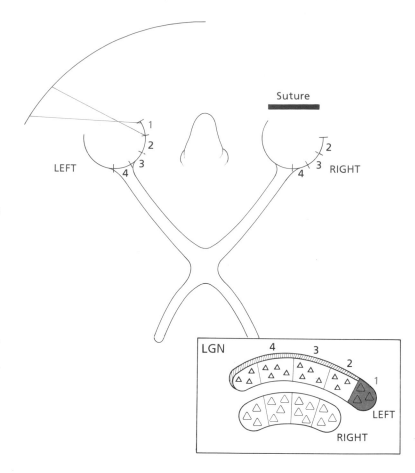

Fig. 22.5 An ingenious anatomical experiment to show that the shrinkage of cells in the lateral geniculate nucleus (LGN) after eye closure is the result of competition for space on cortical cells. For simplicity only two layers of the LGN are shown. The monocular crescent (shown in red) represents a part of the field of view for one eye for which there is no corresponding representation for the other eye. The layer of the LGN in which the monocular crescent for that eye is represented (also shown in red) has no counterpart in the layer representing the other eye. Consequently, when the eye projecting to that layer is sutured, only the cells in it which represent parts of the retina also represented in the other layer shrink. The cells in that part have no corresponding cells in the other layer, and therefore no competition. They do not shrink. (Drawn from the experiments of Guillery, R.W. & Stelzner, D.J. (1972). *J. Comp. Neurol.* **130**, 413–422.)

have suggested that this plasticity, perhaps on a more limited scale than during the critical period, is maintained well into adult life. For example, there is a detailed representation of the hand and the fingers in the somatosensory cortex. In experiments in which a digit was amputated in adult monkeys and the cortical representation of the digits mapped before and after amputation, it was found that the cortical territory occupied by the digit before amputation was occupied by other digits following the amputation.[22] In other words, the cortical space devoted to the healthy digits had expanded to occupy territory belonging to the amputated digit. The fact that such expansion was limited to 600 μm, leaving areas of silent cortex, would suggest that the field of action, or the cortical territory, that a healthy digit can claim is not unlimited, for reasons which we do not understand. Equally, it has been found that, following lesions in area V5 of the monkey, the receptive fields of cells at the borders of the lesion can expand very substantially in all directions, as if the input to them had been modified as a consequence of the lesion.[23] In fact, more recent experiments suggest that the plasticity of the adult brain may be much more extensive than has been supposed.[24] In these experiments, the sensory nerves coming from the forelimbs were severed and the map in the cortex was studied twelve years after severance. It turned out that the representation of the lower face area had expanded into cortical territory that had belonged to the arm and hand, a distance of between 10 and 14 mm.

This evidence suggests, then, that competition between cells for the allegiance of other cells is something that extends well into adult life. It means in effect that cells whose activities are correlated could become linked together to form groups, a supposition[25] which introduces a new and important element into how the visual cortex can function in adult life, a topic which we will return to. What determines the success of one cell over another, or of one group of cells over another, is probably a combination of anatomical variability and correlated responses. The anatomical variability ensures that a cell with, say, a greater axonal spread will have a better chance of contacting another cell than will one with a more limited spread. Two cells which are in better contact will, in turn, have a better chance of 'firing' together and thus becoming further linked. We shall assume, given the developmental evidence, that the linkages may be very strong or very weak and can persist with varying degrees of strength throughout the life of the individual.

The deprivation studies on the visual cortex are but the latest in a form of enquiry that can be traced back scientifically to Freud and Harlow and, in terms of common knowledge about critical periods, to even earlier times. They constitute a marvellous example of the way in which study of the visual cortex can provide us with a vision of brain function and organization. We at least know what plasticity can mean in neurological terms. We know at the very least that deprivation during the critical period can alter the responses of single cells. We have a frame of reference should we want to investigate the susceptibilities of other cortical areas, such as the visual areas of the prestriate cortex or the auditory and somatosensory areas; we can make useful conjectures even about cortical areas involved with language in man. In the not too distant future we shall be able to study these areas in the living human subject during different phases of development with modern techniques such as positron emission tomography. Perhaps no field of endeavour has given us more profound insights into an important aspect of brain organization, an aspect which, as Freud had emphasized, determines our behaviour for the rest of our lives.

References

1 Penfield, W. & Roberts, L. (1959). *Speech and Brain Mechanisms*. Princeton University Press, Princeton.
2 Freud, S. (1935). *An Autobiographical Study*. p. 35. Translated and edited by J. Strachey. W.W. Norton, New York.

3 Freud, S. (1910). *Eine Kindheitserinnerung des Leonardo da Vinci*. (Translated into English by A. Tyson (1964). *Leonardo da Vinci and a Memory of His Childhood*. W.W. Norton, New York.)

4 Harlow, H.F. & Harlow, M.K. (1962). Social deprivation in monkeys. *Sci. Am.* **207**, 136–146.

5 Harlow, H.F. (1959). Love in infant monkeys. *Sci. Am.* **200**, 68–74.

6 Harlow, H.F. (1962). The heterosexual affectional system in monkeys. *Am. Psychol.* **17**, 1–9.

7 Hinde, R.A. & Spencer-Booth, Y. (1971). Effects of brief separation from mother on rhesus monkeys. *Science* **173**, 111–118.

8 Harlow, H.F. (1972). Love created — love destroyed — love regained. In *Modeles Animaux du Comportement Humain*, No. 198, pp. 13–60. Editions du Centre National de la Recherche Scientifique, Paris.

9 Malson, L. (1964). *Les Enfants Sauvages*. Christian Bourgeois, Paris.

10 Itard, J. (1801 and 1806). *Mémoire et Rapport sur Victor de l'Aveyron*. Published as an appendix to Malson, L. loc cit. [9].

11 Zingg, R.M. (1940). Feral man and extreme cases of isolation. *Am. J. Psychol.* **53**, 487–517.

12 Senden, M. von (1932). *Raum- und Gestaltauffassung bei Operierten Blindgebornen*. (Translated into Engish by P. Heath (1960). *Space and Sight*. Methuen & Co., London.)

13 Report in *Vossiche Zeitung*, Berlin (1777), quoted by von Senden [12].

14 Moreau (1913). Histoire de la guérison d'un aveugle-né. *Ann. Oculist. (Paris)* **149**, 81–118.

15 Hubel, D.H. (1978). Effects of deprivation on the visual cortex of cat and monkey. *The Harvey Lectures, Series 72*. Academic Press, New York and London.

16 Wiesel, T.N. & Hubel, D.H. (1974). Ordered arrangement of orientation columns in monkeys lacking visual experience. *J. Comp. Neurol.* **158**, 307–318.

17 Hubel, D.H. & Wiesel, T.N. (1970). The period of susceptibility to the physiological effects of unilateral eye closure in kittens. *J. Physiol. (Lond.)* **206**, 419–436.

18 Rakic, P. (1977). Prenatal development of the visual system in the rhesus monkey. *Philos. Trans. R. Soc. Lond.* B **278**, 245–260.

19 Blakemore, C.B. & Van Sluyters, R.C. (1974). Reversal of the physiological effects of monocular deprivation in kittens: further evidence for a sensitive period. *J. Physiol. (Lond.)* **237**, 195–216.

20 Wiesel, T.N. & Hubel, D.H. (1965). Comparison of the effects of unilateral and bilateral eye closure on cortical unit responses in kittens. *J. Neurophysiol.* **28**, 1029–1040.

21 Guillery, R.W. & Stelzner, D.J. (1970). The differential effects of unilateral lid closure upon the monocular and binocular segments of the dorsal lateral geniculate nucleus in the cat. *J. Comp. Neurol.* **139**, 413–422.

22 Merzenich, M.M., Nelson, R.J., Stryker, M.F. *et al.* (1984). Somatosensory cortical map changes following digit amputation in adult monkeys. *J. Comp. Neurol.* **224**, 591–605.

23 Wurtz, R.H., Yamasaki, D.S., Duffy, C.J. & Roy, J.-P. (1991). Functional specialization for visual motion processing in primate cerebral cortex. *Cold Spring Harb. Symp. Quant. Biol.* **55**, 717–727.

24 Pons, T.P., Garraghty, P.E., Ommaya, A.K. *et al.* (1991). Massive cortical reorganization after sensory deafferentiation in adult macaques. *Science* **252**, 1857–1860.

25 Edelman, G.M. (1987). *Neural Darwinism: The Theory of Neuronal Group Selection*. Basic Books, New York.

Chapter 23: Colour vision and the brain

How does the brain see the colours of the external world? How does it analyze them? Are there colours there to analyze? Is colour a property of the brain or of the world outside? If colour is not a property of the world outside, how can we characterize the properties of objects which allow us to see them in colour? These are fascinating questions. They are, in a sense, questions that are at the interface of biology and physics, and even of philosophy. The answers to them may even give us a clue to a grander problem, namely the brain's knowledge of the external world. In trying to answer these questions we begin, at the very least, to realize two facts of primordial importance for understanding vision and the role of the brain in it, namely that *surfaces are not endowed with codes or labels which allow the brain to analyze them passively with respect to colour and that, consequently, the brain must actively construct the colour of a surface from the information that is available to it.*

The 'paradox' of colour vision

Colour vision is a subject that is burdened with a long and (sometimes) honourable history. It is a subject that has interested philosophers and poets no less than scientists. And among those who have thought and written on the subject of colour are some of the towering geniuses of our civilization — Newton, Young, Clerk Maxwell, Helmholtz, Goethe, Schrödinger and Wittgenstein, to name but a few. In their writings, one will find an attempt to come to terms with a great paradox. The paradox is really created by the fact that the visible spectrum is coloured, lights of different wavelengths having different colours, long-wave light looking red, middle-wave light green and short-wave light blue (Figure 23.1 and Plate 7, facing p. 188). It therefore seems natural to suppose that objects and surfaces acquire their colour by virtue of the dominant wavelength of the light reflected from them, that a red object, for example, looks red because it reflects more long-wave or red light, a green object looks green because it reflects more middle-wave or green light and so on. Indeed, Newton himself so assumed and the assumption has now become part of our cultural tradition. And here enters the paradox. When we view objects in different conditions of illumination, the wavelength composition of the light reflected from them changes. If, for example, one were to

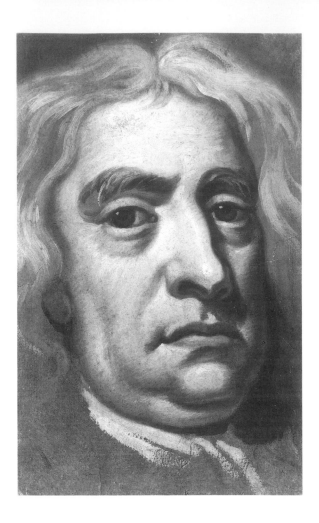

Fig. 23.1 Sir Isaac Newton. (Reproduced by permission of the President and Council of the Royal Society.)

view an orange or banana in a room lit by tungsten light, and then in a room lit by fluorescent light and then, successively, in daylight on a cloudy day and on a sunny day, and at dawn and at dusk, one would find that the orange will continue to look orange in colour and the banana will continue to look yellow. There may be some changes in the shade of yellow and orange, but the colour will remain the same. Yet, if one were to measure the wavelength composition of the light reflected from these surfaces in these different conditions, one will find profound variations. In natural viewing conditions there is thus no prespecified wavelength composition, or code, that leads to a particular colour and to that colour alone. Indeed, if the colours of objects changed with every change in the illumination in which they are viewed, then colour will lose its significance as a biological signalling mechanism since the object could not then be faithfully recognized by its colour any more. Hering put it like this: 'When we think about large...differences in natural or artificial illuminations in which distinct vision is possible, then we really ought to be surprised that we generally take colors as inherent properties of objects rather than as merely accidental and continuously changing properties like, for example, their coldness, coolness, warmth, or heat'.[1]

This property, often called colour constancy, is in fact the single most important property of the colour system, without which colour vision would lose its raison d'être as a biological signalling mechanism. But if such profound variations in the wavelength composition of the light reflected from a surface do not entail a change in the colour of the object being viewed, then we are faced with a paradox, or so it seems. Psychologists reinforce the notion of a paradox by calling this phenomenon 'colour constancy', which implies that there is a colour inconstancy, and by treating the former as a departure from the rule that there is a straightforward and simple relationship between the colour of a surface and the wavelength composition of the light reflected from it. How could such a departure be achieved? Helmholtz[2] tried to account for it by invoking vague factors such as 'discounting the illuminant' through the process of the 'unconscious inference'. Hering thought that the phenomenon could be accounted for by the use of memory, which makes us see the colours 'quite differently from the way we should see them without [the use of our memory]'.[1] But how and under what conditions does one acquire the experience which is used later in life to 'discount the illuminant'? Hering saw the problem and wrote emphatically, 'The physiological mechanisms of regulation are already functioning in the acquisition of these experiences and they provide the means for making these experiences possible to begin with',[1] though he carefully avoided specifying what these physiological mechanisms may be.

There is of course a good reason for this apparent paradox, namely that there is a condition in which the colour of a surface *does* bear a simple and straightforward relationship to the wavelength composition of the light reflected from it. In practice, this is a condition which an organism rarely encounters. Even most humans know nothing of it. The condition is one to be found in laboratories only and is known as a reduction screen or aperture condition. It is one in which a small area is viewed in isolation, and which I shall refer to as a *void viewing condition.* In this condition, a small area illuminated with long-wave light only will look red regardless of its actual colour, one illuminated with equal amounts of lights of all wavelengths will look white, one illuminated with about equal amounts of red and green only will look yellow, and so on. Everything in this viewing condition suggests, then, that the perceived colour of the patch depends upon the wavelength composition of the light reflected from it; everything suggests that the colour of the patch depends upon adding the amounts of light of different wavelength reflected from that patch. But is there a real paradox here, a radical difference between the way we see the colours of surfaces in the void mode and the way we see them when they are part of natural scenes? Can we not derive laws which apply with equal cogency to viewing a small area of a surface in isolation, and to viewing the same area when it is part of a more natural scene? This is worth attempting and leads one to the conclusion that there is no paradox at all.[3]

The Land Mondrian experiments in colour vision

An easy way to understand the problem is to describe a remarkable experiment constructed by Edwin Land.[4] In this, normal human subjects view a multicoloured display made of patches of paper of different colour, pasted together (Plate 8, facing p. 188). The tableau thus produced bears a resemblance to the paintings of the Dutch master, Piet Mondrian, and is therefore referred to as a colour Mondrian. The rectangles composing the scene are of different sizes and shapes, some being rectangular and others square, thus creating an abstract scene with no recognizable objects. This controls for factors such as learning and memory. No patch of the display is surrounded by another of a single colour — the patches surrounding each patch differ in colour. This controls for factors such as induced colours or 'colour contrast' (see Figure 23.2). The patches are made of matt papers which reflect a constant amount of light in all directions so that they can be viewed from any angle without affecting the outcome of the experiment.

This abstract colour display is illuminated by three projectors, each equipped with a rheostat which allows the intensity of the light coming from it to be changed. One projector, which we shall call the *long-wave* projector, is equipped with a filter which passes red light only; the filter on the second, *middle-wave*, projector passes green light only, and that on the third, *short-wave*, projector passes blue light only. For reasons which will become obvious, it is far better to refer to long-, middle- and short-wave light than to red, green and

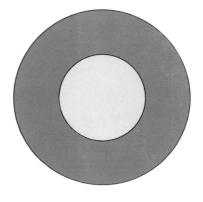

Fig. 23.2 If a neutral, grey, patch is surrounded by a coloured ring, in this case a red one, the central patch acquires the colour of the opponent of the surrounding ring, in this case bluish-green. This is called an induced colour.

blue light. A sensitive measuring device can determine the intensity of light of each wavelength reflected from each patch of the display. The device, a telephotometer, is equipped with an equal sensitivity filter which makes it equally sensitive to light of all wavelengths.

In a darkened room an audience of normal individuals is asked to look at one of the patches of the display, say the green one. The long-wave projector alone is switched on and the intensity of the light coming from it is increased until the telephotometer registers that the green patch is reflecting 60 units of long-wave light.[5] This projector is now switched off, the middle-wave projector is switched on and its intensity increased until the telephotometer registers that the same green patch is reflecting 30 units of middle-wave light, when the projector is switched off. Next, the short-wave projector is switched on and its intensity is increased until the telephotometer registers that the green patch is reflecting 10 units of short-wave light. Now all the projectors are switched on, a condition in which the patch is reflecting 60, 30 and 10 units of long-, middle- and short-wave light, respectively. The audience reports the colour of the patch to be green. Note that the area is reported to be green in spite of the fact that it is reflecting twice the amount of long-wave (red) light than middle-wave (green) light and more long-wave light than short- and middle-wave light combined. *One concludes that, in this condition, the colour of the patch does not correspond to the colour of the predominant wavelength reflected from it.*

The experiment is next repeated with another patch of a different colour, say the blue one. That is, when all three projectors are switched on, the blue patch is reflecting the same triplet of energies as the green patch was reflecting moments before (60, 30 and 10 units of long-, middle- and short-wave light respectively). The audience reports the colour of the patch to be blue. The experiment is now repeated again with patches of other colours, including the black, white and grey patches. Each is made, in turn, to reflect the same triplet of energies, and yet each is found to retain its colour; in other words the orange patch is reported as orange, the red one as red, the white one as white and the black one as black. One concludes from this second experiment that, *when a surface forms part of a complex, multi-coloured, scene there is no simple and obvious relationship between the wavelength composition of the light reflected from that surface and its colour.*

The same experiment is now repeated but with each of the patches being viewed in isolation, in the *void condition* (Hering[1] has described a much simpler version of this experiment) (Plate 9, facing p. 188). When, first, the (green) patch is illuminated with the same triplet of energies as in the experiment above and viewed in the void, the audience reports its colour to be white or a very light grey. When, without changing the energies coming from the (green) patch, the surround is brought into view, the colour of the same patch is immediately reported to be green. When the same experiment is repeated with the other patches, the same result is obtained, that is the (red) patch is seen as white in the void condition and red in the natural mode, the (blue) patch as white and blue respectively, and so on. This experiment leads us to the conclusion that, *in the natural viewing condition, the colour of a patch is determined not only by the wavelength composition of the light reflected from it, but also by the wavelength composition of the light reflected from surrounding surfaces* since the patch had a different colour when viewed in the two conditions.

We next repeat the void and natural experiments with the green patch, placing the green patch in different positions on the display, and thus changing its surrounds with every new position. In every new position, when the green patch is illuminated with the same triplet of energies and viewed in the void condition it is, of course, seen as white; whenever the surround is brought into view, its colour is reported to be green.

We are thus led to the conclusion that the colour of a surface is determined not only by the wavelength composition of the light reflected from it, but also by that reflected from surrounding surfaces, but that it does not bear a simple and obvious relationship to either, since the surround was continually changed in the last experiment.

Yet the colour system is a highly reliable one. Indeed, the above experiments could be repeated with the shutters open for only a fraction of a second, with the same results,[5] thus showing that they cannot be due to factors such as the adaptation of the photoreceptors in the eye, as many have assumed. It would therefore be difficult to imagine that there is no simple and obvious relationship between the physical characteristics of the object being viewed and the colour that the brain assigns to it. Indeed, there is. It lies in a *comparison* of the wavelength composition of the light reflected from a surface and the wavelength composition of the light reflected from surrounding surfaces.

The physical constants of surfaces

The only physical constant of a surface that is of importance, in terms of colour vision, is its *reflectance*. This refers to the percentage of light of any waveband reflected from a surface. It never changes. Thus, a red surface may have a high reflectance for long-wave light, and a low reflectance for middle- and short-wave light. We could be more accurate and say that a given red surface will have a reflectance of 90% for light of 620 nm (long-wave, red light), 20% for light of

520 nm (middle-wave, green light) and 5% for light of 480 nm (short-wave, blue light). If one were to arrange things in such a way that 1000 mW each of long-, middle- and short-wave light are incident on that surface, then it will reflect 900, 300 and 50 mW respectively of long-, middle- and short-wave light (Figure 23.3). If, in another condition, the surface is illuminated by another source of light with the consequence that 300, 400 and 140 mW of long-, middle- and short-wave light are incident on it, the surface will still reflect 90, 30 and 5%, respectively, of light of the three wavebands incident on it; but the actual amounts reflected, and thus reaching the eye, will be 270, 80 and 7 mW respectively of long-, middle- and short-wave light. Note that the reflectance has not changed, and the surface still reflects the same percentage of light of the different wavebands incident on it. But the amounts reflected are now very different. And the only information that reaches the brain relates to these amounts. The brain knows nothing about the reflectances, has no reference for comparison and has never heard of the National Bureau of Standards. It can therefore only register the intensity of light of each waveband reaching it from every surface in the field of view. And the intensities coming from a surface are never constant; they vary with the illuminant in which the surface is viewed. Consequently, to approximate its colour constructs to the true constants in nature, the brain must somehow discard the information relating to the intensities reaching it, and concentrate on the reflectance alone. It must, in brief, reconstruct the

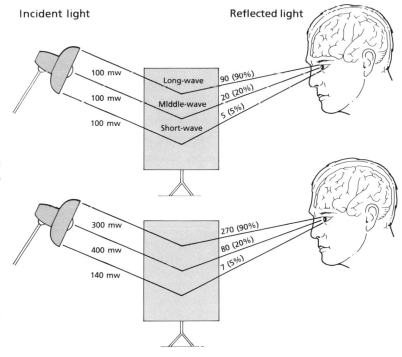

Fig. 23.3 The reflectance of a surface for light of a given wavelength is its efficiency for reflecting light of that wavelength, expressed as the percentage of the incident light of that wavelength which it reflects. The reflectance never changes, although the amounts incident on, and reflected from, the surface change continually. The surface shown here reflects 90%, 20% and 5% respectively of long-, middle- and short-wave light, irrespective of the intensity of the illuminating light.

Incident light — Reflected light

100 mw — Long-wave — 90 (90%)
100 mw — Middle-wave — 20 (20%)
100 mw — Short-wave — 5 (5%)

300 mw — 270 (90%)
400 mw — 80 (20%)
140 mw — 7 (5%)

constant properties of surfaces from the information reaching it which, itself, is never constant. How does it achieve this?

Lightnesses

Obviously the simplest way of doing this would be to *compare* the reflectance of different surfaces for light of the same waveband. Let us begin by considering two surfaces, a red one and a green one (Plate 10, facing p. 188). The red surface will have a high reflectance for long-wave light. It will therefore reflect a large percentage of the long-wave light incident on it. The green surface, by contrast, will have a low efficiency (low reflectance) for long-wave light and will therefore reflect only a small amount of the total that is incident on it. Now, if both surfaces were to be illuminated simultaneously with long-wave light alone, the red surface will appear very light since it reflects a good deal of the light incident on it, while the green surface will appear very dark since it reflects a much smaller percentage of the incident (long-wave) light. If we now increase the intensity of illumination so that a great deal more long-wave light is incident on both surfaces, the red surface will still reflect a good deal more long-wave light than the green surface, and will therefore still look lighter. By contrast, if we were to illuminate both surfaces with middle-wave (green) light, the green surface, having a higher efficiency for reflecting it, will always look lighter, no matter what the actual intensities used. *The biological correlate of reflectance is, then, the lightness record. By determining the efficiency of different surfaces in a scene for reflecting light of a given wavelength, the brain builds a lightness record of that scene for that wavelength.* It is obvious that a lightness record can only be obtained by a comparative process. If the brain does not have a minimum of two surfaces to compare, it cannot compare reflectances and thus construct a lightness record of the scene. In such a case it will have to depend upon intensities reflected from one surface alone. In the above example, if the red and the green surfaces were to be viewed successively in the void mode, the only comparison that is available to the brain is that of the brightly lit patch against a dark background, no matter what the colour of the patch or its reflectance. The area will therefore have a high lightness in both conditions. Hence it would be impossible for the brain to say which area has a higher reflectance for long-wave light. The example given above is for long-wave and middle-wave light only. But short-wave (blue) light will also create its own, and different, lightness record, as will light of any given wavelength.

Even though it knows nothing about the reflectances of individual surfaces but can only register the amounts of light reflected from the two surfaces, the brain has nevertheless obtained information about the reflectance of the two surfaces for long-wave light by comparing the efficiency of the two surfaces for reflecting long-wave light. It has, in brief, gained a knowledge about certain unchanging physical characteristics of the surfaces.

Lightness records

When an entire multicoloured scene is viewed, each surface composing that scene will have a different lightness at every waveband, depending upon its efficiency for reflecting light of that waveband (Plate 11, facing p. 188). The record of that scene, in terms of areas which are lighter or darker, is called its *lightness record*. Since the reflectances of the different surfaces composing that scene never change, even if the intensity of the illuminating light changes, it follows that the lightness record of the entire scene will remain the same for that waveband, regardless of the intensity of the illuminating source. Of course ordinary daylight, as well as tungsten or fluorescent light, contains light of all wavelengths. And each set of wavelengths will produce a separate lightness record. Land's *retinex theory* supposes that what the brain does is to compare the lightness records of a scene, obtained simultaneously in each of three wavebands, regardless of the wavelength composition of the illuminating light and therefore regardless of the relative intensity of the lights of different wavebands. The result of that comparison is the construction of the colour of the surfaces by the brain. For example, in the scene illustrated in Plate 11, the red areas will have a high lightness for long-wave light and low lightnesses for middle- and short-wave light, while the green areas will have a high lightness for middle-wave light and low lightnesses for long- and short-wave light, and so on. Areas which have the lowest lightness for light of all wavebands will be registered as black; those which have the highest lightness will be registered as white, with the rest assuming a different colour depending upon their lightness, which is itself a correlate of their reflectance for lights of different waveband. *In short, colour is the end product of two comparisons: the first one consists of comparing the reflectance of different surfaces for light of the same waveband, thus generating the lightness record of the scene for that waveband, and the second consists of comparing the three lightness records of the scene for the different wavebands, thus generating the colour.*

Colour therefore is a comparison of comparisons. The retinex theory thus differs fundamentally from classical theories in that there is no mixture or addition, but comparison only. It is obvious that, since the lightness is independent of actual intensities and since colour itself is the comparison of the three lightness records, colour itself is also, to a large measure, independent of these intensities.

Now we can see that when the wavelength composition of the illumin-
ant (the light source) in which a surface is viewed is changed, the
intensities of light reflected from all surfaces in the display will
change, but the comparisons will remain the same because the reflec-
tances do not themselves change. Here then is a simple way in which
the brain can 'discount the illuminant'. This ability of the brain to
compare thus makes it independent of the total amount of light
reflected from any given area, since it is only interested in the amount of
light of any given waveband reflected from that area *in comparison*
with light of the same waveband reflected from surrounding areas.

The comparisons and their results are a property of the brain, not
of the world outside, even if all the information needed to undertake
the comparisons is contained in the world outside. Colour then also
becomes a property of the brain, a property with which it invests the
surfaces outside, an interpretation it gives to certain physical proper-
ties of objects (reflectance) and through which it gains a knowledge
about these physical properties. In doing so, it approximates its
interpretation to the true physical constants of surfaces as much as
possible, and therefore makes itself as independent as possible from
the changes in the wavelength composition of the light reflected
from any given area. It is no wonder that Land has said, 'Color is
always a consequence, never a cause'.[6]

Colour is always a consequence, never a cause, because there is no
prespecified wavelength composition (code) reflected from a surface
which would absolutely and uniquely specify the colour of that surface.
Many different wavelength compositions could lead to the perception
of the same colour as a result of the brain's ability to compare the
wavelength composition of the light reflected from that surface with
the wavelength composition of the light reflected from surrounding
surfaces. If there had been a prespecified code, in terms of wavelength
composition, then the brain need not undertake all this comparative
effort. It would be sufficient to endow the organism with a large
number of receptors, each one uniquely tuned to the specified code.
In fact, something very much like this appears to happen with the
sense of smell. An aroma depends upon a particular molecular configuration; unlike colour vision, changing that configuration changes
the aroma substantially. It is as if a particular molecular configuration
specifies uniquely the aroma. It is therefore not surprising to find that
there are many, perhaps thousands, of different smell receptors, each
with a protein structure designed to capture a particular, and more or
less unique, molecular structure.[7] Much of the perceptive work in
smell is therefore done by the receptors in the nose. This is in
contrast to colour vision, where much of the work is done in the
brain.

It is of course difficult to tell whether the interpretation that two different brains give to the same physical constants of surfaces are identical; difficult, in other words, to know whether, experientially, the red that you see is in every way identical to the red that I see. But it is almost certain that the interpretations are very similar. People understand what one means when one says that red is a 'warm' colour, even if they have not been thinking much about colour vision, and common experience tells us that we can use colour codes to convey the same meaning to different people. The subject would be a trite one were it not for the fact that it implies that the anatomical and physiological machinery that the brain uses to construct colours are broadly very similar between individuals. Thus, although we are here dealing with a problem of interpretation, it must be understood as being something a good deal more basic than what is meant by interpretation when it applies to music, for example. It is very simply a construct with which the brain invests certain physical attributes of surfaces and encapsulates its knowledge of them. Philosophers may well object to the use of knowledge in this context. Yet the nervous system assigns the colour red to an object which it knows to have a high reflectance for long-wave light and a low reflectance for lights of other wavebands. It is knowledge which serves it admirably well in its daily endeavours.

Algorithms for generating colours

Land has developed algorithms for how the comparisons can be implemented. The earlier one[8] is perhaps a little too unrealistic for a biological system, for it involves tracing as many as 200 paths to the chosen area of the multicoloured display, taking into account big jumps in reflected energies and discarding them if the differences are small. This is probably much too cumbersome a process for an instantaneous signalling mechanism. The more recent one[9] is physiologically more appealing. In it, the logarithm of the ratio of the light of a given waveband, reflected from a surface (the numerator), and the average of light of the same waveband, reflected from its surround (the denominator), is taken. This constitutes a designator at that waveband. Note the similarity with the receptive field arrangement of the kind of cells one encounters in the lateral geniculate nucleus (LGN) or in the primary visual cortex (V1), where cells have centres and surrounds. The difference is that, in the Land algorithm, the centre can be any size, as can the surround, whereas receptive field centres and surrounds are very limited in size. The process is done independently three times for the three wavebands and the result, entered on the three axes of a three-colour space, gives a remarkably accurate prediction of the colour of the surface. For example, the red surface of a multicoloured display will have a high lightness, and therefore a high designator, in long-wave light and low lightnesses, and therefore low designators, in middle- and short-wave light, while a green surface will have low lightnesses (and thus low designators) for long- and short-wave light and a high lightness (high designator) for middle-wave light.

Why is the spectrum coloured?

We can now begin our enquiry into colour vision in a different way. Instead of beginning with the assumption that a red surface looks red because it reflects more long-wave light, we can ask the question of *why long-wave light itself looks red*. The question is not trivial. Ever since the time of Newton, physicists have emphasized that light itself, consisting of electromagnetic radiation, has no colour. Newton had written, 'And if at any time I speak of light and rays as coloured or endued with Colours, I would be understood to speak not philosophically and properly, but grossly, and according to such conceptions as vulgar People in seeing all these Experiments would be apt to frame. For the Rays to speak properly are not coloured. In them there is nothing else than a certain power and disposition to stir up a sensation of this or that Colour'.[10] Why, then, does light of certain wavelengths look red and that of other wavelengths look green? It would obviously be satisfying to have an account which would apply with equal validity to the perception of a (red) surface that reflects light of all wavebands as red and to the perception of long-wave light uncontaminated by light of any other wavelength as red.

A red area of a multicoloured display looks light in long-wave light, dark in middle-wave light and dark in short-wave light. The nervous system thus assigns the colour red to it, just as it would to any area that shares the property of having a high lightness in long-wave light and low lightnesses in middle- and short-wave light. Now suppose that one looks at a patch illuminated with long-wave light in isolation, in the void viewing mode. The patch produces a high lightness for light of any waveband, since the only comparison that the brain can undertake in these conditions is a comparison of the light reflected from the illuminated patch and the dark surround. The long-wave light thus produces a high lightness while the middle- and short-wave light, being absent, produce no lightness at all. The nervous system thus assigns the colour red to the patch. Let us next look at a patch, once again viewed in isolation, and which is reflecting middle-wave light; it has a high lightness for middle-wave light and no lightness for the other two wavebands. The nervous system thus assigns the colour green to it, just as it would to any patch of a multicoloured display which has a high lightness in the middle-wave record and low lightnesses in the long- and short-wave records.

A slightly more complex situation obtains when the patch is illuminated with roughly equal intensities of light of all wavebands. The perceived colour of the patch is white or a very light grey. How can we account for this in terms of the above description? Recall that the only comparison that the brain can undertake in the void viewing mode is between the illuminated patch and the dark surround. This patch, now illuminated with light of all wavebands, produces a high lightness for each waveband. The nervous system thus assigns the colour white to it, just as it does to a part of the multicoloured display which has the highest lightness in each waveband. An apparently still more complex situation is one in which the patch, viewed in the void mode, is once again illuminated by light of all wavebands, but this time of unequal intensity. Let us suppose that it reflects a small amount of long-wave light and large amounts of middle- and short-wave light. The consequence is that it has a high lightness in all three wavebands, but the highest lightness in the middle and short wavebands. The nervous system thus assigns the colour turquoise to it, just as it does to any patch of a multicoloured display with the same lightness properties.

Colour is the result of comparisons

We thus see that there is no paradox at all. The assumption that there are constant colours and inconstant colours is, in a sense, a byproduct of the history of the subject in which most experiments were undertaken in the aperture or reduction screen mode. The latter in turn reflects the reductionist approach in science, one in which we seek to break down all phenomena to their elements. The brain itself only sees colours; it knows nothing about the sharp intellectual subdivision between constant and inconstant colours.

Notes and references

1 Hering, E. (1964). *Outlines of a Theory of the Light Sense,* translated by L.M. Hurvich & D. Jameson. Harvard University Press, Cambridge.
2 Helmholtz, H. von (1911). *Handbuch der Physiologischen Optik*, 2. Voss, Hamburg.
3 Land, E.H. (1985). Recent advances in retinex theory. In *Central and Peripheral Mechanisms of Colour Vision*, edited by D. Ottoson & S. Zeki, pp. 5–17. Macmillan, London.
4 Land, E.H. (1974). The retinex theory of colour vision. *Proc. R. Instn. G.B.* **47**, 23–58; Land, E.H. (1964). The retinex. *Sci. Am.* **52**, 247–264.
5 In practice, band pass filters have been used in many of these experiments. These pass a broader band of wavelengths than the narrow-band interference filters and it is common to refer to the waveband, by which is meant a band of wavelengths. But the identical results are obtained if interference filters are used instead. In more precise terms, the energies reflected are measured in milliwatts per steradian per metre square.
6 Land, E.H. (1985). Statement made by Land at a Stated Meeting at the American

Academy of Arts and Sciences, Stated Meeting Report, American Academy of Arts and Sciences, April 1985, pp. 7–8.

7 Buck, L. & Axel, R. (1991). A novel multigene family may encode odorant receptors: a molecular basis for odor recognition. *Cell* **65**, 175–187.

8 Land, E.H. & McCann, J.J. (1971). Lightness and retinex theory. *J. Opt. Soc. Am.* **61**, 1–11.

9 Land, E.H. (1983). Recent advances in retinex theory and some implications for cortical computations. *Proc. Natl. Acad. Sci. USA* **80**, 5163–5169.

10 Newton, I. (1704). *Opticks: Or, A Treatise of the Reflexions, Refractions, Inflexions and Colours of Light*. S. Smith and B. Walford, London.

Chapter 24: The cerebral cortex as a categorizer

Is colour vision that unique in principle or can we derive lessons from studying it which are applicable to all vision and, beyond, to the organ responsible for our seeing, namely the visual cortex? There is, in fact, a remarkable lesson to be learned from this study of colour vision, and one which does not figure prominently either in physiological studies or in cortical theories of visual representation, namely that *the function of the sensory parts of the cortex is to act as categorizers of the stimuli in our environment* — according to colour, texture, or sound, and so on. Categorization is, in a sense, the most fundamental problem that the visual cortex has to solve. It leads us to conceive of the visual cortex as a categorizer rather than as an analyzer.

The functions of the visual cortex

We should perhaps begin by asking what the function of the sensory parts of the cerebral cortex in general, and of the visual cortex in particular, is. To many, the answer is simple and straightforward: The auditory cortex allows us to hear, the olfactory cortex to smell, the sensory cortex to feel temperature and pressure and the visual cortex to see. But why do we need to see at all? The obvious answer is: to acquire knowledge about the world in which we live. The only knowledge that the brain is interested in relates to the fundamental, unchanging, properties of objects. It is not interested in the ever-changing information reaching it continually during the day from these objects. Indeed it does all it can to discard such fluctuating and inconsequential information, which is not the same thing as saying that the brain is not interested in change as such, since the latter may itself be the fundamental property of, say, a moving object. This preoccupation with fundamental features perhaps accounts for why it is that the brain has developed so complex and versatile a machinery with which to acquire knowledge through the sense of vision.

In the case of colour vision, acquiring a knowledge about the invariant properties of objects amounts to learning about their reflectances for lights of different wavebands. That knowledge can then be used to categorize the stimuli in our environment perceptually, the task of the category system being '...to provide the maximum information with the least cognitive effort'.[1] Moreover, 'To categorize a stimulus means to consider it, for purposes of that categorization, not only equivalent to other stimuli in the same category but also different from stimuli not in that category'.[1] In a garden on a windy day, when the shape of the vegetation is never static, one should be able to identify certain invariant features of form which allow one to categorize some objects as flowers, instantaneously and effortlessly. One can then (or simultaneously) identify other invariant features, the reflectances for lights of different wavebands, which the brain interprets as colours, and thus be able to categorize the flowers according to colour. Or, in a jungle, a monkey should be able to categorize fruits according to whether they are ripe or not, depending upon the colour, which in turn depends upon the invariant property of reflectance.

In order to be able to extract the invariant features of stimuli and thus categorize objects according to these invariant properties, the brain has evolved the not unreasonable strategy of using different compartments (cortical areas) to identify different invariant attributes of our environment, for example, touch and sound, quite simply because the cortical machinery required to extract the invariant features varies according to the property. The specializations seen in the visual cortex are nothing more than an extension of this strategy into the domain of vision, since the machinery required to extract the invariant features necessary to categorize objects according to colour are different from the machinery required to extract the invariant features which are necessary to categorize objects according to, say, motion. But in trying to identify the stimuli according to their invariant features the brain confronts a major problem, which is that the stimuli are never static, nor do they carry convenient codes or labels. This can be illustrated by many examples. To categorize objects as hot or cold one need not know the precise temperature, which indeed would never be constant. Knowledge of the precise temperature would demand a considerable cognitive effort, in the sense that it would demand access to a thermometer and the knowledge required to read it. But since colour vision is our main theme, we will give our main example from it. The wavelength composition of the light reflected from a surface varies continually, yet the brain is somehow capable of assigning a constant colour to the surface. We shall examine how the brain may achieve this feat in a subsequent chapter. Here, we want to consider this fundamental fact about the world around us in relation to physiological studies of the visual cortex.

To a large extent, physiological studies are static. A light is flashed onto the screen within the receptive field of a cell, or it is flashed off; or a line of a particular orientation may be flashed onto the receptive field of a cell and moved in different directions. Neither the intensity nor the wavelength composition of the stimulus changes during the period of stimulation. With colour studies it is common to flash light of a particular wavelength into the cell's receptive field, but very unusual to mix that light with light of other wavelengths.[2] This static, reductionist, approach is necessary because one wants to isolate the variables that stimulate a cell as much as possible. It is nevertheless from such studies that we have obtained our current picture of how the visual cortex 'analyzes' the visual world. In his book *The Ecological Approach to Visual Perception*[3] James Gibson tells us that the approach used by psychologists is not greatly different from the one used by physiologists and that the assumption is made '...that a picture is formed that can be transmitted to the brain...If the exposure period is made longer, the eye will scan the pattern to which it is exposed, fixating the parts in succession...The investigator assumes that each fixation of the eye is analogous to an exposure of the film in a camera, so that what the brain gets is something like a sequence of snapshots'.

Whether in the hands of the psychologists or the physiologists, there is a fundamental flaw in this approach, for the visual environment is in practice never static; it is usually in a continual state of flux. An object, for example, is commonly viewed from different angles and at different distances — indeed the distance at which it is viewed may, and commonly does, change continually. The pattern of retinal illumination produced by that object will consequently change from moment to moment. Put more simply, *objects in our visual world do not come with a convenient code according to, say, shape or colour, with the function of the visual cortex being nothing more than that of deciphering or analyzing that code.* The word analyze, so commonly used in the physiological and psychological literature alike, itself reveals a powerful misconception about what the visual brain does. To analyze implies to break down, to decompose. Indeed the term is defined in the *Oxford English Dictionary* as, 'To take to pieces, to separate, distinguish or ascertain the elements of anything complex' and analysis is defined as, 'The resolution of anything complex into its simple elements'. The visual cortex is then deemed to 'analyze' the visual image formed on the retina or, more simply still, to analyze the visual environment. The point-to-point connections between the retina and the primary visual cortex no doubt reinforce strongly this notion. But the function of the visual cortex is a good deal more complex and profound than that. To repeat, what the visual cortex has to do is acquire a knowledge about the world through vision and thus be able to *categorize* or classify *objects and surfaces according to vision.* Analysis is a first and important part of this process but the result of an analysis cannot by itself categorize the object. The critical step is for the brain to extract the invariant features of the objects and surfaces in the visual environment from the ever-changing information that is reaching it because '...one purpose of categorization is to reduce the infinite differences among stimuli to behaviorally and cognitively usable proportions'.[1] To do so, the brain must assemble or collate information from large parts of the field of view, not break down a stimulus into its components, but compare its various features to extract its constants for the purpose of categorization. The next step is to generate the constructs which can then be used in the perceptual categorization. How the cerebral cortex is able to achieve this is by no means clear. Indeed, it is not always clear what the invariants are. But colour vision provides good clues to the general principle underlying the operations of the cerebral visual cortex in this process.

Let us consider first what happens when, in studying colour vision, we use the reductionist, analytic, approach, and try to 'break-down' the colour of a surface that forms part of a complex scene into its components. We choose a complex scene for the obvious reason that most scenes in our natural visual environment are complex and the colours in them form part of this complex scene. An obvious way of 'breaking-down' the colour of a given surface is to 'analyze' the wavelength composition of the light reflected from it alone. Let us take as an example the green surface of a colour Mondrian referred to in the previous experiment and suppose that our analysis shows it to reflect 60, 30 and 10 units of long-, middle- and short-wave light respectively (see p. 231). We are naturally interested in analyzing this surface alone, and we can therefore dispense with the rest of the display, in other words view the green area in the void mode. We find, perhaps surprisingly from the viewpoint of an analytic doctrine, that the area looks white. In the process of trying to break down the stimulus into its components, we have actually managed to get rid, at least perceptually, of the colour of the surface, the very attribute which we wanted to 'analyze'. Now the most detailed measurement of the wavelength composition of the light reflected from that surface will not be able to tell what colour the brain will assign to it when it is part of the complex scene.

The general point that this experiment illustrates is that the most detailed analysis of the properties of a surface is useless unless the brain can subsequently compare the result of that analysis with its analysis of the same properties for adjacent surfaces. We shall see in the next chapter how the brain may undertake such a task in colour vision. But this general strategy is not limited to colour vision. The brain has to undertake a comparison continually in constructing all the other attributes of vision. *Thus, far from analyzing the visual image by breaking it down into its components, the brain constructs the visual image by relating the analyzed components to each other and thus extracting the invariant features of objects. These are both stages in the perceptual categorization of objects according to vision, which is what a primary function of the visual cortex is.*

Notes and references

1 Rosch, E. (1978). Principles of categorization. In *Cognition and Categorization*, edited by E. Rosch & B. Lloyd, pp. 27—48. Erlbaum (Lawrence) Associates, London.

2 Physiological studies in colour vision in which a stimulus is continually varied in terms of wavelength composition are rare. Two examples are, Zeki, S. (1983). Colour coding in the cerebral cortex. The reaction of cells in monkey visual cortex to wavelengths and colours. *Neurosci.* **9**, 741—756; Derrington, A.M., Krauskopf, J. & Lennie, P. (1984). Chromatic mechanisms in lateral geniculate nucleus of macaque. *J. Physiol. (Lond.)* **357**, 241—265.

3 Gibson, J.J. (1986). *The Ecological Approach to Visual Perception*. Erlbaum Associates, Hillsdale.

Chapter 25: The retinex theory and the organization of the colour pathways in the brain

Edwin Land used the term *retinex* to describe his theory because he was uncertain of where the critical comparisons resulting in the construction of colour by the brain would be undertaken, although it is now almost certain that they are done in the cortex. The retinex theory came in for a good deal of criticism. There were several reasons for this. The publicity given to Land's early work in magazines such as *Fortune*[1] led to some resentment among scientists who believed, no doubt sincerely, that their much more quantitative work deserved as much, if not more, publicity. The original framing of the findings in terms which suggested that Land's work and ideas had discredited the findings of Newton and Young caused even greater resentment among scientists who had failed to see the originality in Land's work.[2] There was the inevitable argument about priority,[3] with scientists claiming that one of the tenets of Land's theory — that there is a good deal more to colour vision than the activation of specific photoreceptors in the retina by lights of specific wavelength — had already been iterated and reiterated many times. Thomas Young had alluded to it, as had Chevreul, as had Helmholtz, as had Hering, as had many others who had thought about the subject at all. Indeed, even mathematical formulations had been developed to describe the dependence of the colour of a patch upon surrounding surfaces.

These arguments have done nothing to advance the science of colour. Land (Figure 25.1) brought to an intellectual focus a fundamental problem in colour vision, namely *why surfaces and objects retain their colour in spite of wide-ranging changes in the wavelength and energy composition of the light reflected from them*. By labelling this phenomenon 'colour constancy', colour scientists had traditionally treated it more as a 'fancy that' phenomenon and a departure from the more fundamental condition, as they saw it, in which there is a simple and obvious relationship between the colour of a surface and the wavelength composition of the light reflected from it. While paying lip service to the former, their attention was absorbed with the latter. The extent to which this was so is obvious from the fact that most colour science has dealt with the colour of a point or a small area in visual space, and only more recently (in the last decade) has the problem of colour in the natural image assumed greater importance. This is not to detract from the enormous contributions made by classical theory to our understanding of the retinal mechanisms in-

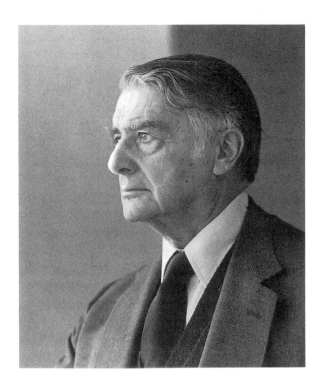

Fig. 25.1 Edwin Land (1909–1991), the American inventive genius and originator of the retinex theory. Was fond of saying that 'there are no second-rate brains in colour vision'. (Photograph by Naomi Savage, courtesy of H. Perry and J. Scarpetti, Rowland Institute, Cambridge, Mass.)

volved in colour and the nature of the inherited colour blindnesses. With this success there also developed a tendency, however, to equate wavelength directly with colour and to try to account for colour vision in general in terms of retinal mechanisms alone, with cortical mechanisms playing a subsidiary role, vaguely defined as the 'unconscious inference' or 'judgement' or 'memory'.

The organization of the visual pathways perpetuated a false view of colour vision

There is perhaps yet another reason, which is rarely advanced, though it is difficult to believe that it did not play a fairly fundamental role in supposing that the brain analyzes and thus determines the colour of a surface by determining the colour of every point in it by an additive mechanism, that is, by gauging the *amounts* of long-, middle- and short-wave light reflected from each point. The reason is to be found in the anatomical connections between the eye and the brain (Figure 25.2). These are organized topographically, with every point in the retina connecting to a corresponding point in the primary visual cortex which, until the last two decades, was considered to be the sole visual perceptive cortex and remains perhaps, even today, the most extensively studied part of the visual cortex. How natural then to assume that the colour of every point is determined independently

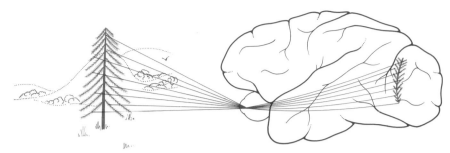

from the rest, by this additive mechanism in the primary visual cortex. Such a supposition would, at any rate, have appeared much less certain if it had been known that there are other visual areas besides the striate cortex, that one of them is specialized for colour while others are specialized for other attributes of vision and that, in the former the retina is not represented in a precise point-to-point manner, but relatively crudely. In an important sense, little recognized by physiologists and unacknowledged by psychophysicists, it was the developments in cortical studies that impressed upon them the importance of studying colour in the natural mode, and attracted their attention to the retinex theory and other, similar, theories. Before that time, most physiologists and psychophysicists were a good deal more concerned with studying colour coming from a point, whereas now an increasing number of scientists, particularly those concerned with neural computation and artificial intelligence, are turning their attention to the problem of how the nervous system uses surface reflectance to assign colours to surfaces. One may be tempted to trace the cause of this to the demonstration of functional specialization, especially one for colour, and the demonstration that the maps in other visual areas are not so neatly arranged as the map in the primary visual cortex. It is likely that this demonstration was the trigger for the questions, 'why should colour be computed separately from the other attributes of vision' and 'how can the brain compute the colour if it needs more than one visual area to do it in?' The real truth is that, more than such specific questions, functional specialization introduced a new way of thinking about what the cortex does. And it made it legitimate to consider problems which, in the day of Helmholtz, were given labels such as judgement and learning, but which today can perhaps be more easily understood in terms of the anatomical connections and physiological properties of particular groups of cells.

Land's theory was in the nature of a computational theory, and included an implementation of how the brain could 'discount the illuminant'. It is for this reason that, in his book, David Marr has described Land's work as the only real attempt at a theory of colour vision, while the others have been descriptions of it.[4] In Land's theory the colour of a point viewed on its own and of a patch which forms part of a complex scene are accounted for by the same laws (see Chapter 23). There is no need to postulate separate elaborate mechanisms such as learning and memory to account for 'colour constancy' as opposed to colour inconstancy. There is, in brief, much that is of interest in Land's theory and techniques for anyone interested in cortical mechanisms underlying colour vision. What is much less certain is whether the brain uses the same implementation procedure as that envisaged by Land to assign colours to surfaces.

The retinex channels and the cone channels

To what extent does the retinex theory correspond to the known physiological facts? Land has supposed that there are three channels, the retinex channels, whose spectral sensitivities correspond loosely to those of the three cone pigments. Each channel is capable of generating a separate lightness record of the visual scene. These three channels are kept separate until the comparison site where they are compared, not mixed.

Each cone type has a pigment which is responsive to considerable parts of the visible spectrum but has a maximal sensitivity at only one part (Figure 25.3). There is a high degree of overlap between the wavelength sensitivity curves of the three pigments and, in particular, between the long- and middle-wave pigments. The consequence is that light of any given wavelength, especially towards the long end of the spectrum, will bleach both the long- and middle-wave pigments. And, given that the two pigments are identical in shape and offset at their peaks by no more than 40 nm, there would be a high degree of correlation between what the channels are transmitting. In other words, an intense long-wave light will bleach both the long-wave and the middle wave pigments. But once bleached, there would be no way of telling the wavelength of the light which induced the bleach. This

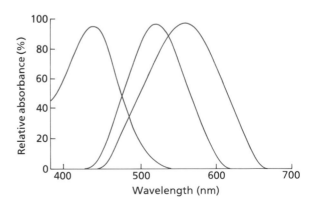

Fig. 25.3 The efficiency with which each of the three cone types absorbs light of different wavelengths.

finding is enshrined in the *principle of univariance*, enunciated by William Rushton,[5] which really states that the pigments differ only in the efficiency with which they can capture lights of different wavelength, that long-wave pigments are more efficient at capturing longer wavelength light but can be induced to capture as much middle-wavelength light by increasing the intensity of the latter by appropriate amounts, and that once a reaction has been set up in the cones one cannot tell the wavelength of the light that initiated the response.

One way of de-correlating the message, and thus increasing the efficiency of transmission, is to render subsequent cells responsive to narrower, or non-overlapping, segments of the visible spectrum. This is done by a system of opponency, whereby an input from one set of cones is opposed by an input from another set of cones, thus leading to cells with narrower wavelength selectivities. Thus the long-wave cones may provide an excitatory input to a subsequent cell in the retina and the middle-wave cones an inhibitory input to the same cell. All the evidence points to the retina itself as the site of this interaction[6] (Plate 12, facing p. 188). The mixing that occurs is not haphazard. The long-wave cones are opposed by middle-wave cones so that a cell may give an ON response to long-wave light and an OFF response to middle-wave light, or vice versa. Such cells are commonly, and mistakenly, referred to as red−green cells. Mistakenly, because implicit in the terminology is the supposition that their reactions themselves lead to the perception of a surface as red or green, a cultural inheritance from the past. As we shall see, this supposition is doubtful. However that may be, and whatever the polarity of the responses, it is through this system of opponency that the range of wavelengths to which a cell will respond with a given polarity is rendered much narrower than that of the cones from which it receives its input. In another group of cells, the long- plus middle-wave cones are opposed by the short-wave cones (Plate 12). The cells will therefore respond with one polarity to short-wave light and an opposite polarity to long- plus middle-wave light. It is obvious that the opponent sensitivities are not equally broad, since the cell in the above example will respond with a given polarity to a large segment of the visible spectrum and with the opposite polarity to a much narrower segment. Such cells are commonly, but again mistakenly, referred to as the yellow−blue cells, since long- plus middle-wave light is commonly thought to be equivalent to red plus green, which gives yellow. A third group of retinal cells receive excitatory inputs from all three types of cone and thus respond maximally when all three cones are excited, that is, they respond best to white light. Opponency, by generating cells with narrower wavelength sensitivities (action spectra) also generates cells with much greater efficiency of coding,[7] in that changes in the intensity of light of a given waveband are much less likely to alter the sensitivity of the cell, since it would not be responsive outside a narrow limit of wavebands. By contrast, changes in intensity of long-wave light would not only excite the long-wave cones but also middle-wave cones, and the greater the intensity of the long-wave light, the greater will be the response of the middle-wave cones. Physiologically, there is therefore little reason to suppose that the output of the cones are kept separate. Beyond the retina, however, there seems to be little further mixture or sharpening of spectral sensitivities,[8] so that the channels that actually feed into the comparator site in the cortex can well be considered to be separate after the retinal stage. Land was therefore right in supposing that the channels which input into the comparison site are not mixed, but he was probably wrong in equating those channels with the cone channels.

The colour channels

How many colour channels are there? Land supposed that there are three and equated these with the three cones postulated by Young and by Helmholtz and demonstrated by spectrophotometric measurements. Does the mixture through opponency, described above, alter the number of channels? It depends on how one looks at it. If one looks at the distribution of the peak sensitivities of the wavelength-selective cells, whether in the optic nerve or the lateral geniculate nucleus (LGN) or the cortex, one finds that it encompasses almost the entire visible spectrum.[9] One could naturally divide these into groups corresponding to long-wave, middle-wave and short-wave groups, as long as it is understood that each may comprise several subgroups. An alternative way of looking at it is to say that there are two times three, or six, channels corresponding to the opponent long−middle (red−green), long plus middle versus short (yellow−blue), and long plus middle plus short versus their absence (white−black). It so happens that these six channels (or three, depending on how one looks at it) correspond rather well to the psychophysical axes of colour established by the German physiologist Ewald Hering and his American successors, Leo Hurvich and Dorothea Jameson.[9] These are the red−green, blue−yellow and black−white pairings, the pairings that have been described as the ones that cannot live with each other and yet cannot live without each other. For a colour cannot be red and green simultaneously, nor can it be yellow and blue, nor black and white (Plate 12, part (b)). And yet, when we look at a red surface for a few seconds and then look at a neutral white or light grey surface, the after-image is green (or vice versa); the after-image of yellow is blue and the after-image of white is black. This is, in a sense, another instance in which the brain 'goes beyond the information given'. For there is no physical law which dictates that certain wavelengths should be opposed only by certain other wavelengths.

Wavelength opponency and colour opponency

The fact that long-wave light excites some cells selectively and also produces the sensation of red, whose after-image is bluish green, the very part of the spectrum that produces an opponent response from the same cell, might tempt one to explain the well-documented opponent colour perceptions in terms of the responses of these cells. But the explanation is not quite so straightforward. In the first place, if such cells themselves determined colour perceptions directly, there would be no need for additional cortical stations dealing with colour. Colour could be determined at the retina or at the striate cortex, the remaining cortical stations being necessary for nothing more than the interpretation, whatever that may mean. In fact, we can conduct perceptual experiments to show that colour opponency does not necessarily correspond to wavelength opponency.[10] Take a colour Mondrian and arrange things such that its green surface reflects more long-wave than middle-wave light. Let us make it that it reflects twice the amount of long-wave than of middle-wave light. Under these conditions, the green surface will look green, even though it is reflecting more long-wave light (see above). When one looks at this green surface for a few seconds and then shifts one's gaze to a neutral, white, surface, the after-image is red. Had the perception been the direct consequence of the responses of the kind of opponent cell described above, the after-image should have been green, since the cell would have been excited by the excess of long-wave light coming from the green surface. Or take a blue surface and arrange things such that the blue surface reflects more long- and middle-wave light than short-wave light, although it still looks blue. If one looks at the blue surface for a few seconds and then looks at a neutral screen, the after-image is yellow. In other words, it would seem that the after-images are generated *after* the colour itself is generated. From which we conclude that *the responses of the narrow-band opponent channels do not correspond directly to the sensation of colour*. Rather, these are the input channels to the postulated comparison site. We can therefore conclude that the input channels do not correspond to the cones. Rather, the outputs of the cones are mixed to create separate, narrow-band channels which must be the equivalent of the retinex channels. These are kept separate until they input into the comparator site.

Where are the lightnesses generated?

In the retinex system, before the colours are generated, the lightnesses must be generated, since it is the comparison of the three lightness records that results in colour. How is this done in the brain, if indeed the brain uses a lightness system as postulated by Land? The answer is that no one really knows. To generate a lightness record of a scene in, say, long-wave light, the brain has to collate information from large parts of the field of view, accepting big changes in brightness and rejecting small differences, and thus registering the relative brightnesses of surfaces in long-wave light. It could do this in stages, but the very minimal requirement to undertake such a task would be a wavelength-differencing stage, in which a cell would have two separate parts to its receptive field, one part of which is excited by long-wave light and a surrounding part which is inhibited by it. In fact, the first stage at which one encounters cells which have both a wavelength specificity and a spatially antagonistic organization is in the LGN. But their properties are disappointing in this respect and no one knows what their function is in terms of colour computations, which indeed suggests that the implementation used by the nervous system to generate colours is somewhat different from what we might believe. These cells give an ON response to long-wave light in the centre and an ON response to middle-wave light in the surround (Plate 13, part (a), facing p. 188), and could not therefore act as a wavelength-differencing system for a given wavelength of light.

The first cells which can genuinely act as a wavelength-differencing system are the double-opponent cells (Plate 13, part (b)), first discovered in the retina of the goldfish,[11] though in the monkey they are first encountered in V1. These cells have a complex functional structure. They have spatially antagonistic centres and surrounds and give an ON response to long-wave light and an OFF response to middle-wave light in the centre and a response of the opposite polarity in the surround. They are therefore well placed to detect the difference in long-wave light between centre and surround. But their receptive fields are much too small. They can therefore undertake such a computation for only very small parts of the field of view. It is, however, interesting to note that these cells ultimately connect to area V4, in a convergent fashion, with the result that the recipient cells in V4 have much larger receptive fields. This, in turn, confers on the latter the ability to undertake a wavelength differencing over much larger regions of the field of view. But this is still hypothetical, and no one really knows how, where and in how many stages the lightness records are generated.

Where is the comparison site?

Wherever they may be generated, the lightness records must be compared to generate the colours, at least in the Land system. Land himself was not certain where the comparison site would be, which is why he coined the term retinex. It is unlikely to be in the retina. The receptive fields of retinal cells are much too small (commonly less than 1°) and such lateral interactions that occur there are limited. The colour system demands that information coming from large parts of the field of view should be compared. What we mean by large cannot be quantified precisely but, in general, anything within 10° of the border of a surface can influence the colour of that surface. Physiological evidence reviewed in the next chapter shows that the earliest possible site is area V4 of the cortex. But there is an experiment,[12] performed after the physiological experiments to be described, which suggests strongly that the comparison site cannot be earlier than V4, assuming that the human brain is similar to that of the macaque monkey.

The experiment is one conducted on normal subjects and on a patient whose corpus callosum (see Chapter 18) had been sectioned to prevent the interhemispheric generalization of epileptic attacks. Recall that when a surface is viewed in the void mode, its colour depends on the wavelength composition of the light reflected from it alone. When, without changing the wavelength composition of the light reflected from that surface, the surround is brought into view, the colour of the surface changes immediately. This is because the brain is now able to compare the wavelength composition of the light coming from that surface with what is coming from surrounding surfaces. In general, the introduction of a surround at a distance of about 7° will alter the colour of the (void) surface. Because the two halves of the brain are connected through the corpus callosum in the normal human subject, the change in the colour of the void surface will occur even if the void surface is presented to one hemi-field and the surround to the other (Plate 14, facing p. 188). But the results are very different in a patient with a severed corpus callosum. Here, if the void is shown to one hemi-field and the surround to the opposite hemi-field, with a separation of no more than 3.7° between the two, the colour of the void surface does not change when the surround is brought in, though it will if the two components are shown in the same hemi-field at the same physical separation. One can conclude therefore that the integrity of the corpus callosum is necessary for the comparison to occur when the two components are presented to the separate hemi-fields.

The interpretation of the experiment in terms of the comparator site in the cortex depends upon a knowledge of the anatomy and physiology of the visual areas in the cerebral cortex (see Chapters 12 and 18). Of the cerebral areas that could be involved, V1 and V2 have wavelength-selective cells, but the callosal fibres connecting them with their counterparts in the opposite hemisphere are limited to the representation of $1-2°$ of the vertical meridian and hence are not extensive enough to connect regions beyond.[13] Areas V3 and V3A are not concerned with colour.[14] The first area to be concerned with colour and to have callosal connections capable of uniting field representations in excess of $5°$ is V4.[13,15] It follows that this is the first possible site of the comparison postulated in the retinex theory. It is a good illustration of what an ingenious experiment can do, and yet another illustration of the many insights into the organization of the cerebral hemispheres that the corpus callosum has given us.

References

1 Bello, F. (1959). An astonishing new theory of color. *Fortune* **59**, 144–206.

2 Walls, G.L. (1960). 'Land! Land!' *Psychol. Bull.* **57**, 29–48.

3 Judd, D.B. (1960). Appraisal of Land's work on two-primary color projections. *J. Opt. Soc. Am.* **50**, 254–268.

4 Marr, D. (1982). *Vision.* MIT Press, Cambridge.

5 Naka, K.-I. & Rushton, W.A.H. (1966). An attempt to analyse colour reception by electrophysiology. *J. Physiol. (Lond.)* **185**, 556–586.

6 Monasterio, F.M. de, Gouras, P. & Tolhurst, D.J. (1975). Trichromatic colour opponency in ganglion cells of the rhesus monkey retina. *J. Physiol. (Lond.)* **251**, 197–216.

7 Buchsbaum, G. & Gottschalk, A. (1983). Trichromacy, opponent colours coding and optimum colour information transmission in the retina. *Proc. R. Soc. Lond.* B **220**, 89–113.

8 Michael, C.R. (1978). Color-sensitive complex cells in monkey striate cortex. *J. Neurophysiol.* **41**, 1250–1266; Zeki, S. (1980). The representation of colours in the cerebral cortex. *Nature* **284**, 412–418.

9 Hering, E. (1964). *Outlines of a Theory of the Light Sense*, translated by L.M. Hurvich & D. Jameson. Harvard University Press, Cambridge; Hurvich, L.M. (1985). Opponent-colours theory. In *Central and Peripheral Mechanisms of Colour Vision*, edited by D. Ottoson & S. Zeki, pp. 61–82. Macmillan, London; Jameson, D. (1985). Opponent-colours theory of the light of physiological finding. In *Central and Peripheral Mechanisms of Colour Vision*, edited by D. Ottoson & S. Zeki, pp. 83–102. Macmillan, London.

10 Zeki, S. (1983). Colour coding in the cerebral cortex: The reaction of cells in monkey visual cortex to wavelengths and colours. *Neuroscience* **9**, 741–765.

11 Daw, N.W. (1984). The psychology and physiology of colour vision. *Trends Neurosci.* **7**, 330–335.

12 Land, E.H., Hubel, D.H., Livingstone, M.S., Perry, S.H. & Burns, M.S. (1983). Colour-generating interactions across the corpus callosum. *Nature* **303**, 616–618.

13 Whitteridge, D. (1965). Area 18 and the vertical meridian of the visual field. In *Functions of the Corpus Callosum*, edited by E.G. Ettlinger, pp. 115–120. Churchill, London; Zeki, S.M. (1970). Interhemispheric connections of prestriate cortex in monkey. *Brain Res.* **19**, 63–75; Zeki, S.M. (1977). Colour coding in the superior temporal sulcus of rhesus monkey visual cortex. *Proc. R. Soc. Lond.* B **197**, 195–223; Van Essen, D.C. & Zeki, S.M. (1978). The topographic organization of rhesus monkey prestriate cortex. *J. Physiol. (Lond.)* **277**, 193–266.

14 Zeki, S. (1978). Uniformity and diversity of structure and function in rhesus monkey prestriate visual cortex. *J. Physiol. (Lond.)* **277**, 273–290.

15 Zeki, S. (1990). Colour vision and functional specialisation in the visual cortex. *Disc. Neurosci.* **6**, 7–64.

Chapter 26: The physiology of the colour pathways

Let us suppose for a moment that there is a straightforward relationship between the wavelength selectivity of a cell and the sensation of colour. There are obvious attractions in such a supposition. After all, when we shine long-wave (red) light onto a screen, we perceive its colour to be red. When we find that that same long-wave light excites a cell, whereas white light or light of other wavelengths does not, we are obviously attracted to the notion that the responses of the cell correspond to the sensation of red. If we subscribe to the doctrine that the colour of a surface is determined uniquely by the wavelength composition of the light reflected from it, we can then even be tempted to jump to the conclusion that this is a cell that codes for red. It is, however, worth testing the proposition.

The Mondrian experiment on single cells

We return now to the standard electrophysiological experiment, described in earlier chapters, in which the responses of single cells in the intact brain are recorded and their reaction to visual stimuli presented on a screen are studied. The difference is that, for this experiment, the stimulus and the 'detectors' are a little more elaborate. The stimulus consists of a multicoloured Mondrian display, in which the squares are of the size of the cells' receptive fields. As with the perceptual experiments described before, the display is illuminated by three projectors, one passing long-wave light, the second middle-wave light and the third short-wave light only. The intensities from each projector can be adjusted and a telephotometer can register the amount of light of any wavelength reflected from any surface of the display. The set-up, in brief, is identical to the Land experiment described earlier (see Chapter 23). A cell can only respond to what is in its receptive field by increasing or decreasing its electrical discharge. It can obviously not 'report' the colour of the stimulus in its field. Nor can the telephotometer, which can only give information on the intensities of lights of different wavebands reflected from the surface in the cell's receptive field. To assign a colour to the surface in the receptive field, a normal human observer with good colour vision is therefore needed. He can then tell what the colour of the patch was when illuminated with lights of different wavelength composition, and when the cell was or was not responding to it. It is only he, in other words a conscious person, who can tell whether the responses of the cell correspond to or correlate with his perception of the colour of the surface. As we shall see, the 'detectors' — the cell, the tele-photometer and the human observer — form a sort of *ménage à trois*, a *ménage* in which strange alliances are formed, depending upon the kind of cell one is recording from.

Let us begin by studying the responses of a cell in area V1[1] (Plate 15, part (a), facing p. 188). The cell is found to have a small receptive field and to respond only when long-wave (red) light is flashed in that field. It is unresponsive to light of other wavelengths and also unresponsive to white light. We can plot its wavelength-sensitivity curve (its action spectrum) by studying the minimum intensity of light of every wavelength to which it will give a response at some arbitrary criterion, say 50% of the flashes. This shows us that the cell is unresponsive to middle- or short-wave light even at the highest intensities available.

Now, when we put the red area of the Mondrian display in the cell's receptive field and ensure that it is illuminated with the standard triplet of energies (i.e. it is reflecting 60, 30 and 10 units of long-, middle- and short-wave light respectively), we find that the cell responds vigorously when all three projectors are switched on simultaneously (Plate 15, part (a)). Next, we put an area of another colour, say green, in the cell's receptive field and illuminate the green area with the same triplet of energies, only to find that it gives an equally good response to the green area. When we put the blue, white and grey areas in the cell's receptive field, and illuminate each in turn with the same triplet of energies, we find that it responds to each with more or less the same vigour. *But when these different areas are put in the cell's receptive field and illuminated in this way, they differ in colour to the human observer. The cell is therefore unable to distinguish the colour of the surface in its receptive field, and its responses correspond with the reading on the telephotometer.* In fact, its responses correspond to the presence and intensity of long-wave light. This can be demonstrated easily, merely by switching off the long-wave light when the cell's response ceases. In this instance, then, the telephotometer and the cell are in alliance against the human observer, who reports that the different patches put in the cell's receptive field differ in colour.

We can now repeat the above experiment, but this time ensure that each area, when put in the receptive field, is seen alone, both by the cell and the human observer. In this void condition, the cell responds precisely as it did when the area in its receptive field formed part of the multicoloured display, i.e. it responds to each area with equal vigour. Here the three detectors in this *ménage à trois* are in full agreement. The cell responds to each area with equal vigour, the telephotometer registers the identical triplet of energies coming from each area and the human observer reports each area, viewed in the void mode, to be identical in colour (a very light grey). *Thus this cell, and many others like it, cannot be registering the colour of the stimulus, a finding which sheds some doubt on the concept that the colour of a surface is analyzed by the primary visual cortex. We should therefore rather think of cells in V1 as analyzing the wavelength composition of the light reflected from surfaces.*

Experiments with colour-opponent cells

This last inference becomes more emphatic when we consider, next, the responses of a colour-opponent cell in V1.[1] This cell gives an ON response to short-wave (blue and bluish-green) light and an OFF response to long-wave (red) light (Plate 15, part (b)). We might begin by supposing, therefore, that it is the kind of cell that underlies our perception of opponent colours, since the opponent of bluish-green is red. When we put a blue area in the cell's receptive field and illuminate the display in such a way that the blue area is reflecting the standard triplet of energies (i.e. 60, 30 and 10 units of long-, middle- and short-wave light respectively) and looks blue to a human observer, we find that the cell does not respond when the lights are switched ON, but only when they are switched OFF. This may seem surprising, since one would a priori expect the cell to give an ON response to the blue area. It can be accounted for by the fact that the blue area is reflecting a lot more long-wave (red) light than it is reflecting middle- or short-wave light, wavelengths to which the cell actually gives an OFF response. To confirm that it is the wavelength composition, not the colour, that determines the responses of this cell, we next arrange for the blue area to reflect more short-wave light than middle- or long-wave light. Let us make it reflect 50 units of short-wave light and 25 units each of middle- and long-wave light. We now find that the area in the cell's receptive field still looks blue to the human observer, but that this time the cell gives an ON response when the projectors are switched on. We get the identical results when we repeat the above experiment in the void mode, that is we ensure that the blue area alone is in the cell's receptive field.

We can now go a step further and ask the question: Since the responses of this cell are dependent upon wavelength composition alone, and not upon colour, can we make it give an ON *and* an OFF response to an area of *any* colour by simply adjusting the wavelength composition of the light reflected from its surface? The answer is yes. The cell described above, and other cells like it, can be made to give an ON or an OFF response to a green, yellow, white, orange or any other surface, depending whether long-wave light is in excess of the light reflected from it. It would thus appear that the responses of cells such as the ones described above cannot be correlated directly with our experience of colour. Something more must happen.

The responses of the double-opponent cells

The initial stage in the implementation of a Land-type algorithm is a wavelength-differencing stage, in which the intensity of light of a given waveband, say long-wave, reflected from one part of the field of view is compared with the intensity of light of the same waveband reflected from another part. The minimum neural requirement to achieve this would be a cell which is able to compare the amount of light of a given waveband, say long-wave light, reflected from one part of its receptive field and light of the same waveband reflected from surrounding parts (see Chapter 25). It should, in brief, be one with a spatially antagonistic surround, the cell giving an ON response to long-wave light in one part of its receptive field and an OFF response in the spatially antagonistic region.

The simplest cell which is able to undertake this task is the double-opponent cell, discovered in the goldfish retina.[2] It is interesting to study the responses of such a cell to areas of different colour.[3] Plate 16 (facing p. 188) shows the responses of a double-opponent cell which gave an ON response to long-wave light and an OFF response to middle-wave light in the centre and the opposite type of response in the surround. Detailed study of the properties of this cell shows that, to respond, it requires a minimum difference in the amount of long-wave light and middle-wave light reflected from its centre and surround. With this stipulation, it is indifferent to the colour of the area in its receptive field. Thus, the cell gave a good response to a red, white, light grey, brown or yellow area in a green surround when each was made to reflect 50, 18 and 6 units of long-, middle- and short-wave light respectively. Under these conditions the surround was obviously reflecting a good deal less of the long-wave light than was the centre. In each case a neutral point could be found when the difference in the amount of long- and middle-wave light reflected from the centre and the surround was such that the cell did not respond, *even if such variations did not change the colour of the areas*. On the other hand, if a white surround was substituted for the green one, the cell's response was greatly reduced.

It is interesting to consider what the common feature was between all the stimuli to which the cell gave a response, since it is obviously not to the colour, and what the different feature was when the cell's response was much reduced. If one were to illuminate a red, white, brown, yellow and light grey area against a green background with long-wave light only (Plate 16), one would find that the green background (which has a low efficiency for reflecting long-wave light) will look dark, whereas the central area will look light (since all the areas with the colours enumerated above have a higher efficiency for reflecting long-wave light). It follows that this is a relatively simple lightness record and that the responses of the cell described above correlate well with a difference in the reflectance of long-wave light between one region and surrounding regions. On the other hand, when the red (or yellow or grey) area is surrounded by white, which has a higher reflectance for long-wave light, the entire scene looks very light, and hence the cell will not respond since it is only interested in differences of sufficient magnitude for a given wavelength between one part of the receptive field and surrounding parts. *It further follows therefore that the double-opponent cell described above, and other similar cells, may be the first stage in the local wavelength differencing which leads to the generation of lightnesses. This must be a first, or initial, stage because, given the small size of the receptive fields of such cells, it is obvious that the wavelength differencing is done at a very local, rather than a global, level.*

In fact, these are not the only kind of wavelength-selective cells to be found in area V1. Another kind of cell, the pseudo double-opponent cell,[4] is one which has a centre receptive-field organization very much like the double-opponent cell described above, but a surround in which light of all wavebands inhibits the cell. It is obvious that such cells would not act as a wavelength-differencing stage for any one given waveband, but for all wavebands. What the role of such cells may be is not clear. There are, moreover, double-opponent cells in area V2[5] but their responses have not been studied in sufficient detail for one to be able to tell whether they are similar to the responses of the counterparts in V1.

The responses of colour cells

Wavelength-selective cells whose responses correlate with the human perception of colours are to be found in area V4,[1] which is not the same thing as saying that all wavelength-selective cells there have this property. But a sufficient number do to suggest that a radical transformation occurs when one moves from areas V1 and V2 to V4. Recall that V4 receives an input from the region of foveal representation in V1, but that its main input is from V2. The input from V2 to V4 is convergent, in that several thin stripes in V2 project to a given small region of V4 (see Chapter 19). If we examine a cell in V4 whose spectral sensitivity profile is very similar to the one which we studied in V1, we will find that there is nevertheless a radical difference between them, not obvious to a more or less casual inspection with spectral lights alone. The sensitivity profile of the cell shows it to be responsive to long-wave or red light only (Plate 17, facing p. 188). When we put a red area, the size of the receptive field, of a multicoloured Mondrian in the receptive field of the cell and illuminate it with the standard triplet of energies, we find that the cell gives a good response to the stimulus. The surprise comes when we put areas of other colour, such as the green, blue and white, and make each area, when in the cell's receptive field, reflect the same triplet of energies. We now find that the cell does not respond to these other areas, even though they are reflecting the identical triplet of energies as the red area, to which the cell responded, was reflecting moments ago. Now the alliances in our *ménage à trois* have changed. This time the human observer and the cell are in agreement with each other, and in disagreement with the telephotometer which is reporting that all the stimuli are identical in terms of wavelength composition when placed in the cell's receptive field. It is obvious that the term 'receptive field' means something more than when applied to cells of the lateral geniculate nucleus (LGN) or of V1. With V4 cells, one commonly finds it difficult to define the surrounds, yet large parts of the surround must be acting effectively to yield the kind of response that is described above.

It is evident from this analysis that the wavelength-selective cells of V1 are really concerned with the component wavelengths reflected from a surface, for example with long-wave light only or middle-wave light only, whereas the cells in V4 are concerned with the colour. We have an interesting example from the motion system which suggests that, in broad outline, a similar strategy is used there.[6] The directionally selective cells of layer 4B of area V1 are also orientation selective. They project to area V5, the motion area where the great majority of cells are directionally selective, commonly without being exigent about the orientation of the stimulus. They also have much larger receptive fields than their counterparts in area V1. Now it so happens that an object consists of many component parts and one cannot determine the precise direction of motion of the object from determining the motion of the component parts over small expanses (see Figure 26.1). It therefore becomes very interesting to note that physiological experiments on the motion system mirror those on the colour system. Cells in area V1 are responsive to the direction of motion of a component of the stimulus (component directional selectivity), whereas there are many cells in area V5 which respond to the overall direction of the entire stimulus (pattern directional selectivity). This distinction is not greatly different from the distinction between the wavelength-selective cells and the colour-coded cells described above, and suggests that the visual system uses a broadly similar mechanism for the motion and colour systems. This illustrates, once

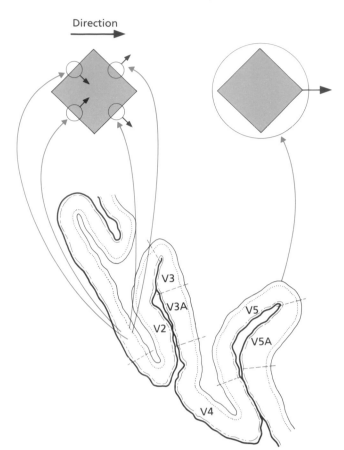

Fig. 26.1 Component motion and overall motion. When an object is moving towards three o'clock, cells with small receptive fields (like the ones in V1), which 'look' at limited regions of the stimulus, will register the component movements in different directions (towards 1.30 and 4.30 o'clock in this case). Physiological experiments show that the directionally selective cells of area V1 register the component directions whereas those of area V5, which 'look' at larger parts of the field of view, register the true, overall, direction. (Redrawn from the work of Movshon, J.A. *et al.* (1985). *Pattern Recognition Mechanisms*, edited by C. Chagas, R. Gattass & C. Gross. Pontifical Academy, Vatican City.)

again, how the study of colour vision reveals general principles about the functional organization of the cerebral cortex.

How are such radical changes brought about? Going back to the Land algorithm, one is obviously driven to suspect that cells in V4 are able to compare the wavelength composition of the light in their receptive fields with that in the surrounding regions. The result of such a comparison enables the cells to 'discount the illuminant' and thus construct the colour of the surface in the receptive field. The cells, in brief, go 'beyond the information given', to quote a title by Jerome Bruner, since the comparison itself is not a property of the stimuli but a product of the activity in the brain. There is, however, nothing mysterious in this and once all the details of the wiring and physiology of the cells in the colour pathways are known, it will almost certainly be possible to account in simple neurophysiological terms for how the brain is able to go 'beyond the information given' in constructing colours. Nor should one conceive of this as an unusual or unique example of going 'beyond the information given'. There are other highly interesting examples. Of these, none is more convincing perceptually than the so-called Kanizsa triangle (Figure 26.2). Here,

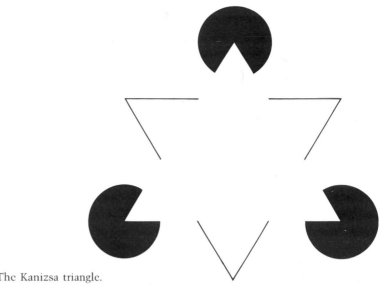

Fig. 26.2 The Kanizsa triangle.

the observer actually undertakes a completion of lines which are not complete, and there are many other such examples. It is of special interest to note that electrophysiological results[7] show that there are cells in V2 which respond to such illusory contours. The mechanism that allows these responses is not known, any more than are the mechanisms which allow cells to respond to an area of a particular colour even in spite of wide-ranging changes in the wavelength energy composition of the light reflected from it. But, at the very least, the presence of such cells allows us to make a beginning in understanding seemingly complex perceptual mechanisms in relatively simple neurological terms.

References

1 Zeki, S. (1983). Colour coding in the cerebral cortex: The reaction of cells in monkey visual cortex to wavelengths and colours. *Neuroscience* **9**, 741–756.
2 Daw, N.W. (1972). Color coded cells in goldfish, cat, and rhesus monkey. *Invest. Ophthalmol.* **11**, 411–417.
3 Zeki, S. (1985). Colour pathways and hierarchies in the cerebral cortex. In *Central and Peripheral Mechanisms of Colour Vision*, edited by D. Ottoson & S. Zeki, pp. 19–44. Macmillan, London.
4 Ts'o, D.Y. & Gilbert, C.D. (1988). The organization of chromatic and spatial interactions in the primate striate cortex. *J. Neurosci.* **8**, 1712–1727.
5 Unpublished results from this laboratory.
6 Movshon, J.A., Adelson, E.H., Grizzi, M.S. & Newsome, W.T. (1985). The analysis of moving visual patterns. In *Pattern Recognition Mechanisms*, edited by C. Chagas, R. Gattass & C. Gross, pp. 117–151. Pontifical Academy, Vatican City.
7 Heydt, R. von der & Peterhans, E. (1989). Mechanisms of contour perception in monkey visual cortex. I. Lines of pattern discontinuity. *J. Neurosci.* **9**, 1731–1748; Peterhans, E. & Heydt, R. von der (1989). Mechanisms of contour perception in monkey visual cortex. II. Contours bridging gaps. *J. Neurosci.* **9**, 1749–1763.

Chapter 27: Some specific visual disturbances of cerebral origin

The anatomical and physiological evidence considered in previous chapters points to a remarkable degree of cortical specificity. Reflecting this, the neurological literature is also replete with highly specific visual syndromes acquired as a result of cerebral disease. Human patients who have suffered cerebral disease are often very difficult to study. The lesions are commonly large, or their extent is uncertain. Indeed, before the advent of modern imaging techniques, one was usually ignorant of the precise position of the lesion unless the brain became available *post mortem*. The consequence of large lesions is a complex of syndromes, often difficult to unravel and separate from one another. Finally, to the clinician, the scientific study of such patients is usually secondary to the desire to rehabilitate them, an understandable and mandatory priority which nevertheless means that the amount of testing that neurological patients undergo is necessarily limited. One can therefore only marvel at the success that students of the human brain have had in charting specific syndromes following cerebral lesions. Some of these syndromes, such as a specific inability to recognize inanimate objects[1] or a specific inability to recognize the faces of animals[2] may strain the imagination of some, while others may think of these as a more generalized disorder of categorization.[3] Other syndromes strained the imagination of earlier neurologists, and chief among these was the syndrome of cerebral achromatopsia. Yet, dramatic though a condition in which one can see everything but not colour may seem, it is nothing more than a reflection of the cortical specificity and the physical segregation of the areas, and subregions of areas, dealing with colour. There is, in other words, a perfectly plausible explanation for it in terms of the anatomical and functional organization of the visual cortex. There is also an equally good explanation, in the same terms, for the syndrome of cerebral akinetopsia, or an inability to see (visual) motion. There are of course other specific syndromes resulting from brain lesions, but it is much less easy to account for them in terms of specific pathways and areas, or at least to account for them in as precise a way as one can for the syndromes of achromatopsia and akinetopsia. This is not because such syndromes are not also the consequence of lesions in very specific regions of the brain but rather because the regions of the brain involved are not nearly so well understood. One good example is the parietal cortex. Lesions here can result in a constellation of bizarre syndromes. These include hemi-neglect of the side contralateral to the lesion, including a neglect of the contralateral field of view; and an inability to localize objects in space or to determine the relationship between objects, a loss of topographical memory resulting in an inability to find one's way home. Interesting though these syndromes are, it is difficult to account for them in terms of specific areas in the parietal cortex or of the pathways leading to them. This is because the areas of the parietal cortex have not been defined with anything like the precision to be found for the prestriate cortex. There is little doubt that, in time, we shall be able to account for parietal lobe syndromes with the same precision with which we can today account for the syndromes of achromatopsia and akinetopsia. The last two syndromes are therefore the ones that I shall concentrate on here, partly because the study of colour and motion vision have laid the foundations for the principle of functional specialization in the visual cortex, and partly because it is easier to show with these, and particularly with achromatopsia, the extent to which the specificity revealed in a study of the normal brain can extend to the pathological brain. Perhaps there is little reason to emphasize yet again what a rich source for exploring brain function colour vision has been.

In discussing visual syndromes of cerebral origin, it is useful to understand the summary diagram of the parallel and specialized pathways leading from the compartments of areas V1 and V2 to the specialized visual areas (Figure 27.1). We use here the diagram obtained from the monkey, making the not unreasonable assumption that the pathways in the human brain are broadly similar, though not identical. At present, the pathways in the human brain are not known in the same detail.

Cerebral achromatopsia

Cerebral achromatopsia is a remarkable condition in which, following cortical lesions, human subjects lose specifically the ability to see the world in colour. In the context of the description given in the previous chapters, pure achromatopsic patients lose specifically the ability to acquire information about certain invariant properties of objects, namely their reflectances for light of different wavelengths. Consequently, they have no knowledge about these properties, which the brain interprets in terms of colour. Theirs is a drab world, almost always described as consisting of 'dirty shades of grey'. Those who are blessed with colour vision are scarcely able to comprehend the condition of such patients, while those who have the syndrome live lives of despair. Perhaps the most humane description of this condition comes from Oliver Sacks.[4] His patient was a successful artist by profession. One day, following a car accident, the patient became

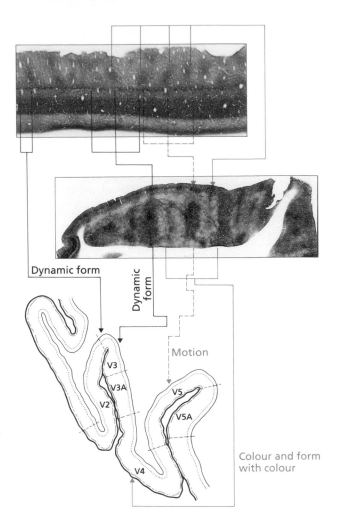

Fig. 27.1 A more formal summary diagram of the connections from the specialized subregions of areas V1 (above) and V2 (centre) to the specialized visual areas of the prestriate cortex. Connections between the latter and the return connections to V1 and V2 are not shown. (Redrawn from Zeki, S. & Shipp, S. (1988). *Nature* **335**, 311–317.)

achromatopsic, a condition which was accompanied by a mild and transient inability to recognize familiar faces and by a transient speech disorder. Adapting to a drab, colourless, world was not easy. Objects could no longer be recognized by their colour, a fact which the rest of us take for granted. Fond of music, he had in the past been in the habit of 'seeing' certain notes in certain colours, a phenomenon known as synesthesia and one which is a characteristic of the cerebral physiology of other artists, notably the French composer and organist Olivier Messian. Painting became difficult, for he could no longer even imagine colours or dream in them. An admirer of Impressionist art, he found each visit to the museum a more painful experience than the previous one. Even trying to interpret the colours of his studio became a painful experience. In despair, he refurnished it in blacks and whites and greys, a therapeutic measure which symbolically also brought to an end a way of life and a blessing.

By any standard, cerebral achromatopsia deserved to be a landmark disease in the study of the brain, but the squabbles of neurologists, described in previous chapters, deprived it of this status. Its very specificity, as well as the specificity of other syndromes affecting colour vision, is testament to the extraordinary specificity of the cerebral cortex. For cerebral achromatopsia is to be distinguished even from the syndrome of colour anomia, in which colours, though recognized, cannot be named. And it has an obverse, a somewhat surprising condition in which colour vision is relatively spared while the other attributes of vision are severely compromised.

The first important point to note about achromatopsia is that the retinal mechanisms mediating colour vision are intact in this condition and all three cone mechanisms are present and functioning normally.[5] The fibres carrying the messages from the retina to the striate cortex are also intact. Hence the defect is entirely central, due to a specific lesion in the cerebral cortex (Figure 27.2 and Plate 18, facing p. 308). *In brief, with achromatopsia, we witness a condition in which the*

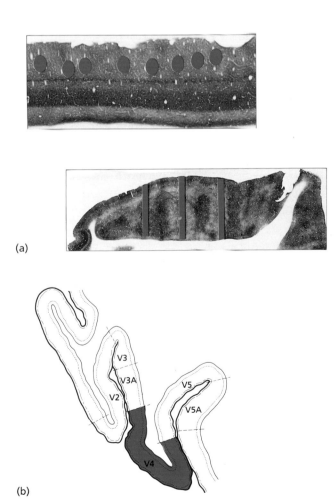

(a)

(b)

Fig. 27.2 Cerebral achromatopsia is caused by a lesion of area V4 (b), which in humans is located in the fusiform gyrus. (a) It could theoretically also be caused if the pathways leading to V4 are destroyed (i.e. the blobs of V1, above, and the thin stripes of V2, centre). See also Plate 18, facing p. 308.

signals relayed to the brain are normal but the mechanism used to construct colours is defective. The second important point, from the viewpoint of functional specialization, is its degree of specificity. Achromatopsic patients can read and write, they can discriminate forms easily and they can detect forms or depths generated from motion (Plate 19, facing p. 308). This is not to suggest that more subtle tests will not reveal some kind of collateral form defect in achromatopsic patients. But their spontaneous complaint is of a loss of colour vision alone and, to a first approximation at least, their defect is selective for colour vision. Moreover, the lesion causing achromatopsia is almost always located in the fusiform gyrus, the very region which is activated with colour stimuli in positron emission tomography (PET) studies. There is only one report[4] of a colour vision defect of cerebral origin which does not obviously involve the fusiform gyrus, but even that is not certain.

Total (bilateral) achromatopsia refers to a condition in which the entire field of view is devoid of colour. The condition is a result of a bilateral damage to area V4 of the human brain, usually the consequence of a stroke (see Figure 27.2). Hemiachromatopsia refers to a condition in which only one half of the field of view is perceived as being devoid of colour, while the other half appears normally coloured. This condition is due to a unilateral damage to area V4 of one hemisphere only, the hemisphere contralateral to the field of view affected (see Chapter 3). An explanation for this is to be found in the results of physiological recordings from area V4 in the monkey brain.[6] These show that the receptive fields of cells in area V4 of the left hemisphere are predominantly in the right half of the field of view, while those of the right hemisphere are predominantly in the left half of the field of view. Consequently, damage to area V4 of one hemisphere should affect the contralateral field of view predominantly.

The form vision of achromatopsic patients

There is a sufficient number of achromatopsic patients with good form vision to convince one that achromatopsia need not be accompanied by an obvious deficit in form vision.[7] This fact requires some explanation. It is difficult to account for it in terms of the physiology of area V4, which shows that there are both wavelength-selective and orientation-selective cells there, though the latter are also wavelength selective to variable degrees.[8] One would therefore expect form vision to be compromised as well, assuming that orientation-selective cells are somehow involved in form vision and that human visual cortex is similar to that of the monkey, at least at this level. Physiological evidence suggests that orientation-selective cells are grouped together within compartments in V4 and that wavelength- and colour-selective cells are grouped in other compartments.[9] It would be difficult to imagine that a vascular lesion, which is usually indiscriminate and does not respect functional boundaries, would selectively spare the orientation-selective cells. Indeed, reflecting the indiscriminate nature of cortical lesions, achromatopsia itself is rarely an isolated syndrome. It is commonly accompanied by a scotoma, due to the involvement of V1. As well, it is commonly accompanied by a prosopagnosia, or an inability to recognize familiar faces, a coincidence which can be explained by the fact that the area of the human cerebral cortex critical for the recognition of familiar faces lies in close proximity to area V4 on the fusiform gyrus. It is therefore commonly damaged along with the latter. Indeed, the literature on prosopagnosia is a rich source of information about achromatopsia. Thus, if lesions of vascular origin affecting V4 spread into neighbouring visual areas, it is difficult to believe that they will selectively spare functional subgroupings within V4 itself. It therefore becomes necessary to search for other reasons, and one can indeed find other, more plausible, explanations for the sparing of form vision in achromatopsic patients.

There is a simple way of accounting for this apparent discrepancy between the experimental results obtained by direct recording from the monkey brain and the characteristics of the syndrome acquired as a result of cerebral disease in man. One can postulate that the process of specialization has proceeded further in the human brain, with the consequence that there are two totally separate areas, one dealing exclusively with colour and the other dealing exclusively with form vision. All that one would then need would be to postulate that cerebral disease can affect one area without affecting the other, which would in turn account for why it is that form vision is unaffected in cases of pure achromatopsia. The simplicity of the explanation is seductive, but it has its drawbacks. In the first place, it is difficult to imagine an area dealing with colour which is not at the same time concerned with form, or at least with boundaries, since boundaries are critical in the generation of colour. Moreover, every object or form in our field of view has a colour, be that colour only a grey. As well, all colours, being confined in space, have a form. The two, form and colour, are therefore not easy to separate. Next, one would have to postulate that, in man, the two areas have become so separated from each other geographically that a vascular lesion could affect the colour area without affecting the form area. At any rate, one would have to postulate that the 'colour centre' and the 'form centre' are much more separated from each other geographically than are the 'colour area' and the 'face area' on the fusiform gyrus, since prosopagnosia is a common byproduct of achromatopsia. They would also have to be much more separate from each other than the 'colour area' and V1, since peripheral scotomas are also a common feature of achromatopsia. Of course, one could argue that the two separate areas are not so distant from each other, that achromatopsic patients frequently do suffer from object agnosia as well. But the latter argument falters because patients with object agnosia commonly have massive lesions, which include area V1 and which affect many other attributes of vision, making it very difficult to argue in favour of the involvement of two separate areas alone.

No total loss of form vision

There is another reason why this argument is difficult to sustain at present. Patients who suffer from form vision defects can never be said to have a total loss of form vision, an interesting finding discussed in greater detail below. They are not therefore 'form blind' in the sense that an achromatopsic patient is 'colour blind'. This is just as true of achromatopsic patients who have some kind of defective form vision which, again, is never total. One reason for this may lie in the fact that orientation-selective cells, presumed to be the basis of form vision, are so ubiquitously distributed in the visual areas of the prestriate cortex. In particular, one finds a massive concentration of them in areas V1, V2, V3 and V3A and a scattering in other areas. Also, there are orientation-selective cells within V4. Here it is important to repeat that the predominant input to the orientation-selective cells of V3 and V3A comes from the 'colour-blind' magnocellular (M) system, a system more concerned with motion. By contrast, the predominant input to the orientation-selective cells of V4 comes from the parvocellular (P) system, a system much more concerned with colour. Reflecting this, the great majority of the orientation-selective cells in V4 have varying degrees of wavelength selectivity, whereas the overwhelming majority of orientation-selective cells in V3 are indifferent to the wavelength of the stimulus. It is for this reason that we consider that there are two more or less distinct form systems. One possible and plausible explanation for why form vision is intact in achromatopsic patients is to suppose that the lesions in such patients spare the other form system, based on V3 and derived largely from the M system.[10] If this is the correct explanation, or at least a partial one, then one should expect to find three features in achromatopsic patients: (1) achromatopsic patients should not be completely 'form blind' and should indeed have relatively good form vision; (2) they should be able to discriminate form better when the forms or objects are moving than when they are stationary; and (3) detailed testing should nevertheless reveal some defect in form vision, particularly the static form vision which entails more detailed examination of objects.

In practice, the first feature — lack of complete form blindness — has been noted so often in achromatopsic patients that it can be considered as established. Moreover, it is a common feature of almost all patients with form vision defects that the defect is never total, suggesting that injury to one part of the cortex dealing with form can be compensated for to a greater or lesser extent by another part of the cortex, also dealing with form.

Now one finds powerful hints, but no proof, that the second feature — better form vision with moving stimuli — may also be true. In the first place, not only can achromatopsic patients discriminate ordinary forms, produced from luminance differences, but they can also discriminate forms produced from movement (structure from motion) as well as depths, all of them functions which almost certainly involve area V3, if the physiology is anything to go by.[11] Next, several studies show that in many subjects, who are both achromatopsic and suffer from form vision defects (the so-called visual form agnosia), the defect in object recognition can be considerably improved if, instead of viewing static forms, the patients view the same forms in motion. Thus, a patient, only able to describe a stationary insect toy vaguely and uncertainly, was almost miraculously able to identify it precisely when it was set in motion for, 'When the toy was put in motion, she correctly identified the figure as a moving toy, "some sort of insect toy"'.[12] Another patient with a similar syndrome improved her recognition of objects significantly when the objects were rotated in front of her immobile head. Moreover, 'from a line-up of 2 very familiar persons and 6 strangers, she could not pick out her sister or the examiner, when they were silent and motionless.... However, [when she] saw her sister walking at a distance of 50 metres [she] recognized her spontaneously'.[13] In another report, a man suffering from a visual agnosia coupled to an achromatopsia, a prosopagnosia and a topographical disorientation, said, 'Generally, I find moving objects much easier to recognise, presumably because I see different and changing views...For that reason the TV screen enables me to comprehend far more of an outdoor scene than, for example, the drawings on my living room walls which I now...cannot recognise'.[14] He was unable to recognize faces and, 'I also have great problems with animals, *particularly if they are not moving*'[14] [my emphasis]. For another agnosic patient, 'moving the object in front of the patient or presenting it from several sides' improved his identification of objects and, 'The patient himself often rotated his head, trying to inspect the objects from various angles'.[15] Yet another agnosic patient who also suffered from Balint's syndrome (i.e. he tended to fixate objects) failed, on static examination, 'to recognize not only letters but also objects' although, 'He identified an ant crawling on the table or a fly in flight but could not recognize visually a spoon or other familiar objects placed before him' (although it should be added that the patient failed to identify objects by slow motion examination).[16] The authors explain that, 'visual recognition consists in fact in the successive and continuous moving of the objects in front of the subject. It is in this way that the patients' ability to recognize visually objects when in motion may be accounted for'.

The above observations are ones which I have gathered from the clinical literature, and there may be many more like them. They are anecdotal asides, often made without comment; they were published long before the revelations of anatomical and electrophysiological experiments on the visual cortex. Paradoxically, they gain added strength because of this very reason, for they were not designed to test any theory in a field in which facts have been dominated by concepts for so long. There has been no systematic or quantitative attempt to study the ability of such patients to discriminate forms in motion, or to compare more systematically their ability to discriminate the same forms in the static and dynamic states. Yet the prevalence of such reports makes it plausible to argue in favour of the supposition that another form system, derived largely from the M pathways, is in operation in such patients. This supposition may also help us to account for why there is no documented case of a subject with a total and selective loss of form vision, and intact vision for other attributes such as motion, colour and depth. The question itself may seem trite, had it not been for the fact that there are other, somewhat unexpected and surprising examples, in which colour vision is more or less select- ively spared (see below). One way of accounting for the absence of a total and selective loss of form vision would be to suppose that to obtain such a loss would require the selective destruction of both the P form system, linked to colour and based on area V4, and the M form system, independent of colour and based on area V3. Consider the extent of the cortical damage that would result in such a loss. Area V3 surrounds area V2 and would be expected to lie both in the cuneus and in the lingual gyrus, the former representing the lower visual fields and the latter the upper visual fields.[17] To obtain a total lesion of V3 would thus entail a destruction which spreads from the cuneus superiorly to the lingual gyrus inferiorly, a destruction that would inevitably involve the lips of the calcarine sulcus (V1) as well and thus lead to a scotoma. Assuming the organization of human V3 to be similar to that found in the monkey, it would stretch posteriorly towards the occipital pole (see Figure 27.3). Hence, a total destruction would involve a considerable portion of the medial surface of the occipital lobe and almost certainly much of V1 as well. To abolish form vision completely would, however, require the further destruction of the fusiform gyrus, where area V4 is located. It is hard to imagine that patients who survived such a destruction would not have much

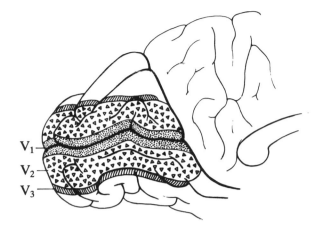

Fig. 27.3 The predicted disposition of area V3 on the medial surface of the human brain. (Reproduced from Horton, J.C. & Hoyt, W.F. (1991). *Brain* **114**, 1703–1718.)

of their occipital lobe, including V1, destroyed and consequently be blind.

The third and last feature mentioned above — that achromatopsic patients should manifest some deterioration in their form vision — has never been systematically studied. But there is at least one study of an achromatopsic patient who found that boundaries between areas in his field of view dissolved with prolonged fixation, suggesting a defect in the P system, and that these boundaries could be rapidly restored if the stimulus was moved, suggesting a healthy and active M system.[18] It is almost certain that the recent advances in anatomy and physiology will lead to a more detailed study of the capacities of achromatopsic patients.

Transient achromatopsia

While post-mortem examination of the brain, or brain scans, reveal lesions in the fusiform gyrus in many cases of achromatopsia, the brain scans of at least one achromatopsic patient[4] revealed nothing. It is possible that the vascular damage could not be adequately imaged by the then available scanning methods. But a study of other types of achromatopsia leads to the conclusion that this condition is not necessarily due to a lesion within V4 itself. It may in fact affect the *input* to V4 at a much earlier stage.

Recall that V4 receives input from the blobs of V1 and the thin stripes of V2. Both have heavy concentrations of wavelength-selective cells, and both are metabolically more active than neighbouring regions. It is this feature which allows one to visualize them at a glance, when sections through the brain are stained with the metabolic enzyme cytochrome oxidase. Because they are metabolically more active, one would suppose that the cells in the blobs and in the thin stripes would be much more susceptible to vascular insufficiency than the metabolically less active subregions such as the interblobs and the interstripes. Thus, in cases of mild vascular insufficiency, one might expect achromatopsia to manifest itself. And if the vascular insufficiency is transient, one might even expect that the achromatopsia itself will also be transient.

This is the very condition that has been described in the literature,[19] although knowing the fate of single-case studies, one naturally interprets this case with diffidence. The case is that of a fifty-four-year-old man who suffered from repeated falling attacks. These attacks were accompanied by a sudden and transient loss of the ability to see the world in colour, the patient now seeing the world in the usual shades of grey. 'Other than this color defect, vision was clear and the objects in the room were correctly identified. About one minute [after the falling attack] he stood up again and was able to discern color. This disorder...persisted for several weeks, 5 to 6 a day, until the institution of treatment'.[19]

Examination of the patient revealed a cerebellar disorder. Both the occipital cortex and the cerebellum receive their blood supply from a common source, the vertebro-basilar artery. Although there was no pathology in this case, and although transient achromatopsia is a very rare syndrome, it is nevertheless worth trying to account for it in terms of the known pathways in the visual cortex. We might suppose, for example, that the metabolically active blobs of V1 and the thin stripes of V2, both of which contain heavy concentrations of wavelength-selective cells, are more susceptible to a decrease in blood levels, and hence to a fall in oxygenation, than are the metabolically less active interblobs or interstripes. Such a supposition would account for the fact that it was colour vision alone which was compromised during these falling attacks, since area V4 would now be deprived of a substantial part of its input (Figure 27.4). This interpretation is not without its difficulties however. Layer 4C of V1, which feeds layers 2 and 3 (and therefore ultimately area V4) as well as layer 4B (and therefore ultimately V3 and V5), is metabolically highly active. One might therefore expect that all visual functions would be compromised in cases of arterial insufficiency and oxygen depletion. This may be due to the fact that layer 4C is still more richly supplied with blood vessels, and hence less susceptible to oxygen depletion, than the upper layers.[20]

The chromatopsia of carbon monoxide poisoning

The interpretation given above runs into difficulties when one considers another somewhat remarkable phenomenon, in which colour vision alone is spared, or at any rate is much less affected than the

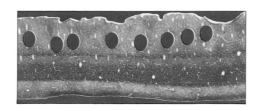

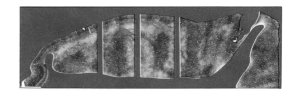

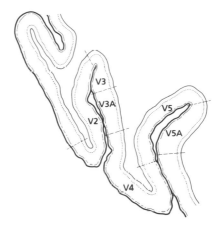

Fig. 27.4 Transient achromatopsia is probably caused by arterial insufficiency which affects the wavelength selective cells in the metabolically active blobs of V1 (above) and thin stripes of V2 (centre) (both shown as red) more than other subdivisions.

other attributes of vision. This is a condition that sometimes results from carbon monoxide poisoning, and was first reported by Wechsler in 1933.[21] His patient was a thirteen-year-old boy of high intelligence who had been admitted to hospital after being overcome by smoke during a fire at his home, a fire which had claimed the lives of five members of his family. He had been unconscious for two hours when admitted. Upon recovery, he was found to be mentally retarded and completely blind. Later examination showed that 'The patient could not recognize small objects, such as a coin, key, pen or watch, and large objects, such as a book, newspaper or telephone, he could distinguish with difficulty'. His depth vision may also have been affected for, 'He groped in trying to grasp objects, and sometimes collided with persons and things, apparently because he could not estimate distance and probably as a result of a defect in visual spatial discrimination.... Color perception, on the other hand, was quick and accurate. He recognized not only all primary colors, but such shades as brown and pink. He knew at once the colors of small objects which he could neither name nor tell the form of. He picked out colors on command'.[21]

To Wechsler, 'the loss of vision...was recognized as cortical because of the preservation of pupillary reflexes, and subsequent absence of optic atrophy'. But how to account for this bizarre syndrome? Wechsler wrote, 'If color vision resides in the cortex and the surface of the brain was destroyed by the pathologic process, color vision should have been lost and not retained. The most probable answer is that either certain parts of the cortex or the layers presumed to perceive and elaborate color vision escaped destruction or they recovered while the visual areas did not. It is barely possible that there are special color-conducting fibers, but all evidence at hand points to the cortex as the seat of color vision. In any event, the case herein presented warrants the statement that color vision and visual acuity can be dissociated in such a way that the former is preserved while the latter is impaired'.[21]

It was, for its time, a remarkable conclusion. Perhaps for this very reason it made not the slightest impression in the neurological world. Those who have since described the same phenomenon have done so without reference to Wechsler, and they in turn have not been referred to by yet others who have described the phenomenon yet again, imagining it to be new. Most authors find it very irritating not being referred to. This is sometimes a sin of ommission rather than one of commission. More often it is a ploy that scientists use, usually to no avail in the end save that of irritating a scientist whom they dislike, probably for no better reason than that he described the phenomenon first. But, in this case, it is more than likely that subsequent authors were completely unaware of Wechsler's description, precisely because, being so bizarre, few took any notice of it. There is one advantage to this, though for the subject, not the author. If a phenomenon has been observed independently by several groups, unaware of each others existence, then it is likely that the phenomenon is real.

Carbon monoxide poisoning is associated with nasty fires and death and it was not long before another, even more tragic, fire was to yield a similar patient.[22] This second patient had been one of the lucky ones. She was among the 132 survivors in a fire which had consumed the Cocoanut Grove nightclub in Boston in 1942, killing 491 souls, many of them servicemen. When the patient appeared in hospital she was totally blind. But after two days she could distinguish white from black. After two weeks she recognized all colours and 'was able to name correctly the colors associated with various objects or the objects which corresponded to colors and could match various shades of the same color. She was able to match colors according to their intensity'. Her ability to recognize pictures and objects remained defective, the patient having 'to recognize by adding up parts instead of by simultaneous perception of all parts'. She 'described pictures as children do, by enumerating details, one after the other'. On the other hand, 'Colored pictures are recognized more easily than uncolored ones because in the former the details are impressed by the difference in color'.[22] Her condition has not changed much over the last forty years.[23]

As with Wechsler's patient, the damage was not limited to vision, the patient suffering from an inability to read (alexia) and to calculate (acalculia) as well. This was much to the liking of Lashley, who was hostile to the idea of a localization for colour and saw in this patient support for his anti-localizationist doctrine. He commented that, 'The development of agnosia in toxic conditions...points to diffuse damage and disorganization rather than to focal lesions'.[24] As a statement, this is unexceptionable. But it nevertheless gives the wrong impression, because colour vision was relatively spared, or at least much less impaired than other attributes of vision, a fact Lashley chose not to mention. Conclusions could have been drawn from this. Wechsler did

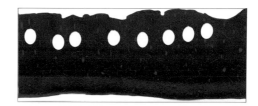

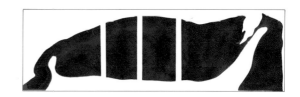

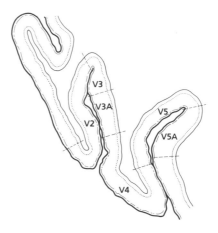

Fig. 27.5 The precise cause of carbon monoxide chromatopsia is not known, but it is reasonably certain that it must spare selectively the compartments and pathways concerned with wavelength and colour, i.e. the blobs of V1 (above), the thin stripes of V2 (centre) and area V4, all of which are shown as white.

so; Lashley did not. But then Lashley had a grand theory of how the brain works and Wechsler did not.

How can one account for this condition? Pathological evidence suggests that layers 2 and 3 are relatively more susceptible to the effects of carbon monoxide poisoning.[25] On the other hand, the most richly vascular parts of these layers are the metabolically active blobs in V1 and the thin stripes in V2. The richer vasculature of these structures may have actually cushioned them from the effects of hypoxia with the consequence that they were relatively spared (see Figure 27.5). At present this explanation is conjectural. Moreover, it is in apparent contradiction to the explanation for transient achromatopsia given above, which supposes that the blobs are more vulnerable to a reduction in blood supply. It is not at present easy to account for this contradiction. But it is important to note that we can speak of these abnormal aspects of colour vision in terms of very precisely defined pathways in the brain.

Phantom chromatopsia

Another syndrome which demonstrates specificity, though one which has made only a very rare appearance in the clinical literature, is the syndrome which I have called phantom chromatopsia.[26] In reality it is not quite as uncommon as the clinical literature suggests, though it is a very awkward syndrome to study because it belongs to the private world of disturbed perceptions. It is, for all that, a very real and distressing syndrome which occurs in patients who are totally blind or nearly so, though painful in a different sense from the usual meaning attached to pain. It drives those who suffer from it to distraction and despair, and even to suicide. In this condition a cortically generated colour, usually golden or purple, enlarges to invade the entire 'field of view'. The phenomenon is more in the nature of an abnormal hallucination. There is, of course, no compelling evidence that the patients actually see the colours since, being blind, they cannot actually be tested. Indeed, three of the patients with this condition whom I have seen suffered a double misfortune — one was the syndrome of phantom chromatopsia itself and the other was the fact that few people believed their descriptions, preferring to consider the syndrome as nothing more than a manifestation of hysterical states. But there is no reason to doubt these stories, which are confirmatory of each other.

To account for this condition is not easy. But there are highly interesting experiments which suggest that actual stimulation of cells in a specialized cortical area may induce perceptual effects which correlate with the properties of the cells.[27] It has been found that microstimulation of small groups of cells, possibly even individual columns of cells, coding for particular directions of motion in area V5 of the monkey, can bias a monkey's judgement of which direction visual stimuli are moving in. This discovery opens up a host of interesting questions and possibilities. Among these is the possibility of abnormal stimulation of cells in the cortex due to some cortical irritation or other, similar, factors. In the experiments reported above, the authors expressed surprise, 'that such large perceptual effects could result from a current level that ostensibly activates a region of cortex whose dimensions approximate those of a single column [of cells]'.[27] Imagine, then, what could happen with abnormally large and more or less chaotic firing of cells in an area. They could generate strange and abnormal perceptual effects. Such abnormal effects have not been reported for motion yet, but phantom chromatopsia provides a good example. There is, however, an interesting example of internally generated colour perceptions, following direct magnetic stimulation of human V4.[28] Plate 20 (facing p. 308) shows the vivid colours generated when human subjects were asked to draw what they 'saw' immediately after such stimulation and to mark on a television screen where in the field of view the percept appeared with respect to a fixation point. There are two interesting features in this figure, in which each drawing is the result of a separate stimulation. Firstly, the fact that the stimulus elicited colour sensations (chromatophenes) and secondly that the extent of the chromatophenes and their position in the field of view bears a strong resemblance to the physiology of area V4. Thus, stimulation of the left hemisphere led to the appearance of chromatophenes in the right hemi-field, and vice versa (see Plate 20). Moreover, the size of the chromatophenes bears a strong resemblance to the size of the receptive fields of single cells in area V4 of the monkey. All this suggests not only that direct stimulation of the specialized areas, by-passing the pathway leading from the retina to them, may be a powerful way of studying the human visual cortex but also that an un-natural stimulation of these areas may itself be the cause of what, until now, have seemed strange visual disorders.

Syndromes such as phantom chromatopsia serve to underline one of the main themes developed in this book, namely that the visual image is a construction of the brain and that it is activity in the cerebral cortex that invests the visual world with some of its properties. Colour, I have argued, is an interpretation that the brain gives to certain physical properties of surfaces and objects, and is entirely the result of brain activity. Another, and different, example may be found in the strong 'illusion' of motion created by some patterns which are strictly static and contain no physical movement whatsoever. The strong motion perception that they induce is almost certainly the result of brain activity, according to rules which we know nothing about as yet. The term 'illusion' is perhaps not the best one to use, for it suggests an element of deception or delusion, a departure from reality, whereas what I mean is that the percept — a result of brain activity — *is* the reality. No patient suffering from the dreadful daily reality of phantom chromatopsia would doubt this statement. But there are other examples, accessible to normal people, and which therefore serve to make this general point more emphatically. A good example is to be found in the work of Isia Leviant, one of which is illustrated in Plate 21, facing p. 308. The work consists of a series of narrow circles and spokes radiating from the centre. Fixation of the centre induces in most, though not all, people a strong perception of motion occurring within the rings. The motion is in opposite directions in different rings and can change direction in any one ring during one, continuous, viewing.

Here then is an example in which one perceives motion which is not physically there in the stimulus that one is looking at. Is this due to activity in a specific part of the brain? My colleagues and I decided to use the PET technique to study the change in regional cerebral blood flow when human subjects viewed the Leviant figure described above. The result was quite remarkable. A specific region of the brain, contiguous and overlapping with V5 but not identical to it, was active when subjects had been viewing the display. It is thus as if the perception of motion in a figure containing no moving component is the consequence of the activity in a specific area of the brain, just as phantom achromatopsia is likely to be the consequence of activity, though an abnormal one, in another part of the brain.

Cerebral akinetopsia

The study of colour and motion vision laid the foundations for the demonstration of functional specialization in the cortex and it seems appropriate that we should find in the clinical literature a syndrome as specific as achromatopsia but this time related to motion vision. Reference has already been made to this syndrome, that of cerebral akinetopsia, of which the best description is to be found in the paper by Zihl and colleagues. This patient had suffered a bilateral cerebral lesion, involving area V5 as demarcated in PET studies but also extending beyond. Her inability has been described earlier (see Chapter 10). Again, the central synthetic mechanisms required to generate a perception of coherent motion, centred on V5, appear to be compromised. The consequence is that the akinetopsic patient has no experience or knowledge of objects when they are in motion, only when they are stationary (Figure 27.6). As with achromatopsia, there are two important points to note, first that retinal mechanisms appear to be intact, and next that the syndrome is highly specific to motion, the patient experiencing no difficulty in seeing colours, forms or depths.

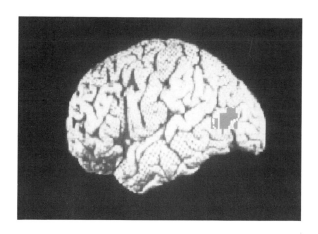

Fig. 27.6 The visual area (V5) compromised in cerebral akinetopsia.

But there is a third important similarity with achromatopsia, namely that motion vision can be spared selectively, a fact first noted by Riddoch[29] and then rapidly relegated to oblivion because of the hostility of Gordon Holmes, the doyen of British neurologists. This too has been described in Chapter 10. Patients with blind fields have been able to detect motion in their scotomatous areas, though without being able to detect any other attribute of the moving stimulus. Recently, it has been shown that lesions within the territory of areas V2 and V3, but not involving V1, also lead to scotomas, and at least one such patient could detect gross motion within the blind field.[30] Unlike the condition of carbon monoxide chromatopsia, it is not easy to account for the selective sparing of motion vision in terms of specific cortical pathways, namely the connections between layer 4B and the thick stripes of V2 and area V5. To do so, especially in patients who had acquired their scotomas as a result of bullet wounds, one would need to postulate that, in V1, the wounds selectively spared not only layer 4B but only the direction-selective cells in that layer, while destroying the orientation-selective cells projecting to V3. If the wound is in V2, then one would have to postulate that it selectively spared the thick stripes, the ones which contain the direction-selective cells. This seems unlikely unless one can show that there are direction-selective-cell-seeking bullets. It is therefore common to ascribe the capacity of such patients to detect motion to subcortical mechanisms, a topic that will be considered in greater detail when we consider the problem of the vision of the blind.

Depth vision

That the ability to see objects in depth can also be selectively compromised following specific lesions in the visual cortex has also been known for a long time, though such reports have made little impact, partly because physiologists do not really understand whether there is any localization for depth perception in the way that there is for colour and for motion. Riddoch[29] described a patient who had an 'inability to appreciate depth or thickness in objects seen...The most corpulent individual might be a moving cardboard figure, for his body is represented by an outline only. He has colour and light and shade, but still to the patient he has no protruding features: everything is perfectly flat'. Depth vision depends upon a disparate input from the two eyes,[31] and one would therefore expect that the cells in the relevant area of the cerebral cortex concerned with depth should be binocularly driven. In fact, the great majority of cells in all the specialized visual areas are binocularly driven.[32] In theory, each should therefore be able to detect depth provided that it receives disparate rather than identical inputs from the two eyes (i.e. that it does not receive input from identical retinal points). Cells tuned to different disparities have been found in area V1.[33] The segregation of such cells has been better studied in area V2, where the majority have been found to lie in the thick stripes,[34] the stripes that derive their inputs from the M layers. Among the visual areas that the thick stripes project to is area V3. This area, together with the adjoining area V3A, has been little studied yet both areas have very interesting features. First, the great majority of cells in them are orientation selective, and next there is a strong suggestion that both areas may be involved in depth perception.[11] One would therefore predict that lesions of area V3 and V3A, or their equivalents in the human brain, will lead to strong defects in form perception as well as in depth perception, but the experiments have not been done. This is not to say that other visual areas, such as V4, may not also be involved in depth perception. The cells of V4 are binocularly driven and lesion experiments show that when the P layers of the lateral geniculate nucleus (LGN) (from which V4 derives its predominant input) are incapacitated,[35] there are defects in fine and, to a lesser extent, coarse depth vision. But the problem has not been addressed in terms of the cortical physiology of area V4 and other P-derived areas.

In summary then, the results of clinical studies mirror those of physiological studies in showing that the remarkably specific areas and pathways of the cerebral cortex can be specifically compromised.

The consequence of experimental lesions in V4 and V5

In theory at least, one might expect that the clinical picture observed in man might be replicated through experimental lesions in specific visual areas in the brain of the monkey. One might then expect that lesions in areas V4 and V5 should lead to very specific visual defects in colour vision and in motion perception, respectively. This is so, although the demonstration has not been as satisfactory in these experimental studies.

Perhaps the first thing to note about experimental lesion work in the monkey is that a monkey is not a man and that the two therefore differ in important respects. While many of the findings gained in studying the monkey brain anatomically and physiologically have been of fundamental importance in understanding the clinical syndromes in man, it does not follow that the two brains will be found to be identical in every respect, even at relatively low cortical levels such as area V1. The next point to note is that it is one brain studying another, and different, brain. Humans arguably know the capacities of other human brains much better than they know the capacities of monkey brains. When one human brain studies the capacities of another human brain, the first can at least determine whether the tasks it asks the second to perform are feasible, whether they are consciously experienced and much else besides. Such a direct comparison is not available with the capacities of the monkey brain. Yet, one cannot help but conclude that many of the paradigms designed to study the monkey brain are derived from a knowledge of the capacities of the human brain. There is no real problem with this if one realizes the limitations of the approach, and realizes, too, that the results may not always be interpretable in ways which apply to both brains. And the last thing to note about experimental studies involving lesions is that they have, in themselves, commonly been a very poor guide to the organization of the visual cortex, at least in the short term, until explanations have been found for them from neuro-anatomy and neurophysiology. For example, extensive lesions of the striate cortex, even nearly complete removal of V1, had only a very marginal, indeed trivial, long-term effect on the discrimination of orientation, a surprising finding given the high concentration of orientation-selective cells there.[36] We may now try to account for this in all sorts of ways. Yet, the fact is that the results seemed not only mysterious when first reported, but also incongruous with the physiological evidence. Equally, removal of the posterior bank of the superior temporal sulcus, where area V5 is located, was originally reported to have had no effect either on movement detection or on movement thresholds,[37] yet again a surprising finding if one assumes that physiological results mean anything at all. Indeed, a reading of the early literature,[38] before V4 was defined, might even leave one wondering whether V4 is a visual area at all. Hence, trying to gain insights into the organization of the visual cortex from the negative results of carefully controlled lesion experiments in monkeys is like trying to read the minds of politicians from what they say to their generals. After all, as late as 1914 French generals had full-drawn plans in their drawers for the invasion of England and, in 1990, Russian generals had equally detailed plans for the nuclear annihilation of Western Europe.

Lesions of area V5, initially found to have no effect at all,[37] were later found to produce a defect in motion perception,[39] but the effects have been transient for reasons which are not entirely clear. One possibility is that the (chemical) lesions in the initial studies were very much subtotal; it has since been reported that larger lesions cause more severe and persistent deficits. It is worth recalling here that the lesion in the 'motion-blind' patient was actually quite extensive and went well beyond the confines of the area which was defined as V5 in the human by PET studies. Another reason may lie in the fact that there is a genuine re-organization of neural tissue within the superior temporal sulcus. Thus, the receptive fields of cells left intact by the chemical lesion were actually shown to increase in size and expand in all directions, presumably compensating thereby for the loss of the (smaller) receptive fields in the lesioned zone.[40] It is worth noting, though by no means as a criticism of these marvellous studies, that the price for the high degree of elegant quantification in them is a sacrifice in repertoire. One wants to know, for example, whether monkeys with V5 lesions are affected in the perception of structure from motion, a condition in which coherent motion is generated first and the form next. One wants to know whether there is any effect at all on the perception of dynamic forms, since they involve movement and since their perception was affected in the 'motion-blind' patient. One wants to learn, in brief, about the full repertoire of behaviour which is affected by such lesions.

Perhaps the most significant result with V4 lesions has been the demonstration of a substantial and long-standing defect in discriminating colours when the wavelength composition of the light reflected from surfaces is changed.[41] In other words, lesions in monkey V4 have resulted in the breakdown of the most important attribute of the colour system, indeed the very biological reason for its existance, namely colour constancy. This has been found to be true even when the V4 lesions were partial and even with colours which are widely separated.[42] This is precisely the result that one might have predicted from a knowledge of the physiology of area V4. Significantly, and reflecting what has been observed in human achromatopsic patients, there was only a minimal effect on wavelength discrimination.[41,43] This is not surprising, given that the cells of area V1 are more concerned with registering wavelengths while those of V4 are more interested in collecting information relating from large parts of the field of view to generate colour (see Chapter 26). There is no good reason why the intact wavelength-selective cells of area V1 should not be — both in V4 lesioned monkeys and achromatopsic patients —

the basis of such a discrimination. Destruction of one area (V4) should still allow the organism to undertake such discriminations as the capacities of the areas left intact by the lesions (V1 and V2) allow (see Chapter 30).

V4 lesions have also produced effects on form vision, more severe in one study[43] with lesions that extended beyond the boundaries of V4 into the inferior temporal cortex and very mild in the other[42] study. That there should be some effect on form vision, though elicitable only when tested in a formal setting, is not surprising since there are orientation-selective cells in the V4 complex and these derive input from the P form system. I emphasize the formal setting because the monkeys are not obviously defective in their ability to see objects and forms in their natural surroundings, or to grasp food accurately and avoid obstacles, a behaviour which suggests that there is at least some substantial element of form vision that is preserved. This is in marked contrast to a syndrome such as achromatopsia where no formal setting is needed to elicit the defect, the patients complaining spontaneously of their inability to see the world in colour.

It is perhaps surprising and a little paradoxical that, although it is experimental work in the macaque monkey that has given us such an insight into the functioning of the human visual cortex and has allowed us to make sense of the bizarre visual syndromes that are the consequences of lesions in the human brain, in the field of lesion work human studies have been a good deal more informative than experimental studies in the monkey.

Notes and references

1 Hécaen, H. & Ajuriaguerra, J. de (1956). Agnosie visuelle pour les objets inanimés par lésion unilatérale gauche. *Rev. Neurol. (Paris)* **94**, 222–233.

2 Assal, G., Favre, C. & Anders, J.P. (1984). Non-reconnaisance d'animaux familiers chez un paysan. *Rev. Neurol. (Paris)* **140**, 580–584.

3 Hécaen, H., Goldblum, M.C., Masure, M.C. & Ramier, A.M. (1974). Une nouvelle observation d'agnosie d'objets. Déficit de l'association où de la catégorization spécifique de la modalité visuelle? *Neuropsychologia* **12**, 447–464.

4 Sacks, O. & Wasserman, R. (1987). The painter who became color blind. *NY Rev. Books* **34**, 25–33.

5 Mollon, J.D., Newcombe, F., Polden, P.G. & Ratcliff, G. (1980). On the presence of three cone mechanisms in a case of total achromatopsia. In *Colour Vision Deficiencies*, V, edited by G. Verriest, pp. 130–135. Adam Hilger, Bristol.

6 Zeki, S.M. (1977). Colour coding in the superior temporal sulcus of rhesus monkey visual cortex. *Proc. R. Soc. Lond.* B **197**, 195–223; Van Essen, D.C. & Zeki, S.M. (1978). The topographic organization of rhesus monkey prestriate cortex. *J. Physiol. (Lond.)* **277**, 193–226.

7 Kölmel, H.W. (1988). Pure homonymous hemiachromatopsia: findings with neuro-ophthalmologic examination and imaging procedures. *Eur. Arch. Psychiatry Neurol. Sci.* **237**, 237–243.

8 Zeki, S. (1983). The distribution of wavelength and orientation selective cells in

different areas of monkey visual cortex. *Proc. R. Soc. Lond.* B **217**, 449−470; Desimone, R. & Schein, S.J. (1987). Visual properties of neurons in area V4 of the macaque: sensitivity to stimulus form. *J. Neurophysiol.* **57**, 835−868.

9 Zeki, S. (1983), loc. cit. [8]; Zeki, S. & Shipp, S. (1989). Modular connections between areas V2 and V4 of macaque monkey visual cortex. *Eur. J. Neurosci.* **1**, 494−506.

10 Zeki, S. (1991). Parallelism and functional specialization in human visual cortex. *Cold Spring Harb. Symp. Quant. Biol.* **55**, 651−661.

11 Zeki, S.M. (1978). The third visual complex of rhesus monkey prestriate cortex. *J. Physiol. (Lond.)* **277**, 245−272; Poggio, G.F., Gonzalez, F. & Krause, F. (1988). Stereoscopic mechanisms in monkey visual cortex, binocular correlation and disparity selectivity. *J. Neurosci.* **8**, 4531−4550.

12 Bender, M.B. & Feldman, M. (1972). The so-called 'visual agnosias'. *Brain* **95**, 173−186.

13 Kertesz, A. (1979). Visual agnosia: the dual deficit of perception and recognition. *Cortex* **15**, 403−419.

14 Humphreys, G.W. & Riddoch, M.J. (1987). *To See But Not To See: A Case Study of Visual Agnosia.* Erlbaum (Lawrence) Associates, London.

15 Ferro, J.M. & Santos, M.E. (1984). Associative visual agnosia: A case study. *Cortex* **20**, 121−134.

16 Botez, M.J. & Sebranescu, T. (1967). Course and outcome of static visual static agnosia. *J. Neurol. Sci.* **4**, 289−297.

17 Horton, J.C. & Hoyt, W.F. (1991). Quadrantic visual field defects. A hallmark of lesions in extrastriate (V2/V3) cortex. *Brain* **114**, 1703−1718; Clarke, S. & Miklossy, J. (1990). Occipital cortex in man: organization of callosal connections, related myelo- and cytoarchitecture, and putative boundaries of functional areas. *J. Comp. Neurol.* **298**, 188−214.

18 Reference is made here to Sacks' patient, whom I have studied.

19 Lapresle, J., Metreau, R. & Annabi, A. (1977). Transient achromatopsia in vertebro- basilar insufficiency. *J. Neurol.* **215**, 155−158.

20 Zheng, D., La Mantia, A.S. & Purves, D. (1991). Specialized vascularization of the primate visual cortex. *J. Neurosci.* **11**, 2622−2629.

21 Wechsler, I.S. (1933). Partial cortical blindness with preservation of color vision: report of a case following asphyxia (carbon monoxide poisoning?) *Archs. Ophthalmol.* **9**, 957−965.

22 Adler, A. (1944). Disintegration and restoration of optic recognition in visual agnosia: analysis of a case. *Arch. Neurol. Psychiatr. (Chicago)* **51**, 243−259; Adler, A. (1950). Course and outcome of visual agnosia. *J. Nerv. Ment. Dis.* **111**, 41−51.

23 Sparr, S.A., Jay, M., Drislane, F.W. & Venna, N. (1991). A historic case of visual agnosia revisited after 40 years. *Brain* **114**, 789−800.

24 Lashley, K.S. (1948). The mechanism of vision. XVIII. Effects of destroying the visual 'associative areas' of the monkey. *Genet. Psychol. Monogr.* **37**, 107−166.

25 Brierly, J.B. & Graham, D.I. (1984). In *Greenfield's Neuropathology*, edited by J. Hume Adams, J.A.N. Corsallis & J.W. Duchen, pp. 125−205. Edward Arnold, London.

26 Zeki, S. (1990). Colour vision and functional specialization in the visual cortex. *Disc. Neurosci.* **6**, 11−64.

27 Newsome, W.T., Britten, K.H., Salzman, C.D. & Movshon, J.A. (1991). Neuronal mechanisms of motion perception. *Cold Spring Harb. Symp. Quant. Biol.* **55**, 697−705.

28 Beckers, G. & Beckers, K. (personal communication).

29 Riddoch, G. (1917). Dissociation of visual perceptions due to occipital injuries, with especial reference to appreciation of movement. *Brain* **40**, 15−57.

30 Horton, J.C. & Hoyt, W.F. (1991), loc. cit. [17].

31 Barlow, H.B., Blakemore, C.B. & Pettigrew, J.D. (1967). The neural mechanism of binocular depth discrimination. *J. Physiol. (Lond.)* **193**, 327−342.

32 Zeki, S.M. (1979). Functional specialization and binocular interaction in the visual

areas of rhesus monkey prestriate cortex. *Proc. R. Soc. Lond.* B **204**, 379–397.

33 Poggio, G.F. (1984). Processing of stereoscopic information in primate visual cortex. In *Dynamic Aspects of Neocortical Function*, edited by G.M. Edelman, W.E. Gall & W.M. Cowan, pp. 613–635. John Wiley, New York.

34 Hubel, D.H. & Livingstone, M.S. (1987). Segregation of form, color and stereopsis in primate area 18. *J. Neurosci.* **7**, 3378–3415.

35 Schiller, P. & Logothetis, N. (1990). The color-opponent and the broad-band channels of the primate visual system. *Trends Neurosci.* **13**, 392–398.

36 Pasik, T. & Pasik, P. (1971). The visual world of monkeys deprived of striate cortex: effective stimulus parameters and the importance of the accessory optic system. *Vision Res.* Suppl. **3**, 419–435; Dineen, J. & Keating, E.G. (1981). The primate visual system after bilateral removal of striate cortex: survival of complex pattern vision. *Exp. Brain Res.* **41**, 338–345.

37 Collin, N.G. & Cowey, A. (1980). The effect of ablation of frontal eye-fields and superior colliculi on visual stability and movement discrimination in rhesus monkeys. *Exp. Brain Res.* **40**, 251–260.

38 Zeki, S.M. (1969). The secondary visual areas of the monkey. *Brain Res.* **13**, 197–226.

39 Newsome, W.T., Wurtz, R.H., Dürsteler, M.R. & Mikami, A. (1985). Deficits in visual motion processing following ibotenic acid lesions of the middle temporal visual area of the macaque monkey. *J. Neurosci.* **5**, 825–840.

40 Wurtz, R.H., Yamasaki, D.S., Duffy, C.J. & Roy, J.-P. (1991). Functional specialization for visual motion processing in primate cerebral cortex. *Cold Spring Harb. Symp. Quant. Biol.* **55**, 717–727.

41 Wild, H.M., Butler, D., Carden, D. & Kullikowski, J.J. (1985). Primate cortical area V4 important for colour constancy but not wavelength discrimination. *Nature* **313**, 133–135.

42 I am indebted to Dr V. Walsh and Professor J. Kullikowski for showing me these results which are being prepared for publication.

43 Heywood, C.A. & Cowey, A. (1987). On the role of cortical area V4 in the discrimination of hue and pattern in macaque monkeys. *J. Neurosci.* **7**, 2601–2617.

Chapter 28: A tense relationship

Anyone studying the cerebral cortex cannot fail to be impressed by its specificity. As we have seen, this is expressed at several different levels:

1 Single cells are highly specific in their responses, responding only when a specific stimulus is presented in a specific part of the field of view in the case of the visual cortex.

2 Cells with common specificities, either with respect to location or to attribute, are grouped together and separated from cells with other specificities, either within an area or between areas.

3 Connections in the cortex are commonly of the 'like-with-like' type, one group of specific cells in one area connecting with their counterparts in another area.

4 This feature is not unique to the visual cortex but characteristic of other cortical areas as well.

If cells with specific functions are forever kept isolated from cells with other specific functions, then it becomes difficult to understand how they might interact to provide us with a unitary visual image. This problem is a more specific version of the problem which Lashley outlined years ago, of 'how the specialized parts of the cerebral cortex interact to provide the integration evident in thought and behavior'. Any insights gained from a study of the integrative mechanisms within the visual cortex might help us to apply them in a study of this more general, and fundamental, cortical problem.

Because of the integration evident in our behaviour, there has been, throughout the history of cerebral studies, a tense and uneasy relationship between the localizationists, those who have tried to chart histologically distinct parts of the cerebral cortex and assign specific functions to each, and the anti-localizationists, those who have remembered that the cortex acts as a whole, in spite of its anatomical and physiological diversity. The localizationists have tended to emphasize the modular structure of the cortex and the subdivision of labour within it; the anti-localizationists have tended to emphasize the fact that these modules, no matter how one defines them, must inevitably interact to provide the integration evident in our behaviour. The pendulum of opinion has swung alternately in favour of one or the other, and each has marshalled arguments which seemed convincing, at least until the other camp got their next blow in. To many surveying the debate from a distance of years, the antagonism may seem bizarre and even fictitious. Functional specialization does not stand in opposition to integration. Rather, integration is a fact which must be explained in terms of functional specialization.

In the days before Broca and Fritsch and Hitzig, the prevalent view was that of the nineteenth century French physiologist Pierre Flourens. He believed that, 'All sensory and volitional faculties exist in the cerebral hemispheres and must be regarded as occupying concurrently the same seat in these structures', in other words that there is no functional localization within the cerebral cortex. With the discoveries of Broca and of Fritsch and Hitzig, opinion swung very much in favour of the localizationists for a long period from the 1860s to the 1920s. It was during this period that anatomists tried to chart histologically distinct parts of the cerebral cortex, relying principally on the cytoarchitectonic and myeloarchitectonic methods, and ushering in what Sholl has called 'an era of feverish map making'.[1] In the period between the 1920s and the 1950s, the localizationist tendency was attacked by Pierre Marie in France, by von Monakow in Switzerland and by Henry Head in England. But the most persistent and forceful attack came from the American neuropsychologist Karl Lashley (Figure 28.1) and helped to create a distinctly anti-localizationist tendency.

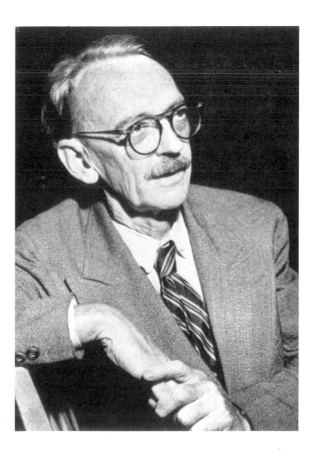

Fig. 28.1 Karl Spencer Lashley (1890–1952), the brilliant American neuropsychologist who was deeply hostile to the idea of a cerebral localization of function. (Reproduced by permission from Polyak, S. (1957). *The Vertebrate Visual System*. University of Chicago Press, Chicago.)

It is important to realize that the anti-localizationists rarely concerned themselves with what they imagined to be simple functions such as vision. They usually dwelt on what they considered to be more complex functions such as speech or memory. It is almost an accident of history that the first clear evidence for localization dealt with aphasia. When neurologists began to question whether so complex a function as speech could be localized, it became an almost fortuitous questioning of the concept of localization, since aphasia was one of the first guides to it. Such complex functions obviously depend upon interactions between several specialized areas, and the problem then becomes one of understanding how the specialized areas interact. When Pierre Marie questioned the validity of the localizationist tendency, he did so on the basis of speech, not of vision, though he had spent much time studying the visual cortex in man. He conceded that aphasia may result from damage to a specific cortical area but took quick refuge in the concept of association cortex, which became a synonym for complexity of function. He wrote, 'We should not forget that this territory is also one which Flechsig considers to be a special associational centre and, in effect, when we examine the psychism of aphasics without preconceived notions we find that in them associational disorders play a major role in disorders of speech'.[2] Note that there is some similarity between the thinking here and that which was so successful in dismissing the notion of a colour centre outside the striate cortex. In both the centre happened to be in what Flechsig had considered to be association cortex, and association cortex could not deal with a single function, or so neurologists believed. Association cortex, in the sense intended by Flechsig, had another function, that of associating the currently received 'impressions' with previous, stored ones. In other words, some kind of integration occurred in association cortex and the anti-localizationists dwelt much on this problem. In his book, *Aphasia and Kindred Disorders of Speech*,[3] Henry Head again considered the complexity of speech and refused to accept the concept of a localized centre for it, while admitting that specific lesions might lead to speech disorders. This notion led him to the concept of 'preferred centres of integration', a formulation which, if one thinks about it, implies localization, at least for integration. Lashley also complained that the localizationist theory did not account for '. . . how the specialized parts of the cerebral cortex interact to provide the *integration* evident in thought and behavior'[4] [my emphasis]. Anxious to emphasize the integrative role of the cerebral cortex, Lashley lost sight of his anti-localizationist stance in vision, even if only momentarily. He wrote that, even admitting the facts of localization, one had to concede that a function like vision '. . . which from an introspective or a behavioristic standpoint is completely integrated turns out, when its pathologic aspect is studied, to be controlled by widely scattered loci contributing quite diverse elements to the whole'.[5] This demanded integration, a notion which those who peddled the concept of functional localization seemed to ignore, so Lashley believed.

Unlike Henry Head or Pierre Marie, who were clinical neurologists, Karl Lashley was an experimentalist who had chosen to study complex functions, but in a simpler organism, the rat. He taught his rats problems which depended upon several sensory cues — visual, somesthetic, proprioceptive, auditory and olfactory. They were, in brief, complex problems, at least in the world of rat ideas. He found that the deterioration in the performance of his rats was proportional to the amount of cortex removed and independent of the actual area removed. This led him to the concept of mass action, a concept which supposed that all cortical areas contribute non-specifically and in more or less equal ways to the efficiency of behaviour, that there is, in other words, no obvious localization of function for more complex tasks.[6] It would be wrong to suggest that the decrement in behaviour was solely a consequence of more specialized areas being involved in larger lesions. Indeed, Lashley believed that cortical areas had functions over and above their sensory or motor ones, vaguely described as a facilitation. He went further and devised ingenious experiments to prove his point. He rendered his rats blind by enucleation and then taught them the maze habits.[7] Once they had learned this, he removed their visual cortex, which was obviously not receiving any visual information in rats whose eyes had been enucleated. Yet the consequence was a sharp decrement in the efficiency of behaviour in the maze habit. This reinforced Lashley's belief that specialized areas of the cortex must have non-specific functions, to the extent that all cortical areas have non-specialized functions. Lashley did not deny the facts of localization in the simpler sense. When making big claims, scientists — or at least the more cautious ones amongst them — prefer to cover themselves with disclaimers, just in case unforeseen facts should compromise their claims. Lashley elevated this art to new heights. He developed a unique style of writing which paid lip service to the idea of localization before savaging it. The complaint that localization theory failed to account for integration was preceded by the statement that, 'No one can today seriously believe that the different parts of the cerebral cortex all have the same functions',[4] while the statement that, 'On anatomic grounds alone there is no assurance that cerebral localization is anything but an accident of growth' is followed by the statement that, 'I do not wish to overemphasize this point. The vast majority of structural elements in the nervous system...look as if they must have some functional value'. This, in turn, is immediately followed by the statement that, '...it is important to realize that this functional value is accepted largely as a matter of faith'.[8] At any rate, through his work and writings, he managed to create an atmosphere that was distinctly hostile to the localizationist school. Indeed, he used tools other than behavioural ones to question the concept of localization. One of these was the cytoarchitectonic method, which he employed and found to be highly unreliable.[9] Through this discovery, his attack on the concept of localization reached new levels. He became hostile to the idea of subdividing the cortex on architectonic grounds, arguing, as we saw earlier, that the cytoarchitectonic areas 18 and 19 (the prestriate cortex) in the monkey should be considered a 'single functional unit'[9] and doubting, on the basis of indifferent evidence, whether complex functions 'like color vision'[10] could be localized in the cerebral cortex.

The problem of complex behaviour revolved, therefore, around the problem of integration. But how was this achieved? One possibility was that it may be done through the system of short transcortical fibres connecting the visual area. But he had '. . . made incisions through the cortex of the rat in every possible plane. . . interrupting transcortical connections, and have been unable to demonstrate any effects of such incisions on maze learning and retention of visual performance',[8] a result similar to that obtained by others in the frontal lobes and motor areas of monkeys. Another possibility was that long association fibres, connecting distant cortical areas and so prominent a feature of the brain, might be used. Lashley dismissed this notion while admitting, in his usual way, that not much was known about them. In the context of the time, this seemed not unreasonable. At the time that Lashley was writing, most track-tracing experiments in the cerebral cortex depended upon the Marchi method, which is based on staining the degenerated myelin of transected nerve fibres. Under the most eminent authorities this method had shown that important visual centres in the cortex were only connected by short fibres. At Oxford, Le Gros Clark had decided from his studies that he could dismiss the conclusions of others regarding long association fibres in the visual cortex. He wrote with some authority that, '. . . we are led to suspect that such long association paths from the visual cortex are completely absent in the monkey and that those which have been described have their origin in inadequately controlled experimental material',[11] a now discredited assertion, though one which Lashley used eagerly to dismiss the role of association fibres in general. Moreover, the most prominent associational system of all, the corpus callosum which links the two cerebral hemispheres, did not at the time seem to have any obvious function, leading Lashley and others to suppose, that its function must be to hold the two sides of the brain together. Lashley concluded that '. . . the absence of symptoms following section of the corpus callosum in man...give no positive evidence as to the function of long association fibers'.[8]

How, then, was this integration achieved? No one knew. Yet everyone sensed that this must be the key to understanding the workings of the cerebral cortex. Perhaps suspecting that he was basing his speculations on a very imperfect knowledge of the anatomy, Lashley wrote, 'I doubt that any real understanding of cerebral integration can be attained until all the details of cellular interactions have been worked out'.[6] This may seem like a truism, but it is nevertheless profoundly true. Recent evidence has shown us how rich the connections between the visual areas are. They have given us some hints as to how integration may be achieved, at least in the visual cortex, and it is to a study of these connections that we shall turn in Chapter 31. Before doing so, however, it is interesting to discuss briefly speculations on integration derived from examining speculations on the modularity of mind.

In his book, *The Modularity of Mind*,[12] Fodor has approached the problem of integration in an interesting way, although he does not refer to it as integration and draws his examples from the philosophy of science rather than from neurological pathways, which is my main concern. The discussion is nevertheless relevant and has truths in it which Fodor, not being an anatomist or a physiologist, is not aware of. In summarizing his view, I am also simplifying it and rendering it much more neurological, and therefore easier to understand.

Fodor puts the question like this: 'Vertical [input] faculties are domain specific (by definition) and modular (by hypothesis). So the question that we now want to ask can be put like this: Are there psychological processes that can plausibly be assumed to cut across cognitive domains? And, if there are, is there reason to suppose that such processes are subserved by nonmodular (e.g. informationally unencapsulated) mechanisms?'. This passage in a sense distils the tense relationship between localization and anti-localization. I shall render it into our language like this: Input systems are domain specific (vision, audition, etc.) and also submodality specific (colour, form, motion, depth in vision). The organization of the cortex is modular, however one defines the module. This modularity correlates well with the specificity of cortical connections, in the sense that subdivisions of one visual area concerned with colour are connected to each other and to other similar subdivisions in other cortical areas, whereas subdivisions concerned with other attributes are connected with their counterparts. It also correlates well with clinical and psychophysical evidence which shows that specific cortical lesions can lead to remarkably specific visual disturbances, such as a specific inability to see colours. Given this, are there any visual processes which can plausibly be assumed to cut across this modularity and thus not be easily localizable? And if there are, is there reason to suppose that such processes are subserved by non-modular connections?

In his discussion of the issue, Fodor coins the terms isotropic and Quineian. Put briefly, these terms imply that everything that the brain knows must be of relevance and importance in determining everything else that the brain ought to believe (isotropy) and 'each hypothesis about "unobservables" must *entail* some predictions about observables' [original emphasis] (Quineianiasm). Translated to the visual cortex, this could be taken to mean that everything that the visual cortex knows must be relevant to its ability to determine that the stimulus before the eyes is a stationary red bus on the other side of the road (isotropy). The hypothesis that this bus is not green and is not moving (both unobservables) must result from the knowledge, due to neural computation, that it is red and stationary (both of them observables). In brief, it must demand a great deal of integration. What kind of anatomical wiring would such an isotropic and Quieneian system demand? It would obviously demand a diffuse system, rather than the 'like-with-like' connectivity which I have been describing. And anatomical evidence shows that there is indeed such a diffuse system.

References

1 Sholl, D.A. (1956). *The Cerebral Cortex*. Methuen & Co., London.
2 Marie, P. (1920). *Traveaux et Mémoires*. Masson, Paris.
3 Head, H. (1926). *Aphasia and Kindred Disorders of Speech*. Cambridge University Press, Cambridge.
4 Lashley, K.S. (1931). Mass action in cerebral function. *Science* **73**, 245–254.
5 Lashley, K.S. (1936). Functional determinants of cerebral localization. *Arch. Neurol. Psychiatr. (Chicago)* **38**, 371–387.
6 Lashley, K.S. (1929). *Brain Mechanisms of Intelligence*. Chicago University Press, Chicago.
7 Lashley, K.S. (1931). Cerebral control versus reflexology: a reply to Professor Hunter. *J. Genet. Psychol.* **5**, 3–20.
8 Lashley, K.S. (1952). Functional interpretation of anatomic patterns. *Res. Publ. Assoc. Res. Nerv. Ment. Dis.* **30**, 429–547.
9 Lashley, K.S. & Clark, G. (1946). The cytoarchitecture of the cerebral cortex of Ateles: a critical examination of architectonic studies. *J. Comp. Neurol.* **85**, 223–305.
10 Lashley, K.S. (1948). The mechanism of vision. XVIII. Effects of destroying the visual 'associative areas' of the monkey. *Genet. Psychol. Monogr.* **37**, 107–166.
11 Clark, W.E. Le Gros (1941). Observations on the association fibre system of the visual cortex and the central representation of the retina. *J. Anat.* **75**, 225–235.
12 Fodor, J.A. (1983). *The Modularity of Mind*. MIT Press, Cambridge.

Chapter 29: A theory of multi-stage integration in the visual cortex

The paradox of vision

The picture that one obtains from studying the visual cortex is one of multiple areas and of parallel pathways leading to them. It is a picture that shows a deep division of labour, the evidence for which is best when obtained from the pathologic human brain. Yet the common, daily experience of the normal human brain stands forever opposed to the notion of a division of labour and of functional segregation. For that experience is one of wholeness, of a unitary visual image, in which all the visual attributes take their correct place, in which one can register the precise position, shape and colour as well as the direction and speed of motion of a bus simultaneously and instantaneously, as if all the information coming from that bus had been analyzed in one place, in a fraction of a second. Nothing in that integrated visual image suggests that different visual attributes are processed in physically separate parts of our cortex. The task, then, is to enquire into how the brain puts the separate attributes together. An initial step in this enquiry is to study the anatomical opportunities that exist for the specialized visual areas to 'talk' to one another. The task, in brief, is to address the problem of integration anatomically. We shall then see that anatomy, in its usual way, gives powerful clues to how the cerebral cortex might be organized to undertake its integrative functions. Moreover, the strategy used by the visual cortex to achieve integration may give us some insights into the even grander problem of cortical integration in general, for the very same problem has to be addressed when studying the cortex at large: how do the specialized areas of the cerebral cortex interact to provide the integration evident in thought and behaviour.[1]

The ghost in the machine

At first glance, the problem of integration may seem quite simple. Logically it demands nothing more than that all the signals from the specialized visual areas be brought together, to 'report' the results of their operations to a single master cortical area. This master area would then synthesize the information coming from all these diverse sources and provide us with the final image, or so one might think. But the brain has its own logic, which only becomes logical after one has discovered what that logic is. In fact, the strategy outlined above faces severe difficulties, of which the most severe is the problem of consciousness, the one that most neurobiologists would prefer to avoid, or at any rate to postpone indefinitely. If all the visual areas report to a single master cortical area, who or what does that single area report to? Put more visually, who is 'looking' at the visual image provided by that master area? The problem is not unique to the visual image or the visual cortex. Who, for example, listens to the music provided by a master auditory area, or senses the odour provided by the master olfactory cortex? It is in fact pointless pursuing this grand design. For here one comes across an important anatomical fact, which may be less grand but perhaps more illuminating in the end: *there is no single cortical area to which all other cortical areas report exclusively, either in the visual or in any other system. In sum, the cortex must be using a different strategy for generating the integrated visual image.*

There is, moreover, another problem which integration, in the way envisaged above, generates. The end result of integration must not lose the components which enter into the formation of the integrated image. As an example, when I perceive a red flower, i.e. both the colour and the form simultaneously, I must nevertheless still be able to categorize that object according to colour alone, or to shape alone. The components forming the integrated image must not be dissolved in the final image.

The three processes of integration

It is obvious, then, that integration is a formidable problem, the end result of which is the construction of the visual image in the brain. We know very little about the strategy that the brain uses to achieve integration, even within the relatively well-studied visual cortex. We can therefore only speculate based on such facts as we possess, which is what the description given below is. The initial point is to realize that, before the visual image can be constructed, its components must be constructed, a process that also requires the brain to undertake a great deal of work. For example, before the brain can label the red rose as having a certain shape and a certain colour, it must assemble together the information which would make of that shape a flower of a particular colour. It would simplify our task if we could therefore think of integration somewhat simplistically, and for descriptive purposes only, as consisting of three interlinked processes, not necessarily occurring contiguously in time, which lead to the integrated visual image in the brain. Each major process involves further subprocesses and can occur at several different levels. The first process involves enlarging the receptive fields of cells so that they are able to respond to, and collect information from, larger parts of the field of view. The second process, which occurs simultaneously with the first, generates cells with more complex and often specific properties, e.g. the orientation selective cells which are generated from the centre−surround cells of the LGN or the directionally selective cells of area V5 generated from V1 cells with corresponding properties; the third process involves the unification of signals from different sources, representing different visual attributes, e.g. form and motion. *By unification, I do not mean that signals literally 'come together' on the same cell; unification could equally well be achieved by distant cells responding in synchrony, a theme developed further below.*

Integration across visual space and enlargement of receptive fields

The need for the first process, integration across visual space, arises from the fact that the receptive fields of cells are limited in size and position, with those in areas V1 and V2 covering only a fraction of the field of view. The visual scene, by contrast, is perceived as a continuous whole, without any breaks. Somehow, the fields of cells must be united to give an uninterrupted panoramic view. Perhaps the simplest way of enlarging receptive fields, and thus achieving integration across visual space, is to connect together cells dealing with a given sub-modality of vision but with non-identical receptive field positions. The cells may merely connect with one another or they may converge their outputs onto another cell which will consequently have a larger receptive field. An example of the first process is found in visual areas such as V1 and V2, where cells representing the vertical meridian in one hemisphere are linked to their counterparts in the opposite hemisphere, without the receptive fields of cells in either hemisphere being thereby enlarged[2] (Figure 29.1). There are several examples of the second process too. The receptive fields of the wavelength-selective cells in V2 are larger than their counterparts in V1, and those of V4 are larger still. This enlargement is a reflection of the anatomical convergence from the blobs of V1 to the thin stripes of V2 and then to V4 and forms a hierarchical chain of increasing size and complexity within a specialized pathway (Figure 29.2). Several blobs in V1 project to a single thin stripe in V2 and several thin stripes in V2 converge onto a given small (ca. $4\,mm^2$) region of V4.[3] Another, separate, example of a hierarchical chain is the projection from layer 4B of V1 and the thick stripes of V2 to area V5.[4] The receptive fields of the directionally selective cells in the latter are considerably larger than their counterparts in the former.[5] Many other similar examples could be given. Interestingly, in each the enlargement of receptive

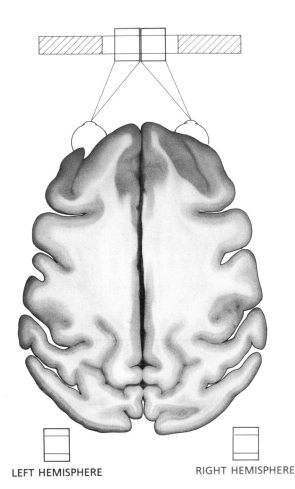

Fig. 29.1 Cells in either hemisphere whose receptive fields include the midline of vision are connected with their counterparts of the opposite hemisphere through the corpus callosum. Their synchronous firing would be one way of signalling that they are responding to the same object.

LEFT HEMISPHERE   **RIGHT HEMISPHERE**

fields does not occur in one step but at several stages, with the smallest receptive fields being encountered in V1 and the largest in the visual areas of parietal and temporal cortex. Clearly, spatial integration is a multi-stage process; it occurs separately in each of the parallel pathways to the extent that, for example, there is a progressive increase in receptive field size in the motion pathways comprising V1 → the thick stripes of V2 → V5, just as there is a progressive increase of receptive field size in the colour pathway comprising V1 → the thin stripes of V2 → V4. What we see in operation here is the principle of *topical convergence*, the convergence that operates within a specialized pathway or system and leads to integration across visual space.[6]

This process of enlarging receptive fields itself creates problems which have to be solved by another form of integration. Cells with large receptive fields are no longer able to signal the precise position of stimuli in the world, or at any rate cannot do so with the same precision that cells with small receptive fields can. The problem has somehow to be solved by relating the responses of cells with large receptive fields to a very precise map of the visual field, such as that

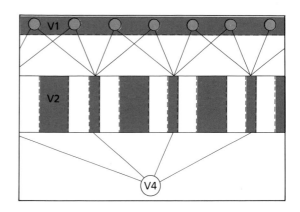

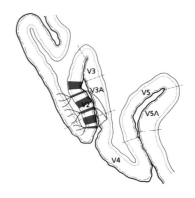

Fig. 29.2 The connections from the blobs of V1 to the thin stripes of V2 to area V4, shown schematically above and on a section through the relevant areas below.

of V1. Tied to this is yet another problem. Suppose that the view in front of you includes a long horizontal line, for example that described by a fence gate. Given its size, the gate will stimulate several orientation-selective cells in V1, in V2 and in V3 with receptive fields in different positions. The nervous system must not only be able to distinguish the fact that the different cells of V1 are being stimulated by the same object but that the cells of area V3, which receives a direct and convergent anatomical connection from V1 and whose cells consequently have larger receptive fields, are also being stimulated by the same object, rather than by different objects, as may happen in conditions when different segments of a horizontal line belong to different objects. This is called the problem of correspondence and identity. As we shall see later, these problems require a different kind of anatomical solution.

The generation of more complex receptive field properties

In generating integration across visual space through this topical convergence, the brain also simultaneously generates cells with more complicated response properties. The progressive elaboration of cells with more intricate properties is probably best worked out in the form system, at least in neurophysiological terms.[7] The geniculate cells not only have smaller receptive fields than the simple cells of the cortex, but also have less sophisticated response properties (Figure 29.3). In the same way, the complex cells have larger receptive fields and more complex properties than the simple cells from which they have been hypothesized to receive their inputs (see Chapter 9). There are many other examples of this, the above being only the best known. We have seen how, in the colour system, the response properties of the colour-coded cells of V4 are a good deal more sophisticated than those of the wavelength-selective cells of V1[8] and how, in the motion system, the directionally selective cells of V5 are able to register the true direction of motion of objects, while their counterparts in V1 can do no better than register the direction of each component.[9]

The generation of 'experiential' cells

Since this second process is linked to the first process, it occurs simultaneously in time and since the first process occurs in several substages, so does the second. This second process may be somewhat loosely referred to as the stage that generates the *experiential cells*. The term experiential is fraught with difficulties and will undoubtedly

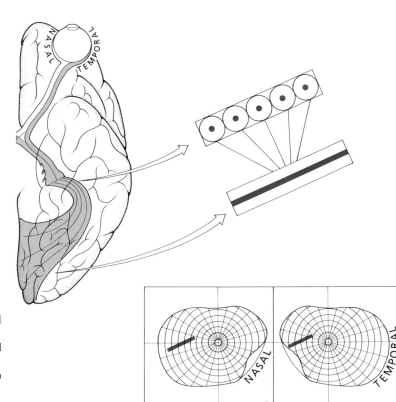

Fig. 29.3 The connections from the centre-surround cells of the lateral geniculate nucleus (LGN) to the cortex are convergent, several LGN cells projecting onto a single cortical cell. This process enlarges the receptive field of the cortical cell and also endows it with more complex properties, enabling it to respond to a line of given orientation in a given part of the field of view.

excite the fury of philosophers. I may be mistaken in using it, but I do so for two reasons. In the first place, it makes it more easy to understand the complex connections of the visual cortex as well as the somewhat bizarre conditions prevailing in conditions such as achromatopsia and akinetopsia, reviewed in the next chapter. Second, it raises a very fundamental question about the visual areas, and indeed all cortical areas: to what extent can the responses of cells in a given area be said to correlate directly with human (or monkey) experience? Can one say that the responses of orientation-selective cells in V1, ones which respond to the vertical orientation, do not correlate with the monkey's experience of a vertical line, indeed contribute directly to that perception? Can one say that the responses of cells in monkey V2 to illusory contours do not contribute directly to, and are the cause of, the monkey's ability to respond to illusory contours? There are many examples one can give in which the response of a cell in the cortex is so specific and correlates so well with a specific visual experience that the question merits serious consideration. If one concedes that the responses of cells in different visual areas may correlate with different kinds of visual experience, that these may in fact be experiential cells, then we begin to understand better not only why integration is a multi-stage process but also why it is that different lesions in the brain result in perceptual deficits of varying complexity.

There is direct evidence to suggest that the responses of cells in area V5 correlate directly with the subjective perception of motion in the monkey.[10] As such, we can think of several levels of experiential cells with differing complexity in the cortical pathways concerned with visual motion. Thus, the response of an orientation- and direction-selective cell with a small receptive field in V1, responsive to motion towards two o'clock, may correlate quite well with my experience of an oriented line moving in the same direction over a small expanse of my field of view. But the responses of such a cell will not correlate at all well with an entire object moving to the right but some of whose components move in the direction to which the above cell is selective, since the motion of the entire object is to the right (see Figure 29.4). The overall motion of the object (to the right) seems to be detected by cells in V5, while the cells of V1 detect the motion of its component parts (which can be in several different directions). To that extent both the cells of V1 and of V5 have responses which are experiential, though those of V5 have more complex experiential properties. To that extent too, both V1 and V5 may be called integrator areas, though the level of integration achieved is different in the two areas.

Two important conclusions follow from this. The first is that *no area of the cerebral visual cortex, including area V1, can at present be said not to contribute explicitly to perception.* In the example given here, both V1 and V5 are considered to contribute explicitly to

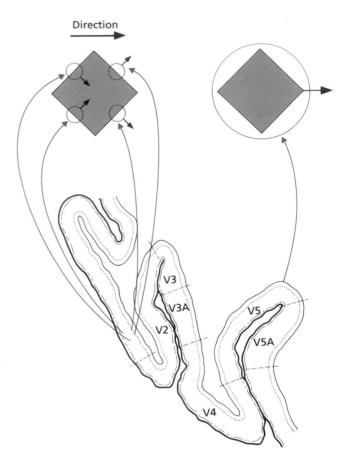

Fig. 29.4 When a complex object such as a diamond is moving to the right, its components move in different directions if viewed through small apertures, corresponding to the receptive fields of cells in V1. The cells of V5, by contrast, are able to register the real motion of the entire object which, in this case, is to the right. (Redrawn from the work of Movshon, J.A. *et al.* (1985). *Pattern Recognition Mechanisms*, edited by C. Chagas, R. Gattass & C. Gross. Pontifical Academy, Vatican City.)

the perception of visual motion, though with varying degrees of sophistication. The second conclusion is that *the severity of the defect following lesions must be related directly to the capacities of the integrator stages left intact by the lesion.* Again, from the example given above, while patients with lesions in V5 should suffer from a profound disturbance in visual motion perception, indeed should have the syndrome of cerebral akinetopsia described earlier, a residual capacity to detect motion based on the capacities of area V1 should remain, which is in fact the case (see below).

The integration involved in the colour system is the same, at least in broad outline. There, the responses of some cells in V4 correlate with my perception of colour whereas the responses of their counterparts in V1 do not. To generate the kind of experiential cell found in V4 requires a good deal of topical convergence, both anatomical and functional. As we have seen, colour vision demands that information coming from large parts of the field of view should be compared and this comparison is presumably integrated into the responses of single cells in area V4. It is only then that the responses of these cells can correlate with the perception of colour. But the fact that the responses of cells in V4 correlate directly with the perception of colours does not mean that the wavelength cells of V1, from which they ultimately receive their input, do not have certain limited capacities in detecting colour stimuli, and may therefore contribute directly to the experience of such stimuli. It should follow from this that patients with an achromatopsia due to lesions in area V4 should nevertheless be capable of some degree of residual colour vision, perhaps of wavelength discrimination, as a result of the activity of cells in area V1, which again seems to be the case (see Chapter 30).

The convergence that results in the generation of orientation-selective cells, and in the enlargement of their receptive fields, occurs between areas (lateral geniculate nucleus to V1) or within an area (simple to complex cells within V1). In fact, intrinsic connections within an area may contribute substantially to this process.[11] But all the indications are that such intrinsic connections obey the 'like-with-like' principle and thus preserve a remarkable degree of specificity. A good example is to be found in the blob-to-blob connections within V1.[12] It turns out that the blobs of V1 can be subdivided into separate groupings, those in which most wavelength-selective cells respond to long-, middle- or short-wave light. Study of the connections of the blobs show, that: (a) cells in blobs connect selectively with other blobs and do not connect with the interblobs; and (b) the cells of any given blob do not connect randomly with any other blob in the vicinity. Instead, they connect selectively with blobs having similar wavelength preferences. For example, a 'long-wave selective' blob will connect with another 'long-wave selective' blob rather than with a 'middle-wave selective' blob. Such is the degree of specificity in cortical connections.[12]

Integration between submodalities: confluent convergence

Once signals dealing with a given submodality of vision, for example colour, are united to allow cells to integrate information coming from large parts of the field of view, the need arises to unite signals belonging to different visual attributes, such as form *and* colour. This can be done by arranging for the specialized areas, or the specialized sub-groupings within an area, to communicate directly with areas or subgroupings which have other specializations. Such connections are known to exist and once again occur at different levels. At the level of areas, V5 has direct outputs to areas V3 and V4, and the latter have links with each other as well as with V5.[6] We note that intrinsic connections within an area may also be of the confluent type, in that they may help to unite signals subserving different submodalities. For example, there are horizontally coursing fibres within area V2. These are of sufficient length to span the territory of the thin, thick and interstripes, subdivisions with different functional cell groupings.[13] They could therefore provide the anatomical opportunity for the sub-divisions to interact with each other, but no one yet knows whether they contribute much to integration. These convergent connections, whether intrinsic or between areas, which might help to unite signals belonging to different attributes of vision, are referred to as *confluent convergence*,[6] to distinguish them from topical convergence.

The confluent, convergent, output to 'higher' areas

Another, and perhaps even simpler, way of uniting signals belonging to different attributes of vision would be to arrange that the outputs of two or more areas converge onto a third area. This is indeed how anatomists thought integration would be achieved.[14] But the problem is not quite so simple. One might suppose that the easiest way of achieving integration through such a confluent convergence system would be for the outputs from two areas with different specializations to actually overlap in the territory of the third. In fact, when one examines such convergent outputs from two specialized visual areas onto a common, third, area one is impressed by how little overlap there is. For example, both V4 and V5 have outputs to a specific part of the parietal cortex lying in the intraparietal sulcus.[15] Equally, parietal and temporal areas have outputs to the same region of the frontal cortex.[16] Yet, when one examines these convergent outputs in greater detail, one finds that they are not really convergent at all, in the sense of being overlapping. Instead, the striking feature is that each area maintains its own territory in the third, and the amount of overlap is minimal.[15,16] Plate 22 (facing p. 308), for example, shows that the inputs from V4 and V5 do not overlap in the territory of the intraparietal sulcus but terminate in contiguous stripes which abut each other only minimally. Areas V4 and V5 also project to the temporal cortex but here again the projections do not overlap directly. Although more examples can be given, the above two anatomical examples illustrate well the extent to which the cerebral cortex uses the strategy of maintaining separate informational systems segregated from each other. This anatomical segregation is perhaps reflected in functional segregation, which may be even more extreme than the segregation into the submodalities discussed so far. One example[16] is found in the frontal cortex. Physiological evidence shows that cells dealing with different kinds of rapid eye movements (saccades) are grouped together, that these different functional subgroupings are separated from each other and that their distribution is systematically related to an anatomical feature of the frontal cortex. Thus cells dealing with vertical saccade are grouped together and separated from horizontal saccade cells. A study of the distribution of the two types of cells in relation to the interhemispheric (callosal) fibres connecting the two hemispheres shows that this differentiation can be related directly to differences in interhemispheric connectivity. Vertical saccade cells are concentrated within the callosally connected patches of the frontal cortex and horizontal saccade cells are concentrated within the callosal-free zones. Another interesting example of cortical separation and segregation is derived from the study of patients with lesions.[17]. Clinical evidence shows that lesions which lead to the syndrome of prosopagnosia, the inability to recognize familiar faces, can nevertheless spare the recognition of the expression on a face which, itself, is not recognized.[18] This implies that the recognition of familiar faces and the recognition of facial expression are two different things which, because of functional specialization in the brain, depend on two different neural systems, each of which can be specifically compromised. It is no doubt only a question of time before these differences will be found to be reflected in anatomical differences in connectivity and perhaps even in architecture. But from the point of view of integration, each of the two neural systems of recognition — the one dealing with the recognition of the face as belonging to a given individual and the other with the more general features of facial expression — have to be integrated with the image of the face constructed by the visual cortex.

To all intents and purposes, therefore, present evidence suggests that a direct convergence of inputs onto single cells from different sources, registering different attributes of the visual scene, is not the predominant or preferred approach that the cortex uses to unite signals coming from these different sources. This is not to suggest that such direct convergence does not occur, but only that it is not the predominant mode of integration. For example, it has been shown[19] that there are cells in an area of the brain, known as the polysensory area, which respond to visual, acoustic and somesthetic stimuli. But these cells are in a minority and their properties may be generated by local circuits rather than by direct convergence of outputs from specialized areas. Even in the polysensory area, however, most cells are exclusively visual. If the cortex does use such a strategy of direct convergence, it must do so sparingly.

The degree and extent of separation discussed above and elsewhere in this book naturally raises the fundamental question of how and where the inputs finally overlap, or indeed whether they overlap at all. It is, after all, possible that the cortex uses a more subtle strategy for uniting signals belonging to different attributes. It is obvious from this description, too, that the integration brought about by confluent convergence is also a multi-stage process and involves interactions at several different levels.

The integration of perceptually explicit signals

The anatomical picture that we are beginning to obtain is highly complex. One might well want to learn why it is that the visual areas connect directly with each other, as well as through higher and lower areas (see below). More simply, one would like to know why the anatomical pathways serving integration are not deferred until *after* the stage of the specialized visual areas. One obvious answer to this question lies in the fact that there are several stages in each of the specialized visual pathways. For example, the colour pathways in the cortex include subdivisions within areas V1 and V2, as well as area V4. Similarly, the motion pathways include areas V1, V2 and V5, and several other areas besides. Although the responses of cells at each level of the pathway may be used at subsequent levels to achieve spatial integration and generate more complex properties through the process of topical convergence, it nevertheless remains that the responses of cells at each level of the pathway, even early ones, may contribute to perception explicitly. These explicit responses, i.e. ones which require no further processing, must then be integrated with explicit contributions derived from other sources. If one had to wait until the final stage, whatever that may be, the output of the cells may be further transformed and the signal may no longer be explicit, but only implicit in the response of the cell. Let us suppose, for example, that the visual field in front of you contains a single, oriented line which is red in colour and moving to the right perpendicular to the axis of the line. There is no good reason why the orientation and direction of motion of such a stimulus should not be detected by the direction-plus orientation-selective cells of layer 4B of V1, and its colour determined by the cells of V4. The simultaneous and synchronous firing of the relevant cells in the two areas could then specify the properties of the visual stimulus. It is not obvious why the output from layer 4B should be relayed to V5 to be able to detect such a simple stimulus, especially since the output of the cell may be integrated with the outputs of other cells projecting to V5 and thus be specialized to signal a more elaborate moving stimulus. It is therefore sometimes an advantage to achieve integration at earlier, rather than later, stages. The simplest way of doing this is to allow integration to occur at that stage rather than at a later stage, when the output of the cells may have been further transformed. Hence signals must be accessible to integration at every stage. And integration is therefore itself a multi-stage process.

The catalogue given above leaves out of account another anatomical system which may serve to unite signals from diverse sources. This is the system of reciprocal connections or back (re-entrant) projections considered in Chapter 31. What becomes obvious from considering the anatomy of connections between the visual areas is that the anatomical opportunities for integration are manifold. They also lead us to a theory of multi-stage integration in the visual system.[6,20] This theory supposes that integration is not achieved in a single step through a convergent output to a higher area or set of areas. It supposes, instead, *that integration is achieved at different stages, including stages where functional specialization is first established in the visual cortex, i.e. areas V1 and V2.* In its curious way, anatomy has always led the field in suggesting how the brain does things, probably much to the chagrin of other neurobiologists who have traditionally despised the field of neuro-anatomy. What the anatomical evidence tells us in this instance is that the brain has solved the problem of integration in a very different way from the one which common sense might have dictated.

References

1 Lashley, K.S. (1931). Mass action in cerebral function. *Science* **73**, 245–254.

2 Hubel, D.H. & Wiesel, T.N. (1967). Cortical and callosal connections concerned with the vertical meridian of visual fields in the cat. *J. Neurophysiol.* **30**, 1561–1573; Zeki, S.M. & Sandeman, D.R. (1976). Combined anatomical and electrophysiological studies on the boundary between the second and third visual areas of rhesus monkey cortex. *Proc. R. Soc. Lond.* B **194**, 555–562.

3 Zeki, S. & Shipp, S. (1989). Modular connections between areas V2 and V4 of macaque monkey visual cortex. *Eur. J. Neurosci.* **1**, 494–506.

4 Shipp, S. & Zeki, S. (1989) The organization of connections between areas V1 and V5 in the macaque monkey visual cortex. *Eur. J. Neurosci.* **1**, 309–332; Shipp, S. & Zeki, S. (1989). The organization of connections between areas V5 and V2 in the macaque monkey visual cortex. *Eur. J. Neurosci.* **1**, 333–354. Zeki, S.M. (1976). The projections to the superior temporal sulcus from areas 17 and 18 in the rhesus monkey. *Proc. R. Soc. Lond.* B **193**, 199–207.

5 Zeki, S.M. (1974) Functional organization of a visual area in the posterior bank of the superior temporal sulcus of the rhesus monkey. *J. Physiol. (Lond.)* **236**, 549–573; Albright, T.D. & Desimone, R. (1987). Local precision of visuotopic organization in the middle temporal area (MT) of the macaque. *Exp. Brain Res.* **65**, 582–592.

6 Zeki, S. & Shipp, S. (1988). The functional logic of cortical connections. *Nature* **335**, 311–316.

7 Hubel, D.H. & Wiesel, T.N. (1962). Receptive fields, binocular interaction and functional architecture in the cat's visual cortex. *J. Physiol. (Lond.)* **160**, 106–154.

8 Zeki, S. (1983). Colour coding in the cerebral cortex: the reaction of cells in monkey visual cortex to wavelengths and colours. *Neuroscience* **9**, 741–765.

9 Movshon, J.A. *et al.* (1985). The analysis of moving visual patterns. *Exp. Brain Res.* Suppl. **11**, 117–151.

10 Logothetis, N.K. & Schall, J.D. (1989). Neuronal correlates of subjective visual perception. *Science* **245**, 761–763.

11 Gilbert, C.G. & Wiesel, T.N. (1979). Morphology and intracortical projections of functionally characterised neurones in the cat visual cortex. *Nature* **280**, 122–125; Gilbert, C.G. & Wiesel, T.N. (1981). Laminar specialization and intracortical connections in cat primary visual cortex. In *Organization of Visual Cortex*, edited by F.O. Schmitt, F.G. Worden, G. Adelman and F.G. Dennis, pp. 163–191. MIT Press, Cambridge; Gilbert, C.G., Hirsch, J.A. & Wiesel, T.N. (1991). Lateral interactions in visual cortex. *Cold Spring Harb. Symp. Quant. Biol.* **55**, 663–677.

12 Ts'o, D.Y. & Gilbert, C.D. (1988). The organization of chromatic and spatial interactions in the primate striate cortex. *J. Neurosci.* **8**, 1712−1727; Matsubara, J., Cynader, M., Swindale, N.V. & Stryker, M.P. (1985). Intrinsic projections within visual cortex: evidence for orientation specific local connections. *Proc. Natl. Acad. Sci. USA* **82**, 935−939.

13 Rockland, K.S. (1985). A reticular pattern of intrinsic connections in primate area V2 (area 18). *J. Comp. Neurol.* **235**, 467−478.

14 Jones, E.G. & Powell, T.P.S. (1970). An anatomical study of converging sensory pathways within the cerebral cortex of the monkey. *Brain* **93**, 793−820.

15 Unpublished results from this laboratory; see also, Zeki, S. (1990). The motion pathways of the cerebral cortex. In *Vision: Coding and Efficiency*, edited by C. Blakemore, pp. 321−345. Cambridge University Press, Cambridge.

16 Goldman-Rakic, P. (1984). Modular organization of prefrontal cortex. *Trends Neurosci.* **7**, 419−429.

17 Damasio, A.R. (1990). Category-related defects as a clue to the neural substrates of knowledge. *Trends Neurosci.* **13**, 95−98.

18 Tranel, D., Damasio, A.R. & Damasio, H. (1988). Intact recognition of facial expression, gender, and age in patients with impaired recognition of face identity. *Neurology* **38**, 690−696.

19 Bruce, C.J., Desimone, R. & Gross, C.G. (1981). Visual properties of neurons in a polysensory area in superior temporal sulcus of the macaque. *J. Neurophysiol.* **46**, 369−384.

20 Zeki, S. (1990). A theory of multistage integration in the visual cortex. In *The Principles of Design and Operation of the Brain*, edited by J.C. Eccles & O. Creutzfeldt, pp. 137−154. Pontifical Academy, Vatican City.

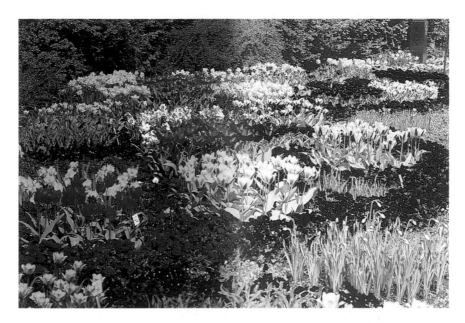

Plate 18 Because it is the contralateral field of view which is represented in each hemisphere, a unilateral lesion in V4 causes hemiachromatopsia, when only one half of the field of view is seen in colour. (Reproduced by permission from Zeki, S. (1990). *La Recherche* **21**, 712−721.)

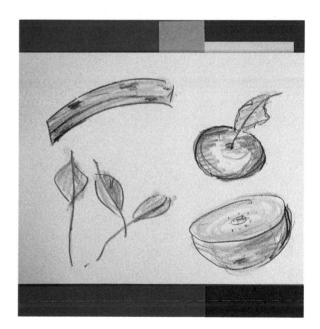

Plate 19 The drawings of an achromatopsic patient from memory show how well his form vision is preserved and how deeply his colour vision is affected. Clockwise from the upper left these are drawings of a banana, a tomato, a cantelope, and some leaves. This patient is described in greater detail by Sacks, O. & Wasserman, R. (1987). *New York Review of Books* **34**, 25−33.

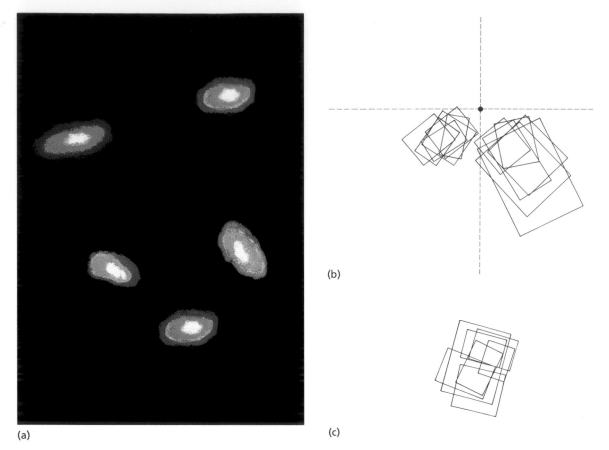

(a)

(b)

(c)

Plate 20 (a) The chromatophenes produced by unilateral stimulation of human area V4. (b) The chromatophenes thus produced have sizes which resemble the receptive field sizes of single cells in monkey area V4 (c). Stimulation of left human V4 produced chromatophenes in the right hemi-field and vice versa (b), suggesting a resemblance between the organization of human and monkey V4. (Photographs (a) and (b) courtesy of K. & G. Beckers.)

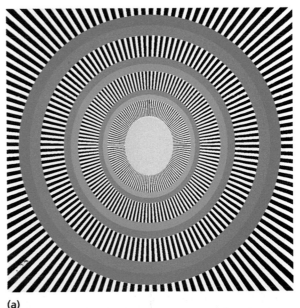

(a)

(b)

Plate 21 When most human subjects view the figure shown in (a) (entitled *Enigma* and executed by Isia Leviant) and fixate the centre, they perceive movement in the circles. Positron emission tomographic studies (b) show that this perception is correlated with increased activity in a region of the prestriate visual cortex corresponding largely to area V5 and its immediate vicinity (regions of highest activity shown in white and red). In (b), (A) shows horizontal slices through the averaged brain, to indicate the active regions when human subjects looked at a pattern in motion (arrows point to area V5). (B) shows the regions of the most significant blood flow changes (arrows) when the same human subjects looked at Enigma.

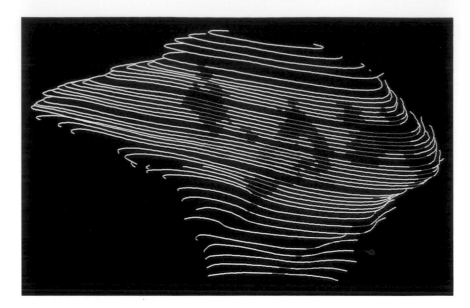

Plate 22 A computer-aided reconstruction of a small region of the parietal lobe to show the distribution of inputs to it from area V4 (red) and area V5 (green). The region where the outputs of the two areas in the parietal cortex overlap is shown in yellow. Notice that each area largely maintains its own territory within the parietal cortex and the amount of overlap is relatively small.

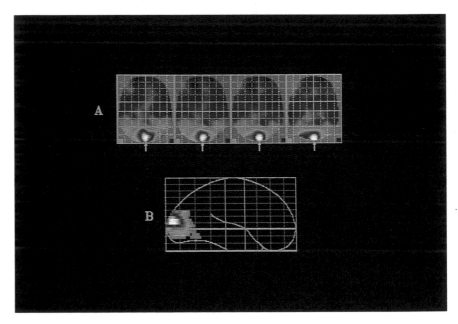

Plate 23 The horizontal brain slices in (A) show the activity in the human brain, measured by changes in regional cerebral blood flow, when human subjects looked at displays of structure from motion (for details of the paradigm see Figure 31.2). The maximum activity occured in area V1 (arrows). (B) The regions of significant change projected onto a profile of the brain.

Chapter 30: The disintegration of cerebral integration

The best evidence for integration does not come from the diseased, pathologic brain. It comes instead from the normal brain and is an experience which each one of us has continuously during the day and even at night when we dream. There are good reasons for this. Integration is a diffuse and multi-stage process, involving all the submodalities of vision and all visual areas. It uses the *reciprocal* (*re-entrant*) connections between the specialized areas as well as the *re-entrant* projections from the specialized areas to the areas which feed them (see below). It follows that discrete lesions in the brain do not interfere with the processes of integration to nearly the same extent as they do with the processing of particular submodalities of vision, such as colour. For example, an achromatopsic patient with a lesion restricted to the fusiform gyrus may not see the world in colour, but the other visual areas are functioning normally and the signals in them can be integrated with signals in other intact areas.

It is nevertheless interesting to consider here whether there are any neurological cases in which, following a cerebral injury, patients are specifically unable to undertake the kind of integration discussed above, whether topical or confluent, and to consider the extent to which such neurological cases support a theory of multi-stage integration. *Implicit in this theory is the supposition that each stage of the visual pathways, including area V1, contributes explicitly to perception.* One would therefore predict that where the processes of topical convergence are compromised, a patient should be able to detect the kind of stimuli that the cortical stages leading to the injured area are capable of and should also be unable to detect the kind of stimuli that the injured area, and the ones it feeds into, are specialized in constructing. Here, as elsewhere, the neurological literature is murky but enough is known to suggest that, in broad outline, something of this kind does happen.

The residual vision in cerebral akinetopsia

A good example to begin with is the akinetopsic patient of Zihl described earlier (see Chapter 10). Because of a bilateral lesion involving area V5, this patient is unable to see objects in motion but can see them when they are stationary. The kind of integration that would enable the brain to detect the phenomenal motion of an entire object is severely compromised in her because her area V5, where such an integration apparently takes place, is damaged. This does not mean that she is unable to detect the presence of motion *per se*. Indeed, a recent study of this patient concludes that 'the overall deficit...is characterized by a large discrepancy between detection [of motion], which is relatively unimpaired, and discrimination, which can be severely impaired'.[1] This same study showed that the patient is able to detect certain kinds of simple, slow motion, presumably those mediated by the direction-plus orientation-selective cells of her intact area V1, cells whose properties are the result of a topical convergence and therefore an integrative machinery. Though the authors do not consider the possibility that intact motion mechanisms in V1 may mediate this residual capacity to detect motion, their own description is revealing. They write, 'Thus, the overall results suggest that the local component information necessary for the derivation of motion is intact and thus the anomaly occurs at a later stage, where a more global analysis takes place'.[1] But if the anomaly occurs at a later stage, why suppose that the intact motion-detecting cells of V1, with their limited capacities, are not the ones that contribute directly to the limited experience of motion which this patient has? There is at present no obvious reason why the intact cells of area V1 should be excluded from providing a perceptual contribution. This has not been shown conclusively; indeed the question itself has not been asked. But until definitely excluded, the possibility must be considered, if only because it provides a simple explanation for the residual motion vision in a 'motion-blind' patient. (It is important to emphasize here that, even if area V1 is intact, it does not follow that its cells remain totally unscathed by the lesion. It is almost certain that the re-entrant input from V5 to V1, discussed below, will also be damaged, and hence that the intact V1 of a patient lacking an area V5 is not quite as intact as that of an individual who has both areas. These same comments apply to achromatopsia and will be considered in more detail below).

The residual vision in achromatopsia

A parallel example is found in achromatopsia. Here a principal centre of integration, area V4, is usually compromised, with area V1 being either partly or completely intact. Here again, patients appear to be able to detect differences in wavelength but cannot use the signals to construct colours. Their knowledge, in brief, is limited to such capacities as the wavelength-selective cells of V1 and V2 have. For example, an achromatopsic patient with a partially intact V1 whom I studied with Wolfgang Fries could discriminate wavelength differences of 10–20 nm, although he described them all in terms of shades of grey. Not all agree that the intact cells of V1 may contribute explicitly to such perceptual capacities as these patients have. Two recent studies[2,3] describe cases of achromatopsia, one of them incomplete,[2] in which the patient could undertake certain kinds of colour discriminations. These are so bizarre as to seem surprising at first. In particular, in one of the studies[3] the patient was able to detect the boundaries between two stimuli which differed in colour only (i.e. they were isoluminant) and which were therefore perceptually identical to him, provided that the two stimuli abutted each other. In other words, like the akinetopsic patient, the deficit in this one is also characterized by 'a large discrepancy between detection, which is relatively unaffected, and discrimination, which can be severely impaired'.[1] The authors of this study reject any explanation in terms of V1, which was partly intact in both patients. Instead, they seek to account for this observed, apparently bizarre, behaviour in more complex terms, supposing that there are two specialized prestriate areas, one specialized for the conscious perception of colour and the other for extracting contours from colour. Noting that the patient could discriminate the two isoluminant stimuli 'by detecting an edge between two stimuli that were, to him, perceptually identical', they suggest that, 'achromatopsia is the result of damage to regions of extrastriate cortex that are indispensable for the conscious appreciation of hue as opposed to using chromatic differences to extract contour [shape]'.[3] But such an argument soon lands one in difficulties, for it implies that there are two cortical stages for the appreciation of colour, one conscious and the other unconscious, and that each is tied to a separate cortical area, an argument with which I have little sympathy. To me, only a conscious brain can construct colours and only a conscious brain can gain a knowledge about the reflectance properties of objects and interpret these properties in terms of colour. Moreover, as we have seen, *the construction of colour itself requires boundaries between regions that have different reflectances for lights of different wavelengths*. To discriminate wavelengths and to construct colour are two different things (see Chapter 26). To suggest that there may be prestriate cortical centres which extract contours from colour, distinct from areas which use contours to generate colours, is to go well beyond the evidence at present available. Perhaps a more plausible explanation would be to try and account for the perceptual capacities of such patients by reference to the capacities of the intact cells of V1. There is reason to believe that the orientation-selective cells of the interblobs of V1 could be the source of the information that achromatopsic patients use to detect boundaries between isoluminant stimuli. These cells can respond to the boundaries between two isoluminant stimuli without being particularly selective to the colour of either of the two patches forming the boundary.[4] This is precisely what the patient could discriminate, without being able at the same time to detect the difference between the two stimuli, just like a V1 interblob cell. It is not that such a patient sees colours but is not conscious of them, as the authors imply, or that he sees colours but does not understand them. It is just that he sees and understands what the limited capacities of his V1 cells enable him to see and therefore to understand, namely a border between two isoluminant patches and nothing else. Such an explanation would be in accord with the known physiology of area V1 and also consistent with the supposition that the activity of cells in area V1 may contribute explicitly to perception. It is also consistent with the view that integration is a multi-stage process, with each stage making a direct, and perceptually explicit, contribution.

Failure of integration in visual agnosia

By far the most interesting examples of a failure of integration are to be found in patients with visual agnosia. Neurologists commonly speak of such patients as if they are 'form blind', suffering from 'object agnosia'. But opinion on the subject has been divided, at least in part because the syndrome itself is complex and manifests itself with variations in different patients. Patients may be able to recognize some objects, but not others; they may not recognize an object at one examination and yet be able to do so at a subsequent one. Some may be able to read while others cannot.[5] The lesions are commonly large, often associated with scotomas and some, but not all, patients suffer from problems of amnesia, aphasia and general mental deterioration. All this makes it difficult to relate a specific impairment to a specific cerebral defect. Indeed, some neurologists have vigorously championed the view that agnosia is nothing more than the consequence of a failing visual apparatus.[6] Yet there exists a sufficient number of patients whose eyes are normal, who are not aphasic and who do not suffer from mental deterioration to testify to the fact that there is a syndrome in which patients can apparently see objects, or at least parts of objects, and yet be unable to recognize what the objects are. It is but one jump from this demonstration to the supposition that there is some mysterious disease in which patients see but do not understand, a disease which has its anatomical and physiological basis in the supposed subdivision of the visual cortex into parts that 'see' and parts that 'understand' what is seen.

In fact, an examination of the literature reveals that cases of total loss of form vision do not exist, save perhaps in cases of carbon monoxide poisoning (discussed below). Why is this so and why are there so many degrees of severity in object agnosia compared with achromatopsia? Leaving aside the possibly important contribution to the recognition of dynamic forms that the V3 form system can make (see Chapter 27), I suggest that many of these agnosic patients are not agnosic at all in the classical sense of the term; it is not that they see but do not understand, but rather that they understand what they see and do not understand what they do not see. In other words, there is no sharp distinction between the faculties of seeing and of understanding, as the literature on agnosia would have us believe. Put otherwise, they are only incapable of seeing forms which demand a higher and more complex level of integration, while those demanding simple integrative processes are intact. Since integration itself is a multi-stage process, one should not be surprised to find that there are degrees of agnosia, ranging from the severe effects of carbon monoxide poisoning, due to damage of V1 itself, to the relatively mild ones due to damage of more central visual areas. Of course, integration can also operate in the opposite direction, 'top-down' in fashionable neurological parlance, and patients as well as ordinary, healthy, people can be made to see things once they have understood them but not until then.

The form vision of carbon monoxide poisoned patients — a breakdown in early levels of integration

Carbon monoxide poisoning has catastrophic effects on vision. Patients are left with nothing more than a rudimentary sense although, significantly, colour vision is relatively spared.[7] It is at least plausible to argue that V1 itself is damaged through this poisoning, which is not to say that the damage does not attain other cortical areas as well. The fact that colour is relatively spared argues strongly in favour of a differential effect on the functional subdivisions within V1 and their prolongation into the visual areas of the prestriate cortex; one would expect, in brief, that the blobs of V1 → thin stripes of V2 → V4 system will be relatively spared compared with the other systems also emanating from V1, and described earlier.[8] But if the damage occurs at the level of V1 and has a predeliction for the interblobs and for layer 4B, where orientation-selective cells abound, then one can expect the consequences of the damage to be very severe indeed. Just how severe it can be is illustrated in Figure 30.1. Here, even the ability to see single lines is compromised, presumably because even the relatively low level of integration that V1 is capable of — the generation of cells which respond to lines of specific orientation — is compromised.

The effects of carbon monoxide poisoning can also vary somewhat in severity, but they are nevertheless severe in all cases. Carbon monoxide poisoning has generally been considered to result in an agnosic syndrome. But I suggest that this, at least, is one group of

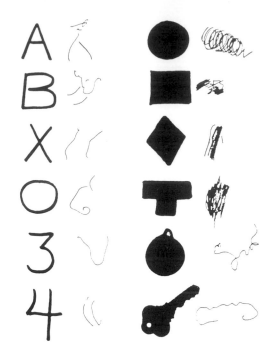

Fig. 30.1 The severe agnosia of a patient suffering from carbon monoxide poisoning is evident in his inability to copy simple letters or shapes. (Reproduced by permission from Benson, D.F. & Greenberg, J.P. (1969). *Arch. Neurol. (Chicago)* **20**, 82−89.)

patients from whom the mystique of a separation between seeing and understanding, implicit in the term agnosia, could be removed. Because of the severe damage to area V1, the brains of such patients are not capable of the elementary integration which is subsequently used by the specialized visual areas of the prestriate cortex. They neither see nor understand even elementary forms. They have, to use Hughling Jackson's term, an imperception.

The syndrome is different when the agnosia is the result of damage to more central visual areas and either spares V1 or involves it only partially, so that a good deal of it is left intact. This happens commonly in cases of strokes. Here we find that although the defect can be severe, it is not nearly as severe as in patients with carbon monoxide poisoning. There are many objects which they can both see and name and their performance commonly improves with time. Indeed, at first sight one may not even be aware of any defect in form recognition. One reason which had led neurologists, since the time of Lissauer, to the view that such agnosic patients can see but cannot understand is that they can commonly draw even complex figures, though without being able to make any sense of the figure they have drawn, or to understand it (Figure 30.2). Yet how is it that these patients draw? There is good agreement in the literature that the drawing is piecemeal, small segments of the picture or of its outline — segments that the patient can see and understand — being drawn one after another. Once drawn, the patient can still only recognize small segments of the drawing and not its entirety. The patient's report of the process itself

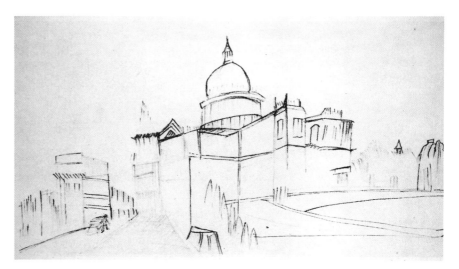

Fig. 30.2 The drawing of St. Paul's Cathedral, London, by an 'agnosic' patient. (Reproduced by permission from Humphreys, G.W. & Riddoch, M.J. (1987) *To see but not to see*. Erlbaum, Associates, Hillsdale.)

is more or less uniform. One patient stated that when he copied a complex figure, 'all he saw was a complex pattern of lines, which did not correspond to a particular object'. This is well reflected in his description of the difficulty of recognizing common objects, 'I have come to cope with recognising many common objects, if they are standing alone...When objects are placed together, though, I have more difficulties'.[9] The latter is possibly an example of what has been called simultagnosia, or an inability to perceive more than one object in the field of view at a time. It is the simple components of a figure that the patients are able to see and to understand because the integrative mechanisms necessary to construct simple forms, such as lines, are intact while those needed for more complex forms are compromised. Indeed the authors of this fascinating report state that the patient 'has intact registration of form elements (single lines and edges), but...his ability to integrate these elements into "perceptual wholes" is in some way impaired. The intact information about the local form elements enables him to make accurate copies of stimuli he cannot identify'.[9] Note the close similarity between this statement and the description of the achromatopsic patient as one who could detect 'an edge between two stimuli that were, to him, perceptually identical'.[3] In the former case, the patient should have been able to use the information provided by his intact orientation-selective cells to detect single lines and edges, but would not be able to integrate the information into a whole form; in the latter, the patient should have been able to detect the boundary between two isoluminant stimuli through his intact interblob cells of V1, but would not be able to use that information to generate colours. In both the integrative mechanisms which are the responsibility of higher visual areas are compromised. And note, too, the similarity with the description of the akinetopsic patients in whom, 'the overall deficit . . . is characterized by a large discrepancy between detection [of motion], which is relatively unimpaired, and discrimination, which can be severely impaired'.[1] Once again, one can postulate that the integration necessary to discriminate the coherent direction of motion over a large part of the field of view is compromised after damage to V5 but that the intact cells of V1 are capable of signalling the presence of motion. Nor are these isolated cases. The patient of Adler,[10] for example, described her experiences in very similar terms. Shown a green battleship, she mistook it first for a fountain pen, then for a green knife before identifying it as 'a boat'. She explained, 'At first I saw the front part. It looked like a fountain pen because it was shaped like a fountain pen. Then it looked like a knife because it was so sharp, but I thought it could not be a knife because it was green. Then I saw the spokes and that it was shaped like a boat, like in a movie where I had seen boats. It had too many spokes to be a knife or a fountain pen'. Another patient, 'When looking at a picture . . . could identify individual detail but could not appreciate the significance of the entire scene'.[11] These descriptions are so representative that they apply to most agnosic patients.

In principle, one should be able to account for some of these so-called agnosias by appealing to the physiology of the visual pathways, and in particular the capacities of different areas involved in the integration of the visual image. This is not an easy task because the visual areas which are involved in the recognition of even simple objects, as well as the details of the integrative processes, are not known, especially in man. But there are occasional cases which provide insights into the kind of explanation which one might use to account for some aspects of agnosia or, to use Hughling Jackson's much better term, imperception. An interesting case is that of an artist who became agnosic after a cerebral vascular accident and whose agnosia was accompanied by mental deterioration and, more significantly, a restricted scotoma.[12] The scotoma can be attributed to involvement of V1 and possibly also of V2. In any case, if V1 is involved, then V2 would be deprived of its input, at least from the affected area. One of the interesting features of this artist was his failure to see subjective contours, for example the Kanizsa triangles, described earlier. When shown the triangle in Figure 30.3 he described it as 'a three cornered thing . . . I see three edges and three circles'. The authors explain that the patient's 'descriptions and drawings focused on the individual elements physically present, omitting, despite probing, any reference to the subjective occluding figure'.[12] The patient, in brief, was not able to 'fill in' perceptually the gaps in the Kanizsa triangle. This failure is similar to the agnosic patient described above, in whom the failure of integrative mechanisms was such that he commonly failed

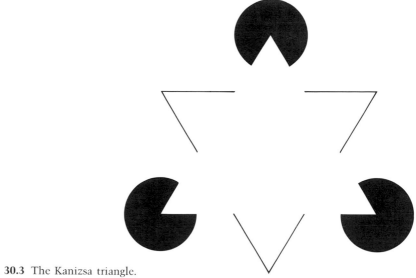

Fig. 30.3 The Kanizsa triangle.

to 'fill in' or complete a missing part, presumably because 'a patient using unintegrated information about form may...faithfully reproduce a gap in the figure because the information about the overall form is not available to "drive" the filling-in process'.[9] What, in neurological terms, constitutes the 'drive' or the 'filling-in' process is not known. But a reasonable hypothesis has been presented about the kind of activity in areas V1 and V2 which may lead to it. Although it is not certain that these are the actual neural mechanisms used, it is entirely plausible to suppose, in the light of the physiological evidence, that the kind of cells in area V2 which respond to virtual lines[13] are damaged, or that the inputs to them are disrupted. At any rate, such an explanation is as plausible, or even more so, than one which postulates a mysterious breakdown in 'understanding' what was seen.

More problematic is confluent convergence. Here one would wish to know whether there is any example of a patient who can, for example, see motion and colour but cannot integrate the two, with the consequence that the colour of a moving object is not seen in register with the motion. To my knowledge such a syndrome has not been described. The reason is simple. If the brain is intact enough to register both the colour and the coherent motion, it follows that both areas V4 and V5 must be intact, and therefore probably the connections between them as well. If one of them is compromised, or if the connections between the two are compromised, then no confluent convergence, and hence no submodality integration, can occur, a condition which has been described. One agnosic woman, for example, 'saw part of a whole picture such as a jockey but not the horse upon which the jockey was sitting...even though she could identify the correct colour of the horse';[14] in other words, she could not tag the colour to the correct form. Another patient, a professor of art, whose visual fields 'appeared to be normal for motion and recognition of gross objects' nevertheless 'could not group together all triangular shaped objects, but he could match and segregate the patterns according to the colours'.[14] A more severe dissociation between colour and object vision has been described,[15] but the pathology is still too uncertain to draw definite conclusions. Thus, Gelb's patient[15] saw the colours detach themselves from objects and appear in different distances from the eye in a step-like (*treppformig*) manner, the patient feeling as if he could dip his fingers into the series of coloured layers. As well, von Senden[16] quotes Grafé on the appearance of sensations following operations for congenital cataract: 'To begin with, the newly-operated patients do not localize their visual impressions...they see colours much as we smell an odour of peat or varnish...but without occupying any specific form of extension in a more exactly definable way'.

We do, however, possess a somewhat remarkable case of negative integration, one in which an abnormality in colour vision actually affects severely the perception of other attributes of vision through an inhibition.[17] This is, in a sense, the obverse of integration. The patient is a young man who, at the time of examination, had no medical history of note save a trivial appendicectomy. There was no evidence of any brain damage and the disease is considered to be of metabolic origin, though no one can tie it to a specific pathway of the brain. The patient's abnormality manifests itself whenever red appears in his field of view and, to a lesser extent, the same is observed with green and blue. The inhibition spreads for about 4° from the edge of the red surface or object and creates a sort of dynamic scotoma, so that the patient is unable to see the shape of objects or their movement in the scotomatous field — indeed he is unable to see any objects at all in the affected region. I have had occasion to study this patient. Testing showed that the inhibition was not due to the presence of long-wave (red) light as such. This is because the inhibition was not there when a scene which lacked red surfaces (e.g. a black, white, grey scene) was illuminated with light containing all wavelengths, including long-wave (red) light, even if the scene was arranged to reflect more long-wave light than light of other wavelengths. On the other hand, whenever a red or orange surface was present in a scene illuminated with the same projectors, the inhibition manifested itself instantly. The effect could be transferred from one eye to the other, suggesting that the inhibition occurs in an area central to V1, where there are strong monocular preferences. Since the effect also spreads for about 4° across the vertical meridian, it also follows that the inhibition must be central to V2, whose callosal connections are limited to the central $1-2°$. V4 therefore seems likely to be the first possible site of such an inhibition.

I do not wish to give the impression that all the many manifestations of agnosia can be accounted for by reference to the known visual pathways in the brain. This is far from so. We have little clue to the pathways involved in face recognition and still less to those involved in the recognition and categorization of faces according to expression, another syndrome which has been described. Nor yet do I wish to give the impression that all these syndromes can be accounted for purely and simply as a failure in integration, that there are no problems of memory and access to it that are involved, or of a defect in categorization which has also been described. Indeed, we shall discuss in the next chapter the critical role that memory plays in recognition, through re-entry. But the boundary that separates integration from categorization is imprecise — the second process cannot be undertaken without the first. And we know that the second process can remain intact when the first is compromised. Patients who are agnosic and therefore unable to recognize and categorize some objects visually are commonly able to do so by appealing to another sense, for example that of touch or of sound. The faculty of categorization is not impaired; the faculty of visual categorization is, precisely because the integrative mechanisms which are the necessary base for undertaking such a categorization are themselves impaired. But this is not to suggest that there may not be good clinical cases in which the faculty of categorization is itself impaired. My aim here has been simply to show that there is another way of looking at these defects, and that the result of such an enquiry leads us to the view that seeing and understanding merge into one another, and are not discrete activities localizable to different parts of the cerebral cortex.

In summary, clinical evidence suggests that many examples of form agnosia can be considered to be failures of the integrative mechanisms in the brain, leading the patient to both see and understand only in relation to the capabilities of the intact parts of the brain. This is not to suggest that one can account for all cases of what has been called visual agnosia in these relatively simple terms. But, if there is a case for separating the two processes of 'seeing' and 'understanding', that case has not yet been made convincingly.

References

1 Hess, R.H., Baker, C.L. & Zihl, J. (1989). The 'motion-blind' patient: low-level spatial and temporal filters. *J. Neurosci.* **9**, 1628–1640.
2 Victor, J.D., Maiese, K., Shapley, R., Sidtis, J. & Gazzaniga, M.S. (1989). Acquired central dyschromatopsia: analysis of a case with preservation of color discrimination. *Clin. Vis. Sci.* **4**, 183–196.

3 Heywood, C.A., Cowey, A. & Newcombe, F. (1991). Chromatic discrimination in a cortically colour blind observer. *Eur. J. Neurosci.* **3**, 802–812.

4 Gouras, P. & Kruger, J. (1979). Responses of cells in foveal visual cortex of the monkey to pure color contrast. *J. Neurophysiol.* **42**, 850–860; Thorell, L.G., De Valois, R.L. & Albrecht, D.G. (1984). Spatial mapping of monkey V1 cells with pure color and luminance stimuli. *Vision Res.* **24**, 751–769.

5 Critchley, M. (1964). The problem of visual agnosia. *J. Neurol. Sci.* **1**, 274–290.

6 Bay, E. (1953). Disturbances of visual perception and their examination. *Brain* **76**, 515–550.

7 Wechsler, I.S. (1933). Partial cortical blindness with preservation of color vision: report of a case following asphyxia (carbon monoxide poisoning?) *Archs. Ophthalmol.* **9**, 957–965; Adler, A. (1944). Disintegration and restoration of optic recognition in visual agnosia: analysis of a case. *Arch. Neurol. Psychiatr. (Chicago)* **51**, 243–259; Adler, A. (1950). Course and outcome of visual agnosia. *J. Nerv. Ment. Dis.* **111**, 41–51. The following papers describe cases of carbon monoxide poisoning: Hécaen, H., Angelergues, C., Bernhardt, C. & Chiarelli, J. (1957). Essai de distinction des modalités cliniques de l'agnosie des physionomies. *Rev. Neurol. (Paris)* **96**, 125–144; Benson, D.F. & Greenberg, J.P. (1969). Visual form agnosia: a specific defect in visual discrimination. *Arch. Neurol. Psychiatr. (Chicago)* **20**, 82–89; Abadi, R.V., Kulikowski, J.J. & Meudell, P. (1981). Visual performance in a case of visual agnosia. In *Functional Recovery from Brain Damage*, edited by M.V. van Hof & G. Mohn, pp. 275–286. Elsevier, Amsterdam; Campion, J. & Latto, R. (1985). Apperceptive agnosia due to carbon monoxide poisoning. An interpretation based on critical band masking from disseminated lesions. *Behav. Brain Res.* **15**, 227–240; Milner, A.D., Perrett, D.I., Johnston, R.S. *et al.* (1991). Perception and action in 'visual form agnosia'. *Brain* **114**, 405–428.

8 Zeki, S. (1990). A century of cerebral achromatopsia. *Brain* **113**, 1721–1777.

9 Humphreys, G.W. & Riddoch, M.J. (1987). *To See But Not To See. A Case Study of Visual Agnosia.* Erlbaum Associates, Hillsdale.

10 Adler, A. (1944). Disintegration and restoration of optic recognition in visual agnosia: analysis of a case. *Arch. Neurol. Psychiatr. (Chicago)* **51**, 243–259.

11 Gomori, A.J. & Hawryluk, G.A. (1984). Visual agnosia without alexia. *Neurology* **34**, 947–950.

12 Wapner, W., Judd, T. & Gardner, H. (1978). Visual agnosia in an artist. *Cortex* **14**, 343–364.

13 Heydt, R. von der (1987). Approaches to visual cortical function. *Rev. Physiol. Biochem. Pharmacol.* **108**, 69–150.

14 Bender, M.B. & Feldman, M. (1972). The so-called 'visual agnosias'. *Brain* **95**, 173–186.

15 Quoted by, Critchley, M. (1965). Acquired anomalies of colour perception of central origin. *Brain* **88**, 711–724.

16 Senden, M. von (1932). *Raum- und Gestaltauffasung bei Operierten Blindgebornen.* (Translated into English by P. Heath (1960). *Space and Sight.* Methuen & Co., London.)

17 Hendricks, I.M., Holliday, I.E. & Ruddock, K.H. (1981). A new class of visual defect: spreading inhibition elicited by chromatic light stimuli. *Brain* **104**, 813–840.

Chapter 31: The anatomy of integration

Problems generated by integration

The anatomical pathways and processes of integration discussed above result in severe problems. The enlargement of receptive fields, a necessary step in the integrative process, means that a cell becomes less efficient at pinpointing the precise position of a stimulus. This is because it will respond with nearly equal vigour throughout its receptive field, which may be several degrees across. Somehow the activity of cells with such large receptive fields, say in area V5, must be referred back to an area with a very precise topographic map, such as V1, so that the precise positional information, lost during the process of receptive field enlargement, can be recovered. Next, there is the question of uniting explicit signals from two very different sources, at different stages of two parallel pathways. Suppose that the need arises to unite the perceptually explicit signals of cells in the thick stripes of area V2 with the perceptually explicit signals from cells in area V4 so that, let us say, the simultaneous and synchronous firing of a cell registering the orientation of a stimulus located at a certain distance from the organism and a cell registering the colour of that same stimulus, between them specify the properties of the object. This would demand that cells in the thick stripes connect with cells in area V4. But anatomical evidence shows that in the forward pathway from V2 to the specialized visual areas of the prestriate cortex, the cells of the thick stripes are connected with V3 and V5, not with V4. An alternative way of uniting explicit signals in the two stations would therefore be for area V4 to back connect with the thick stripes of V2. There is, next, what is commonly referred to as the *binding problem*, a critical problem for visual physiology. The problem is that of determining that it is the same (or a different) stimulus which is activating different cells in a given visual area or in different visual areas. Suppose that three cells in area V3, all responsive to the horizontal orientation but with adjacent rather than overlapping receptive fields, are activated by the same horizontal stimulus, for example the upper edge of a fence gate. Suppose further that these three cells receive inputs from twelve cells in area V1 with a corresponding orientation which, in turn, are responding to the same stimulus. The task here is to ascertain that the three cells in V3 and the twelve cells of V1 are all responding to the same, and not to different, stimuli (see Figure 31.1). One way of achieving this would

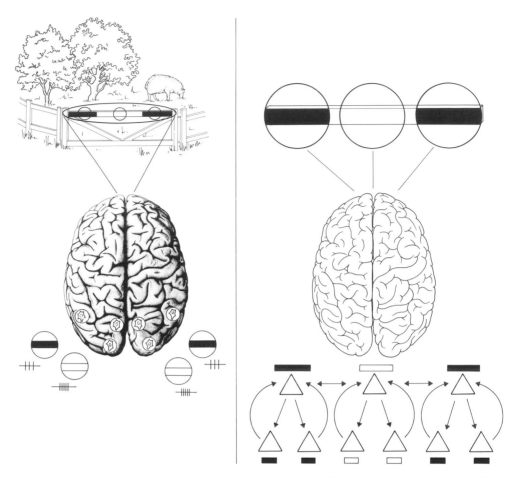

Fig. 31.1 Some mechanism must ascertain that cells in the cortex responding to the same orientation but with different receptive fields are responding to the same object. This figure shows one possible system of connections to ensure this. The cells of V1 (bottom row, right) registering the horizontal orientation but with non-overlapping receptive fields communicate with one another, and also with cells in V3 (top row, right) registering the same orientation. The latter not only communicate with each other but also have a return input back onto the cells of V1 which feed them.

be for the responses of the three cells of V3 to correlate in time, to fire together in temporal synchrony, to oscillate together.[1] But what or who in the cortex monitors the fact that the cells are firing in temporal synchrony and therefore correlate in time? It is no good pleading for a higher, master cell; one would then be stuck with the problem of who monitors the activity of the master cell. A solution would be for the cells in V3 to project back to the cells of V1 which feed them, and fire in temporal synchrony with the latter. The determination that all these cells are responding to the same horizontal line then becomes a function of whether the entire network is firing in temporal synchrony or not.

It is but one step from this problem of identity, of determining that cells in different areas are responding to the same, rather than to different, stimuli within a small part of the field of view, to the larger problem of the finished, integrated, visual percept of a whole visual scene, and the conscious awareness of it. For here again intrudes the binding problem, in the sense that there must be some signal, some indication, that the colour signalled by cells in one area belongs to the same object as the shape discriminated by those of another and the movement indicated by a third. There is, in brief, the binding problem writ large. This might be achieved by the responses of cells in one area correlating in time with those in another, once again raising the problem of who monitors the synchrony and of who, finally, is conscious of the end product.

I have limited myself to three areas in this description, but this is for descriptive purposes only. Many more areas are involved when we look at a complex scene, but the description applies equally to multiple areas. This naturally raises the question of how the cells responding to the same object in the same, as well as in different, areas come to fire in temporal synchrony. It is a subject about which we know very little in physiological terms. But a necessary prerequisite would be that the cells are anatomically connected with one another reciprocally. That is, the output from a cell, or a group of cells, to another group should be reciprocated by a return output from the latter to the former.

There are other problems which can be solved, or at least more efficiently solved, by an anatomical arrangement which permits visual areas which undertake given tasks to make the results of their operations known to the visual areas which feed them.[2] One is the problem of *conflict*, where the cells in an area signal an attribute of a stimulus which is different from the attribute signalled by the cells of another area, from which they receive their input. The example has already been given of an object moving to the right but whose components move in a variety of different directions (Figure 29.4, p. 302). The direction signalled by the cells of V5 is now in conflict with the direction signalled by the cells of V1, from which V5 is receiving its input. Somehow, signals from V5 must be re-entered to the appropriate cells of V1 to resolve the conflict. Re-entry might also be important in another kind of integration, one which involves the translation of one kind of visual stimulus into another. The term translation is vague, because no one really knows what the underlying neurological mechanisms may be. Whatever one might call it, it nevertheless leads to a coherent percept. For example, instead of generating forms from luminance contrast (such as a black bar against a white background), one could generate it from a pattern of moving textures (Figure 31.2). No bars will be detected when the entire texture is made to move coherently in one direction alone. But when different segments of

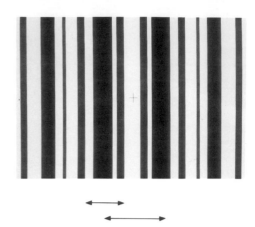

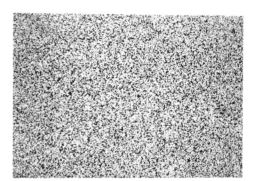

Fig. 31.2 The generation of structure from motion. (Above) A series of vertically oriented lines generated from luminance differences (white lines against a black background). (Below) Lines of the identical size and orientation can be generated if different segments of the texture are made to move in different directions, for example if segments corresponding to the black background move to the left and those corresponding to the white lines move to the right.

the texture move in different directions, forms become immediately visible. In other words, form becomes visible through motion. Here the brain must detect the coherent motion first, a function of area V5. The coherent motion, thus generated, must then somehow be translated to excite the same orientation-selective cells in areas V1 and V3 which are excited by the bars generated from luminance contrast, or at least cells with a similar kind of orientation preference in the two areas. There are many other examples to show that one attribute of vision can be created from another, shape from shading and depth from motion being commonly quoted examples. They all require that one attribute be generated first, and that the second one be generated from the first. One may suppose, then, that when we look at a visual scene the final visual image in the brain is a synthesis, not only of the synchronous and simultaneous activity of the cells in all the specialized visual areas and the further areas to which they project, but also, through the return connections, of the activity of areas such as V1 and V2 which feed them.

Dreams and hallucinations

In fact, an external visual scene is not necessary for generating a visual image. An image can be generated with the eyes completely shut, as in dreams, or in states of blindness. Powerful centrally generated images can also be perceived in the absence of a corresponding visual stimulus, even when the eyes are open, as occurs commonly in visual hallucinations. Dreams and hallucinations are not subjects which most visual neurobiologists would wish to concern themselves with. But any theory of integration must take them into account, for both consist of integrated visual images, with the difference that they are entirely centrally generated. It is worth discussing these problems briefly, if only to pinpoint features which are relevant to understanding normal physiology.

The most obvious example of a centrally generated visual image in the absence of all immediate stimulations occurs in dreams. Dreams have been analyzed in great detail by all manner of psychologists and psychiatrists, and many theories have been built around them. They may give powerful indications of a person's wishes and desires; they may be psychologically bizarre, even pathological; they may be in the form of nightmares or of pleasant remembrances of things past; one may attribute biological functions to them.[3] What is not in doubt is that they are usually *visually normal and derived from normal visual experience*. In the words of one psychoanalyst, '. . .it is entirely possible that the dream work cannot compose a new visual structure anymore than it can a new speech'.[4] Indeed, it is because of this very normality that the psychoanalyst is able to interpret them at all. By normality I mean nothing more than that the visual image which appears in dreams is coherent, that one sees people in places as they might appear normally. It is very unusual to see a person with a head in one place, a torso in another and the limbs in a third, as in some surrealist painting, unless of course one is dreaming of a particularly gruesome murder, which then becomes visually coherent; it is most unusual to hear of dreams in which one end of a bus moves in one direction and the other in the opposite direction, or of a dream in which the wings of a plane fly in one direction and the fuselage in another, or of one in which the colour of an object appears in one place and the object itself in another. It is this element of visual normality, of verisimilitude, that gives dreams their reality. This may all seem obvious and yet it requires a great deal of accounting for in neurophysiological terms. Although we have no precise knowledge of what triggers dreams,[5] it is almost certain that it must involve the simultaneous activity of several visual areas and that these areas must interact to provide the integration that is evident in dreams, since the coherent visual image is itself the product of the simultaneous activity of many separate areas. The result of this interaction must then somehow be re-entered into the cortex, as if it were coming from the outside.

As compelling are the visual hallucinations. These, once again, may be defined as perceptions in the absence of a visual stimulus. It is common to find that the objects and people in a hallucinatory episode are somewhat distorted, being for example much smaller (micropsia) or much larger (macropsia) than in real life. But otherwise their hallmark is that of a visually normal scene, indeed one that is commonly, though not always, reported to be quite a pleasant one.[6] They are commonly of people, sometimes of charming ladies, sometimes of warriors, often of animals in jungles and forests, scenes that are reminiscent of the paintings of Le Dounier Rousseau. They are commonly in vivid colours. Their normality is such that Thomas Huxley wrote, 'There can be no doubt that exactly those parts of [the] retina which would be affected by the image of a cat . . . or the portions of sensorium with which those organs of sense are connected, were thrown into a corresponding state of activity by some internal cause'.[7] Hallucinations, like dreams, are therefore *visually normal*.

The visual normality of dreams and hallucinations, their sense of reality, is so intense and compelling that all of us have experienced situations which we subsequently find difficult to ascribe to dreams or to reality. It is therefore difficult not to conceive of them as internally generated images which are re-entered into the cortex as if they were coming from the outside. If this were so, one would naturally expect that the primary visual cortex might be involved, if only because in normal vision (to which dreams bear such a strong resemblance) the first cortical stage which the incoming visual signals enter is area V1. Indeed, evidence suggests that during dreaming there is a massive increase in cerebral blood flow not only in the visual areas of the prestriate cortex, but also in the striate cortex itself, and probably in area V2 from which it is difficult to separate in the low-resolution positron emission tomography (PET) scans.[8] There is another reason for this interest in V1 and the adjoining area V2. These are the two areas with the highest precision of mapping, in the sense that they contain highly detailed maps of the retina and hence of the field of view. In dreams and hallucinations, just as in normal vision, objects maintain their topographic position. One might expect therefore that, wherever the images in dreams and hallucinations are generated, they must be re-entered into an area with high topographic precision.

Integration through re-entry

We may here consider re-entry, and the integrative mechanisms which it may be responsible for, in the context of object agnosia in general and of prosopagnosia in particular, to illustrate a more general point about re-entry, namely that it must be operative in many other integrative processes. Prosopagnosia is a disease in which, following cerebral lesions, human subjects are unable to recognize familiar faces. It has some fascinating features. Most prominent among these is that *prosopagnosic patients have not lost the concept of a face*. They know what a face is. Indeed, they even know that they are looking at a face, but cannot recognize it as a particular face. There are many interesting accounts of this, even occasions when a prosopagnosic patient could see but could not recognize his own face in a mirror. An interesting insight is given by a patient. He explained that, '...I have never been able to recognise any person by sight alone. I cannot recognise my wife except by the sound of her voice...I have learned that to recognise people its often easiest to use non-facial [visual] clues'. In answer to the question. 'Are you able to recognise yourself in a mirror?', he answered, 'Well, I can certainly see a face, with eyes, nose and mouth etc., but somehow it's not familiar; it really could be anybody. I can also see enough to decide whether my now-limited hair is in need of a brush, but at the same time as this I don't seem to have enough detail to know whether...my face is dirty'.[9] There is one extraordinary and somewhat frightening description of the process of dissolution of facial recognition,[10] as it occurred. It is the record of a patient who, while talking to his physiotherapist, suddenly exclaimed, 'But Mademoiselle, what is happening is that I can no longer recognize you'. He knew who she was, knew her to be there, physically present, knew that he was talking to her, but he could no longer recognize her face. Given this, it should come as no surprise to learn that prosopagnosic patients can easily recognize many features of a face, for example, the eyes, ears and nose.[11] A prosopagnosic patient once related how, 'I can see the eyes, nose and mouth quite clearly but they just don't add up. They all seem chalked in, like on a blackboard'. Perhaps a little more surprising is that the memory trace of the familiar face is there in some, but not all, prosopagnosic patients. Thus, prosopagnosic patients report that they can close their eyes and 'see' the familiar face, for example that of their children.[11] A prosopagnosic patient related that, 'I can shut my eyes and can well remember what my wife looked like or the kids'.[11] All this suggests that some kinds of prosopagnosia at least are not necessarily due to a defect in the cerebral mechanisms required to construct faces. Instead, the memory traces of particular faces cannot be tagged onto the constructed images to identify them as particular faces, belonging to particular individuals, either because of a breakdown in the forward input from the cortical area critical for the construction of faces to the memory trace, wherever that may reside, or because the memory traces cannot be re-entered onto the constructed images.

The failure of re-entry in prosopagnosia

The syndrome of prosopagnosia has acquired a great deal of interest in recent years because of the discovery[12] that in the macaque monkey there is a specific region of the cortex which contains cells whose optimal responses are to faces. The area is located in the temporal lobe, at some distance from the specialized visual areas which have been our main concern. One could then suppose that prosopagnosia is nothing more than yet another manifestation of the specificity of the visual cortex. One may suppose also that it is a consequence of a failure of integrative mechanisms operating at a higher level to construct faces from the incoming visual signals, in an area specialized for faces and through neural mechanisms about which we know nothing. A manifestation of the specificity of the brain it certainly is, as well as being a failure in integrative mechanisms and also an expression of the importance of faces in our daily life. But there may be more to it than that; it may indeed be a good subject to consider from the point of view of re-entry, even if many specialists in the field might disagree with such an analysis. I do not pretend that this is the correct way of looking at prosopagnosia; it is certainly not the only way. But it is worth considering.

Some authorities[13] maintain that prosopagnosia is not a specific failure to recognize faces, but rather a more general disturbance in the recognition of individual members of the generic class. They do not agree that there is such a radical distinction between object agnosia and prosopagnosia; '. . .it has not been noted', they say, 'that if instead of being asked to identify, say, a "book" or "chair" the patient is asked "whose book" or "whose chair" it is, the patient will fail to answer'.[13] This very interesting observation leads them to the equally interesting supposition that, '. . .true prosopagnosia is a memory disorder, and the major factor in its appearance is a disturbance in the mechanism that allows an ongoing correct visual percept to evoke its appropriate, previously acquired context'.[13] This formulation, which could apply equally to some, but not all, cases of what has come to be called visual object agnosia (the inability to recognize previously familiar objects) merits consideration in terms of re-entry. It is as if the memory store of a familiar face or a familiar object, wherever that may reside, must be re-entered onto the parts of the cortex which have constructed the face, resulting in the recognition of that face as belonging to a given individual. In the absence of that re-entry, the face is seen as a face and is understood to be a face, but is not seen as a particular face, nor is it recognized as a particular face, because the re-entrant neural mechanism required to integrate the incoming signals with the memory trace is defective. In brief, it is not that the prosopagnosic patient cannot see the face, nor is it the case that he does not understand that it is a face. It is simply that he cannot relate it to a given individual face. *Prosopagnosia can then be considered to be the manifestations of a breakdown of integrative mechanisms due to a failure of forward and re-entrant mechanisms.*

There are several interesting observations which suggest that the memory system itself may be modular, with the nervous system allocating different memory compartments to different features. It is of particular interest to note that such a conclusion had been reached a long time ago from a consideration of visual memory and hallucinations.[14] Thus, Ormond wrote as long ago as 1925 that, 'Past visual impressions are arranged in definite groups within the visual memory areas, so that one or more of these groups may disappear without any interference with the others...It is probable that the visual memory centres for objects, places, forms and colour are in different areas from those for visual memory of words, letters and figures but that they are contiguous'. More recent studies take this conclusion a step further. In particular, the demonstration that the recognition of a face as a familiar face can be compromised independently of the recognition of the expression on that face,[13] or that the recognition of a person by his gait can also be specifically compromised, suggests that the memory systems are themselves highly specific and that it is these specific systems that have to be re-entered onto the constructed image.

The anatomy of integration in the visual cortex

One of the more remarkable aspects of the connectivity of the cerebral cortex is the fact that when a given area A sends an output to area B, area B sends a return output back to area A,[15] an arrangement which is best referred to as re-entry.[16] This is such a ubiquitous arrangement that there are only a few exceptions to it.[17] It constitutes a powerful means by which one area can influence the area it receives an input from, perhaps even modifying the responses that it will receive before it receives them. A typical arrangement might be that illustrated in Figure 31.3. The cells of area A which project to area B are situated predominantly in the upper cortical layers, though a few are also

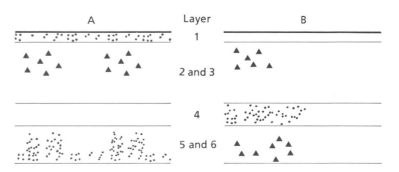

Fig. 31.3 A simplified schema to show the distribution of cells (triangles) and fibres (dots) in two areas connected to one another.

present in the lower cortical layers. The fibres of these cells terminate predominantly in layer 4 of area B. The cells which project back from area B to area A are situated predominantly in the lower layers of area B, while their fibres terminate in the upper and lower layers of area A and spare to a large extent layer 4. It is noteworthy that although the projecting cells and the return fibres occupy different layers in each of the two areas (i.e the projecting cells are layer asymmetric with respect to the re-entrant fibres), the total extent of the (tangential) distribution is much the same.

In the visual system a unique re-entrant system connects the specialized visual areas with areas V1 and V2. As we have seen, the output from these two areas is highly segregated, with specific functional and anatomical subdivisions of each area projecting to specialized visual areas whose functional properties correspond to that of the specialized groupings from which they receive their input. For example, the thin stripes of V2 project to V4, whereas the thick stripes project to V3 and to V5 (Figure 31.4). *Yet the return input to V1 and V2 from the specialized visual areas is diffuse.* The re-entrant input from any given specialized visual area is not segregated nor is it restricted to the territory of cells in V1 and V2 that project to that area. A good example is found in layer 4B of V1. If one were to label the cells of this layer projecting to V5, one would find them to be clustered together and separated from each other by unlabelled cells, and therefore cells which project to destinations other than V5. If one were to study the re-entrant input from V5 to layer 4B of V1, one would find that its distribution, by contrast, is not clustered and is not restricted to the territory of the cells projecting to V5, but covers the spaces in between as well[18] (Figure 31.4). In short, the re-entrant input into layer 4B distributes not only to the territory of cells projecting to V5 but also to the territory of cells projecting elsewhere. Since, besides projecting to V5, layer 4B projects to V3 and to the thick stripes of V2, *it follows that, through this reciprocal projection, V5 has the anatomical opportunity of influencing not only cells in layer 4B of V1 projecting to it, but also those projecting to other areas as well.* We note here that layer 4B belongs predominantly to the magnocellular (M) system, so that this reciprocal input is a means of uniting the two different branches of the M system — V3, which is concerned predominantly with form, and V5 concerned with visual motion. It follows that the principles of topical and confluent convergence are both involved in this re-entrant pathway; topical convergence serves to return signals from cells with the large receptive fields in V5 back to the cells of layer 4B, and may actually enlarge the receptive fields of cells in the latter layer,[19] while confluent convergence helps to unite the motion signals returning from V5 with signals relating to form and the V3 system.

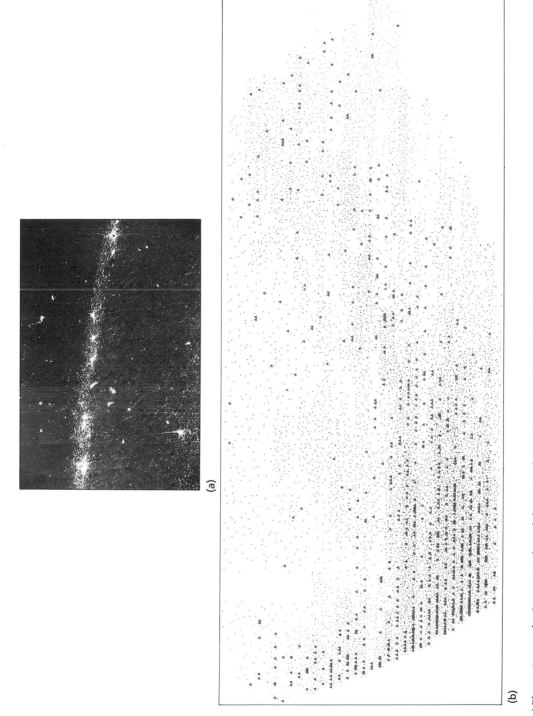

Fig. 31.4 (a) Photomicrograph of a section through layer 4B of a monkey in which area V5 had been injected with a tracer that labels the cells projecting to it as well as the destination of the fibres leaving it. Notice that the cells projecting to V5 (shown as white dust) distribute throughout and include the territory of the cells as well as that between them. (b) A reconstruction taken from many sections such as the one shown in (a) and aligned with respect to one another. Labelled cells are shown in triangles while the fibres from V5 are shown in stippling. Notice the distribution of fibres in a wider territory, one which includes the region between the labelled cells.

Much the same picture obtains when one considers V2. Recall that this area is characterized by a special architecture consisting of thick stripes, thin stripes and interstripes. The thick stripes belong predominantly to the M system since they receive input from layer 4B (which receives its input from the M layers of the lateral geniculate nucleus [LGN]) and the cells in them project to areas V3 and V5. The thin stripes and the interstripes belong predominantly to the parvocellular (P) system since they receive their inputs from layers 2 and 3 of V1, which is fed by the P layers of the LGN. The output from V2 to V5 is from the thick stripes. But the return output, from V5 to V2, is widely distributed within V2 and, although densest in the territory of the thick stripes, it also includes the territory of the thin stripes and the interstripes.[20] It follows that through this return input V5 is able to influence not only the cells of V2 that project to it, but also the cells of V2 that project elsewhere. In other words, the arrangement of this re-entrant projection allows motion signals from V5 to influence the colour signals in the thin stripes of V2, which connect with V4.

In summary, the arrangement of these return connections gives us the strong impression that they may constitute one of the anatomical pathways involved, not only in integrating the visual image in the cortex, but also in generating one visual construct from another, for example form-from-motion.[16,18,21] In the latter example, one might expect that, when a structure is generated from coherent motion, the motion must be generated first in V5, and the results communicated to V3, both directly and via V1 and V2, to stimulate the form selective cells there. Indeed, computer simulations using the pathways which we have described suggest that this is more than plausible.[22] The anatomical system linking V5 and V3, through V1 and V2 therefore seemed to us to be an excellent one to study directly in the human brain, with the PET method. The paradigm we used to study the interaction of these areas is breathtakingly simple and was inspired by the anatomical pathways between the visual areas which we had unravelled.

Simple forms, ones which we know from our physiological experiments would activate the cells of area V3, can be generated from luminance differences. The forms may consist, for example, of a set of white bars against a black background, as shown in Figure 31.2. Bars of the identical width and disposition can also be generated, however, from moving textures. Thus, if a moving texture pattern such as the one shown in the upper part Figure 31.2 is divided into zones which correspond with the width of the bars in the lower part of Figure 31.2 and if the motion of the texture within the bars is in a direction different from the direction of motion in the regions surrounding the bars, then one can see the same bars with the same orientations as when the bars were generated from luminance differences. One may suppose that the same simple forms, though this time generated from coherent motion rather than from luminance differences, would also activate the cells of V3. But the neural route used this time must be more circuitous. This is because, whereas the bars generated from luminance differences can activate the orientation selective cells of V3 by activating first the orientation selective cells of V1 (and V2), the route taken when the bars are generated from motion is somewhat different. Now coherent motion must be generated first, by feeding signals from V1 to V5 (since coherent motion is a function of V5) and the result of the operation performed by V5 fed back to V3, either through the pathway linking V5 with V3 directly or through the one linking it via V1 and V2, through the re-entrant connections. If this reasoning is correct, then one should observe some very interesting results when studying the activity of visual areas to such stimuli, as can be done by observing the blood flow changes in these areas when human subjects view the stimuli described above. In particular, one might expect that the increase in blood flow through V1 and V2 would be substantially greater when humans look at forms produced from motion than when they look at the same forms produced from luminance differences. Because of the re-entry to V1 and V2 necessary to activate the orientation selective cells by coherent motion, activity in these areas would be substantially greater when human subjects view forms generated from motion than when they are generated from luminance differences alone, since the latter does not involve interaction between the V3 and the V5 systems through V1 to nearly the same extent as does the former.

The experiment was worth trying at any rate. Consequently, we compared[23] the activity in the brain of human subjects when they viewed (a) a set of vertically oriented bars generated by luminance differences (form); (b) two sheets of moving textures, moving in two opposite directions (motion); and (c) a set of vertically oriented bars identical to (a) except that they were generated from the moving textures, the textures within the bars moving in a direction opposite to the texture between the bars (form-from-motion). The results we have obtained, using six subjects, were very consistent with the re-entrant analysis I have given above and elsewhere. Thus, a comparison of the brain activity when subjects had been viewing the form-from-motion stimulus with the brain activity when they had been viewing the form stimulus alone or the motion stimulus, showed that there was a highly significant increase in local cerebral blood flow (and therefore activity) within areas V1 and V2 when subjects had been viewing the form-from-motion stimulus compared to the weighted mean activity when they were viewing the motion stimulus alone and the form stimulus alone (Plate 23, part (b), facing p. 308).

The above results are consistent with the interpretation I have been giving in this chapter, that the re-entrant input to V1 and V2 from the specialized visual areas is critical for the generation of at least some visual percepts. But I do not mean to suggest that integration occurs solely in V1 or that the percept is in V1. It is rather the dynamic interaction between these areas that is essential for the perception of form-from-motion. There may of course be other interpretations of the results I have given above, for example that the form-from-motion stimulus employed in our study is a more potent stimulus than either form alone or motion alone in activating the cells of V1. We have discounted this explanation because the residual activity left, after subtracting the form *and* the motion component, is greater in V1 and V2 than in other areas of the visual cortex. While I still remain diffident in asserting that the interpretation given here is the only one, it is certainly an interpretation. Moreover, it shows how one can use ingenious paradigms, themselves the outcome of experimental anatomical studies, to study the organization of the human brain.

In anatomical terms, a similar re-entrant pathway connects area V4 with area V2. V4 receives its input from the thin stripes and the interstripes of V2. But the return projection from V4 to V2 includes the territory of all the stripes.[24] Hence, through this return projection, V4 is able to influence not only the cells of V2 that project to it, but also cells that project elsewhere. The re-entrant pathway constitutes, in brief, another system for uniting signals belonging to form, colour and motion.

It follows therefore that the re-entrant pathways are not modular and not easily localizable.

We now extend our conclusion from the previous chapter and say that the integrated visual image in the brain is the product of the simultaneous activity of several visual areas and pathways, including areas such as V1 and V2 which receive their input from the LGN, distribute them to the specialized visual areas and are re-entrantly linked with the latter.

As the re-entrant pathways are diffuse, non-modular and not easily localizable, and the opportunities for integration are many and integration itself is a multi-stage process, it follows that integration is a diffuse and not easily localizable process. We can now answer Fodor's question (see Chapter 23) as far as vision is concerned: 'Are there psychological processes that can plausibly be assumed to cut across cognitive domains? And, if there are, is there reason to suppose that such processes are subserved by nonmodular...mechanisms?' The answer to both questions is yes. The psychological process is that of integration, and integration is non-modular in character.

The diffuse, non-modular and multi-stage character of integration leads us to the plausible conclusion that the operation of the visual cortex is both isotropic and Quineian, in the sense used here and modified after Fodor, that everything that the visual cortex does must be of relevance to its ability to determine the precise characteristics of a visual stimulus, a theme taken up again in the next chapter.

Notes and references

1 Milner, P.M. (1974). A model for visual shape recognition. *Psychol. Rev.* **81**, 521–535; Malsburg, C. von der & Schneider, W. (1986). A neural cocktail-party processor. *Biol. Cybern.* **54**, 29–40.

2 For a more general discussion of re-entry see Edelman, G.M. (1978). Group selection and phasic reentrant signalling: a theory of higher brain function. In *The Mindful Brain*, edited by G.M. Edelman & V.B. Mountcastle, pp. 51–100. MIT Press, Cambridge. Re-entry is conceived of more as a dynamic process, which nevertheless would have to depend upon the kind of anatomical connections that I describe here, i.e. the return connections from one area to the area feeding it. These reciprocal connections must not be confused with the process of re-entry though they are the basis for it.

3 Crick, F. & Mitchison, G. (1983). The function of dream sleep. *Nature* **304**, 111–114.

4 Fisher, C. (1954). Dreams and perception. *J. Am. Psychoanal. Assoc.* **2**, 389–445.

5 Hobson, J.A. (1988). *The Dreaming Brain*. Penguin Books, London.

6 Flournoy, H. (1923). Hallucinations Lilliputiennes atypiques chez un vieillard atteint de cataracte. *Encéphale* **18**, 566–579.

7 Huxley, T.H. In *Elements of Physiology*. (Quoted by D.H. Tuke (1889). Hallucinations and the subjective sensations of the sane. *Brain* **11**, 441–467.)

8 Heiss, W.-D., Pawlik, G., Herholz, K., Wagner, R. & Wienhard, K. (1985). Regional cerebral glucose metabolism in man during wakefulness, sleep and dreaming. *Brain Res.* **327**, 362–366.

9 Humphreys, J.W. & Riddoch, M.J. (1987). *To See But Not To See. A Case Study of Visual Agnosia*. Erlbaum Associates, Hillsdale.

10 Lhermitte, J., Chain, F., Escourolle, R., Ducarne, B. & Pillon, B. (1972). Étude anatomo-clinique d'un cas de prosopagnosie. *Rev. Neurol. (Paris)* **126**, 329–346.

11 Pallis, C.A. (1955). Impaired identification of faces and places with agnosia for colours: report of a case due to cerebral embolism. *J. Neurol. Neurosurg. Psychiatry* **18**, 218–224.

12 Gross, C.G. (1972). Visual functions of infero-temporal cortex. In *Handbook of Sensory Psysiology*, Vol. 7, Part 3, edited by R. Jung, pp. 451–482. Springer-Verlag, Berlin; Perrett, D.I., Rolls, E.T. & Caan, W. (1982). Visual neurones responsive to faces in the monkey temporal cortex. *Exp. Brain. Res.* **47**, 329–342; Perrett, D.I., Mistlin, A.J. & Chitty A.J. (1987). Visual neurones responsive to faces. *Trends Neurosci.* **10**, 358–364.

13 Tranel, D., Damasio, A.R. & Damasio, H. (1988). Intact recognition of facial expression, gender, and age in patients with impaired recognition of face identity. *Neurology* **38**, 690–696.

14 Ormond, A.W. (1925). Visual hallucinations in sane people. *Br. Med. J.* **2**, 376–379.

15 Gilbert, C.D. & Kelly, J.P. (1975). The projections of cells in different layers of the cat's visual cortex. *J. Comp. Neurol.* **163**, 81–105; Rockland, K.S. & Pandya, D.K. (1979). Laminar origins and terminations of cortical connections of the occipital lobe in the rhesus monkey. *Brain Res.* **179**, 3–20; Felleman, D.J. & Van Essen, D.C. (1991). Distributed hierarchical processing in the primate cerebral cortex. *Cerebral Cortex* **1**, 1–47.

16 Zeki, S. & Shipp, S. (1988). The functional logic of cortical connections. *Nature* **335**, 311–317.

17 Jones, E.G. (1984). Connectivity of the primate sensory motor cortex. In *Cerebral*

Cortex, Vol. 5, *Sensory Motor Areas and Aspects of Cerebral Connectivity*, edited by E.G. Jones & A. Peters, pp. 113–183. Plenum Press, New York.

18 Shipp, S. & Zeki, S. (1989). The organization of connections between areas V5 and V1 in the macaque monkey visual cortex. *Eur. J. Neurosci.* **1**, 309–332.

19 Allman, J., Miezin, F. & McGuiness, E. (1990). Effects of background motion on the responses of neurons in the first and second visual cortical areas. In *Signal and Sense: Local and Global Order in Perceptual Maps*, edited by G.M. Edelman, W.E. Gall & W.M. Cowan, pp. 131–141. Wiley-Liss, New York.

20 Shipp, S. & Zeki, S. (1989). The organization of connections between areas V5 and V2 in the macaque monkey visual cortex. *Eur. J. Neurosci.* **1**, 333–354.

21 Zeki, S. & Shipp, S. (1989). Modular connections between areas V2 and V4 of macaque monkey visual cortex. *Eur. J. Neurosci.* **1**, 494–506.

22 The computer experiments were inspired by and use the very pathways described here. They evolved from joint discussions held at this laboratory and at the Neurosciences Institute, New York. See Finkel, L.H. & Edelman, G.M. (1989). Integration of distributed cortical systems by reentry: a computer simulation of interactive functionally segregated visual areas. *J. Neurosci.* **9**, 3188–3208. See also Tononi, G., Sporns, O. & Edelman, G.M. (1992). Reentry and the problem of integrating multiple cortical areas: simulation of dynamic integration in the visual system. *Cerebral Cortex* **2**, 310–335.

23 The experiments described here were performed jointly with Richard's Frackowiak's laboratory.

24 Zeki, S. & Shipp, S. (1989). Modular connections between areas V2 and V4 of macaque monkey visual cortex. *Eur. J. Neurosci.* **1**, 494–506.

Chapter 32: Further unsolved problems of integration

What is the value of having so extensive a system of reciprocal connections and what problems does it solve? The answers to these questions are by no means obvious but the kind of solutions that they might provide become clearer if we consider some aspects of visual physiology. We shall then see that although several visual processes might demand reciprocal connections, the presently known organization of the reciprocal pathways does not provide anything like a satisfactory solution.

The representation of space

We have already discussed how the visual cortex must be concerned with spatial integration to give a visual percept which is spatially continuous. Within this panorama one can nevertheless still pinpoint with an extraordinary accuracy the position of objects and stimuli in visual space. How can this be done? It would obviously require that there must either be cells with very small receptive fields located in a cortical area with a very precise topographic map in it, or that cells with larger receptive fields should have 'hot spots' within their fields, spots where a stimulus would evoke the maximal activity. An examination of receptive field sizes of cells in different visual areas of the cortex shows that the smallest are those of areas V1 and V2. Moreover, it is in these latter areas that the retina, and by extension the field of view, is most precisely mapped. Field sizes are much larger and topography is much less precise in the specialized visual areas. Sizes become especially large and topography almost non-existent in the visual areas of the parietal cortex and the inferior temporal cortex.[1] This enlargement of receptive fields is probably a necessary step in the computational process employed by the brain because, for each attribute, the brain has to compare what is happening in one small region with what is happening elsewhere. But it creates problems. Many cells with large receptive fields in V5, for example, respond very well when spots of light are moved in the appropriate direction, but not to movement in the opposite, null direction. But their response in the preferred direction is equally vigorous no matter where the stimulus is in the receptive field. Moreover, one does not have to start stimulation at one end of the receptive field to obtain an optimal discharge. A spot flashed in the centre and moved in the appropriate direction will elicit as good a response. Therefore, what one gains in terms of selectivity (to direction of visual motion in this case), one loses in terms of topographic precision. In brief, such a cell would not be able to signal the precise location of a stimulus in visual space. Some cells in the parietal cortex do have 'hot spots', but these are themselves so large as to be of little use in signalling the precise position of objects.[2] Yet the organism is able to locate the precise position of objects, even moving ones, with a remarkable precision, which is one good reason why games such as tennis and cricket are so popular. In the very same way, one is able to locate the position of a small coloured object very precisely, even if the determination of the colour of that object depends upon information coming from relatively wide parts of the field of view. Hence, some referral system with a good representation of space co-ordinates is needed. Of all the visual areas the one with the most precise representation of visual space is area V1, and the next most precise is area V2. Anatomical studies show that all the specialized prestriate visual areas have return inputs to V1 and V2.[3] Hence it seems possible that a return input may be used to refer the position of an object whose properties have been computed to a precise location in visual space. This is a suggestion derived purely from anatomy and no experiments to test it have been undertaken. We still have no clue as to how the brain is able to recover the local sign, once that information is lost in the larger receptive field of a cell within a specialized cortical area, or within an even higher visual area. Almost certainly there are several solutions to the problem that computational neurobiologists can point to and, equally probably, the brain will be found to use none of these but a more ingenious one instead. What is important here is that the anatomical machinery for connecting cells with large receptive fields to ones with small fields is available through this return path in the cortex and the suggestion is therefore anatomically plausible.

In fact, of course, the location of the precise position of objects in visual space cannot be achieved without reference to the observer. It is very interesting to find therefore that there are cells in the visual cortex whose responses are gaze-locked, in the sense that they will respond only if the organism is gazing in a particular direction and not in other directions. These cells were first discovered in the parietal cortex of the awake, behaving monkey. That such cells should be located here is of great interest since lesions of the parietal cortex in man cause bizarre syndromes, of which the most prominent is disordered space perception. This disorder can take a variety of forms and include such things as spatial disorientation, spatial hemi-neglect and a disordered perception of the relationship between objects in visual space.

In experiments which use the awake, behaving monkey, the animal is taught to fixate a small spot of light flashed on a screen facing it for a limited period of time. The receptive field of the cell is plotted while the animal fixates the spot (e.g. point D in Figure 32.1). When the animal fixates, next, point C, the receptive field position of the cell on the screen should move as well, to the position marked C. In fact, one finds that one can only plot the receptive fields of such gaze-locked cells when the animal is fixating spots at certain positions on the screen. In the example given in Figure 32.1 the receptive field of the cell could only be plotted when the animal was fixating a point in the region D of the screen. In other words, the cell is only responsive when the animal is gazing in certain directions and not in others, even if the appropriate stimulus is present in the null-fixation positions.

When first discovered in the parietal cortex[4] these cells were found to have very large receptive fields, commonly spanning both hemi-fields. Moreover, the part of the parietal cortex in which they were located does not receive a direct input from V1 and V2, and does not have a direct re-entrant input to these areas either. Consequently, it must communicate with areas V1 and V2 indirectly, either through

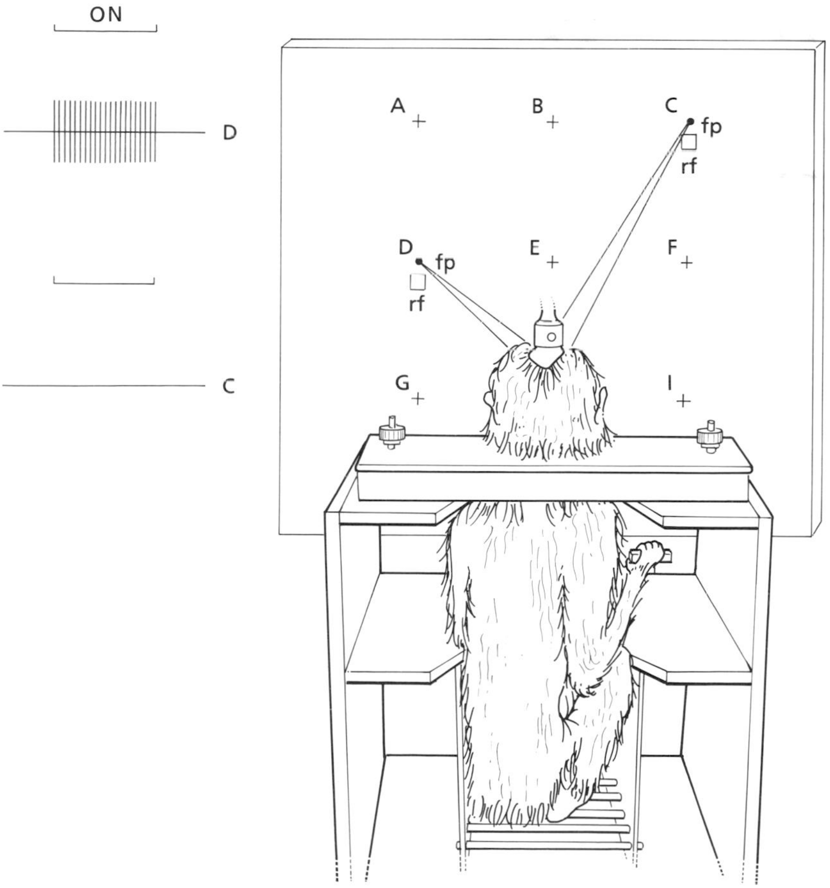

Fig. 32.1 The responses of a 'gaze-locked' V3 cell recorded from an awake, behaving, monkey. When the monkey fixates a point fp situated immediately under D, the cell gives a good response when stimulated with the line of the appropriate orientation in its receptive field (rf). When, however, the monkey fixates a point fp situated just underneath C, the cell is no longer responsive to the same stimulus flashed in the position which the receptive field should occupy. The horizontal bar indicates when the stimulus was in the receptive field. (Modified from Galletti, C. & Battaglini, P.P. (1989). *J. Neurosci.* **9**, 1112–1125.)

other cortical areas or through subcortical centres. But, more recently, gaze-locked cells have been discovered in areas which receive a direct input from V1 and V2 and send a re-entrant input to them, namely areas V3 and V3A.[5] The receptive fields of cells in both are considerably smaller than those of cells in the parietal cortex. The fact that at least some of the cells in the third visual complex are gaze-locked invests the area with a new role, that of locating the position of objects in visual space. This is particularly interesting because such gaze-locked cells are also orientation selective, and therefore involved in form vision as well.

No one knows the anatomical machinery which generates the gaze-locked cells, nor the dynamics of the connections between area V3 and areas V1 and V2. But the discovery of such cells in an area (V3) with a return input to V1 and V2 makes the suggestion that one role of such an input is to help locate the position of objects in space, by referral to the areas which have the most detailed topographic maps in them, even more plausible. Plausible but by no means proven, and indeed unable to give a complete description of the anatomy and functioning of the system for visual spatial localization. For it is also important to be able to determine the absolute position of objects in egocentric space. For example, if you see a telephone in front of you, the position of that telephone will remain the same when you move your head or eyes. The brain should be able to register the position of the telephone with respect to you when that happens. In fact, just such cells have been discovered in area V6 of monkey parietal cortex.[6] Using the awake, behaving, monkey once again, it has been found that some cells of V6 are gaze-locked while others have even more complex properties (Figure 32.2). A cell might, for example, be visually responsive to bars moving towards 11 o'clock and have a well-defined receptive field in the lower right contralateral quadrant when the animal is made to fixate a spot (spot 7 in Figure 32.2). But when the monkey is asked to fixate a spot in a new position (e.g. points 1−6 of Figure 32.2), one would either expect the receptive field position on the screen to change, or the cell not to respond at all if it is gaze-locked. One would certainly not expect the receptive field to occupy the same position on the screen that it did when the monkey was fixating position 7. In fact, that is precisely what happens, no matter where on the screen the monkey is made to fixate. In other words, the cell is able to detect the absolute position in egocentric space. It is worth mentioning that at least some of these cells are orientation selective. Once again, this underlines the fact that there is no strict dichotomy between the 'what' and 'where' systems in the cortex.

It is not clear whether area V6 has direct connections with V1 and it is certainly not known whether the connections are re-entrant. It does seem to have weak connections with V2. It is, however, known

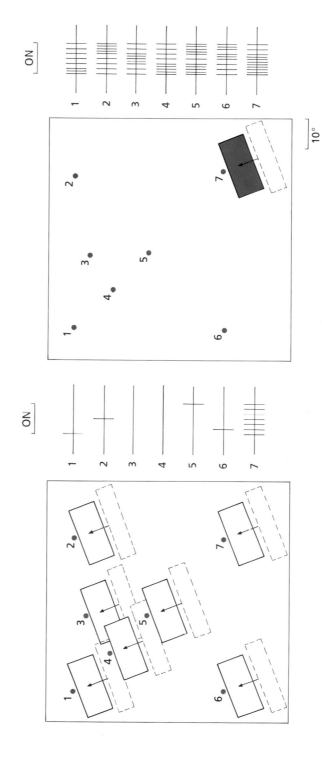

Fig. 32.2 The responses of a real position cell in area V6 of the awake, behaving, monkey. (Left) When the monkey fixated position 7, the cell responded well to an oriented bar moving upwards towards 11 o'clock. When the monkey fixated positions 1–6 and the positions which the receptive field should have occupied were stimulated in the same way, the cell was unresponsive. (Right) When the monkey fixated positions 1–6 and the receptive field at position 7 was stimulated, the cell gave a good response. ON indicates when the stimulus was in the receptive field. (Drawn by permission from the data of Galletti, Battaglini and Fattori, University of Bologna, Italy.)

to have reciprocal connections with V3 and V3A and the former of these has re-entrant connections with V1. It is therefore possible that the latter areas are intermediaries in this spatial location machinery.

Thus, the precise machinery used for locating objects in space is far from being known, but some of the anatomical pathways for doing so have been unravelled. This is an area rich in rewards for future studies and will almost certainly provide important insights into the role of the return connections into areas V1 and V2 from the specialized visual areas.

Dreams, hallucinations

We have already alluded to the visual normality of most dreams and hallucinations, to the fact that they are integrated, centrally generated, images which must somehow be re-entered into the cortex as if they were coming from the outside. If dreams and hallucinations depend upon re-entry into V1 or V2, the above assumption can be readily tested, at least in patients with a damaged V1 and V2, or so one would imagine. Unfortunately the task is not that simple and direct proof of this supposition is in fact lacking.

From an analytic point of view, hallucinations may well be preferable to dreams for the purposes of such an analysis, since humans are perfectly conscious of their hallucinations and can describe them in great detail while they are occurring. In order words, a hallucination can be reported immediately and not, as happens commonly with dreams, several hours or even days after. There are many features of hallucinations, of which the following are the most interesting in the context of this enquiry:

1 They can occur in subjects who have been completely blinded by retinal disease.

2 They can occur in subjects who are only partially blind.

3 In the partially blind the hallucination may occur in the blind field, or it may occur in the visually normal field.

4 There are reports of hallucinations in subjects with lesions in area V1.

5 There is at least one report of a somewhat abnormal hallucination following a tumour in a visual area well-removed from areas V1 and V2.[7]

These features are worth analyzing briefly.

That hallucinations occur in subjects who are completely blind tells us, of course, that these are internally generated images which are more or less normal and depend upon the integrity of at least some of the visual areas. Blindness can have many causes. If it is due to damage to the eye or the retina, there is no reason why the cortex should not operate normally, as it would in a dream situation. If the damage is more central and actually involves the visual pathways, the cortex could again operate with a greater or lesser degree of normality. The more interesting cases are ones in which the cortex itself is damaged. It is in fact extremely difficult to determine from the clinical literature whether hallucinations obtain in people with a completely damaged area V1. There is one report of a patient with a damaged striate cortex but who was subject to hallucinations.[8] Yet we have no knowledge of whether the damage was complete in this patient and, more significantly, whether area V2, another area which is the recipient of a diffuse, return input from the specialized visual areas, was also damaged.

If it can be shown that formed visual hallucinations are possible in the absence of areas V1 and V2, then the implications from the viewpoint of a cortical neurobiology of vision are very important. For such a demonstration would imply that integration and the maintenance of the topographic relationships that are such important features of hallucinations could be established without reference to areas with a highly detailed map of the retina, that the topographic precision is a feature of the activity of the specialized visual areas, even though all the physiology suggests that such areas have at best a very crude topographic map of the retina, relative to the ones in areas V1 and V2. If, on the other hand, it can be established that either area V1 or area V2 are necessary for formed hallucinations to occur at all, then another function of re-entry into these areas will have become clear. Either way, it goes to show that dreams and hallucinations, up until now the preserve of the psychoanalyst, are legitimate areas of enquiry for the neurobiologist, even though most would shrink with horror at the thought of investigating what appears so impenetrable a problem.

I do not suggest that the problems outlined above are in any sense minor problems. They are critical and fundamental to an understanding of how the visual cortex functions. Re-entry is as necessary to provide an adequate solution to preserving the local sign and to interpreting dreams and hallucinations as it is for the integration discussed in earlier chapters. The need for it is dictated by an awesome problem, that there is no ghost in the machine, no homunculus noting carefully what each part is doing. It is a problem that takes us to the very borders of consciousness.

References

1 Gross, C.G. (1972). Visual functions of infero-temporal cortex. In *Handbook of Sensory Physiology*, Vol. 7, Part 3, edited by R. Jung, Springer-Verlag, Berlin; Mountcastle, V.B., Motter, B.C., Steinmetz, M.A. & Duffy, C.J. (1984). Looking and seeing. The visual functions of the parietal lobe. In *Dynamic Aspects of Neocortical Function*, edited by G.M. Edelman, W.E. Gall & W.M. Cowan, pp. 159–194. Wiley, New York.

2 Mountcastle, V.B., Motter, B.C., Steinmetz, M.A. & Duffy, C.J. (1984). loc. cit. [1]; Andersen, R.A. (1987). Inferior parietal lobule function in spatial perception and visuomotor integration. In: *Handbook of Physiology*, 5(2), edited by V.B. Mountcastle, F. Plum & S.R. Geiger, pp. 483−518. American Physiological Society, Washington, D.C.

3 Perkel, D.J., Bullier, J, & Kennedy, H. (1986). Topography of the afferent connectivity of area 17 in the macaque monkey: A double-labelling study. *J. Comp. Neurol.* **253**, 374−402.

4 Andersen, R.A. & Mountcastle, V.B. (1983). The influence of the angle of gaze upon the excitability of the light-sensitive neurons of the posterior parietal cortex. *J. Neurosci.* **3**, 532−548.

5 Galletti, C. & Battaglini, P.P. (1989). Gaze-dependent visual neurons in area V3A of monkey prestriate cortex. *J. Neurosci.* **9**, 1112−1125.

6 Battaglini, P.P., Fattori, P., Galletti, C. & Zeki, S. (1990). The physiology of area V6 in the awake, behaving monkey. *J. Physiol. (Lond.)* **423**, 100P.

7 Mooney, A., Carey, P., Ryan, M. & Bofin, P. (1965). Parasagittal parieto-occipital meningioma with visual hallucinations. *Am. J. Ophthalmol.* **59**, 197−205.

8 Lance, J.W. (1976). Simple formed hallucinations confined to the area of a specific visual field defect. *Brain* **99**, 719−734.

Chapter 33: Consciousness and knowledge through vision

When and at what stage of the visual pathway do we become conscious of seeing an object and when are we conscious of the characteristics of that object? At what stage of the visual pathway does the nervous system acquire knowledge about the unchanging properties of objects and surfaces in terms of their reflectances for lights of different wavelengths and interpret these properties as colour? Are there conditions in which we can pay attention to a visual stimulus, see it and yet not be conscious of having seen anything at all? These are philosophical questions in a sense, but the more plausible answers to them and to many other questions like them do not come from philosophical speculation alone but rather from the hard science of experimentation.

There is a great deal that has been written about consciousness and about the so-called mind—brain problem. Is there such a duality? Does the brain cause the mind? Or is the brain the mind? One can discuss such questions endlessly, as philosophers like to, though without resolving the problem, a state of affairs that is probably much to the liking of philosophers. A sensible attitude is to be found in the work of John Searle.[1] He considers that mind and intentionality are certain properties of neural systems, including the cells that compose them, just as certain physical attributes are properties of the lattice structure of crystals. The micro-properties of the system invest it with certain macro-properties. There is an important question of causality here, for the micro-properties do not cause the macro-properties; rather, the macro-properties are features of objects which have molecules with given micro-properties. In the same way, neurophysiological events in the brain do not cause mental events, but rather mental events are a feature of neurophysiological systems with certain properties. We can therefore say that colour vision, for example, is a feature of a neural circuit with certain properties, that motion is a feature of other neural circuits with other properties and that consciousness is also a feature of many neural organizations with certain properties. To return to the example of physical objects, one might say that solidity (a macro-property) is a feature of a certain kind of lattice structure of crystals (micro-property), though one would not then go on to say that the molecules, which are components of that lattice, themselves possess solidity. In the same way, colour vision (a macro-property) is a feature of certain neural organizations (micro-property), though it does not follow from this that individual neurons within that organization are capable of seeing in colour. Similarly, motion vision is a feature of certain other neural organizations, though individual cells composing that neural organization cannot be said to perceive motion. Beyond that, consciousness is a feature of both types of neural organization and of many other, though not all, neural systems as well. There is no colour unless I see it; I cannot see it unless I am conscious. There is no conscious awareness unless certain neural organizations are intact and functioning normally, and it is a feature of such neural organizations that they possess consciousness. The important task then becomes that of determining what kind of neural organization (micro-properties) would have features which could plausibly be said to embody the minimum necessary for, say, colour vision, motion vision (macro-properties) and indeed for consciousness, since it is a feature of a system that can see and experience colour that it is conscious.

At first sight one might consider it more than a mouthful to tackle the problem of colour vision alone, without adding the extra and seemingly insuperable burden of consciousness. There is a little, though not much, that we know about the kind of micro-properties that would lead a neural system to have colour vision as one of its features. We could point to a fairly elaborate cortical machinery, the details of which are given in earlier chapters, and then add a catalogue of things which we know nothing about, which is enough to occupy several generations of neurobiologists yet to come. Given this vast lacuna, does one have to tangle with problems such as consciousness at all?

Unfortunately, yes. Colour vision is a system for acquiring knowledge about certain unchanging physical properties of objects, namely their reflectance for lights of different wavelengths. Knowledge cannot be acquired without consciousness. We can therefore now extend our description and say that consciousness and the acquisition of knowledge are features of certain neural organizations concerned with colour vision.

This may seem far-fetched had it not been for clinical evidence which strongly suggests that something of this kind must occur. It is perhaps relatively easy to account for a syndrome such as akinetopsia by supposing that the final integrative machinery required to collate information from large parts of the field of view is compromised, with the consequence that patients with lesions in V5 cannot acquire the knowledge about the coherent motion of objects in particular directions. Much more difficult to account for are conditions when patients can 'see' the directional motion but have no conscious awareness of having seen anything at all. Such a syndrome may seem surprising, but it is now a well-documented one in the literature.

Blindsight

For a long time it used to be thought that a lesion of the striate cortex causes total blindness in a corresponding part of the field of view, large (hemianopic) if the lesion is large and small (scotomatous) if it is small. One who had half-heartedly dissented from this view was Riddoch (see Chapter 10). He had observed that some of his scotomatous patients could detect motion in the field of view, although they appeared to be blind to everything else. This led Riddoch to consider movement as a special form of vision. He believed that it was a result of spared mechanisms within V1, though without detailing what these mechanisms might be. Studies in the early 1970s confirmed the observations of Riddoch. They also extended them by showing that not only are blind fields due to cortical lesions not necessarily completely blind but that cortically blind patients can 'see' a good deal more in their blind fields than even Riddoch had believed. The phenomenon is now aptly termed *blindsight*.[2] Note that blindsight results from a cortical lesion, not a lesion of the retina or of the optic tract, the consequence of which is total blindness. Moreover, not all patients with a cortical lesion have blind-sight; whether a patient has blindsight or not (i.e. whether he is completely blind or not) depends, according to a recent study,[3] on the amount of occipital cortex spared, a total lesion of occipital cortex leading to a total blindness. However that may be, the point of interest is that, although blindsight patients can 'see', at least in a rudimentary way, in their blind fields, they are nevertheless not consciously aware of having seen anything at all. Their vision is therefore useless; they cannot acquire any knowledge about the world through it.

How is this possible? A standard method of studying this phenomenon is to force the patient to guess whether something was occurring in his blind field. It turns out that blindsight patients are surprisingly good at reporting correctly what was in the blind part of their field of view, in other words that their 'guesses' are significantly correct. They can thus detect the presence and the direction of motion, can make simple pattern discriminations and can even detect and discriminate wavelengths.[4] One wonders how Henschen would have reacted to this discovery. In dismissing the evidence for a colour centre outside the striate cortex, he had said that if such a centre did exist, then a patient with a damaged striate cortex but with an intact fusiform gyrus 'would have to be absolutely blind and yet be able to see colours, which makes no sense'.[5] In fact, just this improbable scenario occurs in blindsight with the difference that although the patients can 'see', they are not consciously aware of having seen, just as in Eliot's poetry, 'When, under ether, the mind is conscious, but conscious of nothing'. Indeed, they are not aware of any visual experience at all, often protesting that they had seen nothing. It is as if the integrity of the primary visual cortex were necessary for the *conscious* experience of vision.

The question that arises here is whether the information contained in the visual stimuli presented in the 'blind' field, stimuli which the patients can discriminate but cannot 'see', reaches the cortex at all. The answer is that it is likely that it does. There is a direct, though sparse, route from the lateral geniculate nucleus (LGN) to the visual areas of the prestriate cortex.[6] The precise extent of the termination of this pathway in the prestriate cortex is not known, but it is known that V4 is definitely among the recipient areas, as is V5. If such a projection also exists in man, then we would have a means of accounting for the ability of patients with blindsight to discriminate the direction of motion and perhaps wavelengths. That such a pathway may exist in the human brain and that signals presented in the blind field actually reach the cortex is strongly suggested by evidence which shows that, when visual stimuli are presented to the blind field of blindsight subjects, evoked potentials can be picked up directly from the cortex.[3] There is reason to believe that subcortical structures such as the pulvinar or the superior colliculus are involved in such discriminations as blindsight patients are capable of because even hemispherectomised patients are capable of some residual vision. There is however every indication that the visual signals from the blind field reach the cortex and that, in spite of this, patients are not consciously aware of having seen anything at all.

It is not easy to account for this phenomenon in neurophysiological terms in anything other than a sketchy and somewhat speculative way, though there are enough facts to make at least part of the account plausible. If we concentrate on motion vision, the first important point to note is that not only is the integrity of the specialized visual areas (in this case V5) necessary for the conscious perception of this attribute of vision but also the integrity of the areas feeding them (areas V1 and V2). Thus, a patient with a lesion in area V5 is not able to see objects in motion, except to a very limited extent (akinetopsia). But a patient with a lesion in area V1 and with an intact V5 is also not consciously aware of having seen objects in motion, even if visual signals are reaching V5 directly, through the pathway linking the LGN to V5, and even if the patient can guess correctly, when forced, the direction of motion of the moving signals. In neither case is the patient able to acquire any knowledge about the visual world in motion. One can therefore postulate that the integrity of both V1 and V5 is necessary for the conscious perception of motion. It is possible that the integrity of V2 is also necessary. Lesions in V2 almost certainly cause blindness[7] but the phenomenon of blindsight has not been studied with hemianopias created by lesions restricted to V2.

The facts given above imply that, to gain a conscious awareness of having seen and therefore to acquire knowledge about the world through the sense of vision, signals must be processed in V1 first, before they are relayed to V5. Alternatively, whatever operations V5 may undertake, the results of that operation must be re-entered into V1. Of course, both processes may come into play, and both may be critical for the conscious awareness of having seen and hence of the acquisition of knowledge.

The more interesting of these two processes is the one relating to re-entry, partly because the solution to several other problems, including that of consciousness, is made easier by postulating that areas such as V1 and V2 are informed of the results of operations undertaken by areas such as V5, through the return projection from the latter to the former. Consider first the problem of conflict, referred to earlier. An example of this is the condition in which the direction-plus orientation-selective cells of V1 signal local directions of motion. These directions are in conflict with the global direction of motion of the same object signalled by the cells of V5. A necessary step in resolving the problem would be that the signals from V5 should be re-entered into V1. Or consider the problem of the illusory Kanizsa contours. The cells of V2 will respond as if there is a line there (i.e. they will respond to the illusory contour), but the cells of V1 (from which V2 receives its input) will not respond to the illusory contour and would therefore not signal the presence of a contour. Once again, this generates a conflict which can be best resolved by the two areas in collaboration.[8]

But re-entry by itself does not resolve these problems. For we become faced immediately with the binding problem, that of determining that the object which the cells of V5 signal as moving to the right and the cells of V1 as moving in all possible directions, is actually the same object in spite of the conflict. The problem could be solved by having the relevant cells in both areas fire more vigorously than other cells. But identification on the basis of strength of response creates problems. A cell specific for the vertical orientation might respond more vigorously to a telegraph pole, for example, because the part of the pole falling within its receptive field is brighter than the parts falling on the receptive fields of other cells selective for the same orientation. One way of solving this problem is to arrange that all the cells responding to the same object should fire in temporal synchrony. Note that the synchrony itself will demand re-entry, for otherwise we are faced with the same old problem of who it is that determines that the cells are firing synchronously (see Chapter 31).

Next, we face the problem of consciousness. At what stage of the visual pathway do we become consciously aware of the presence of a visual stimulus (assuming us to be attending to it). It makes little sense to say that the areas must report to a higher area, for here we visit yet again the old problem of who the higher area reports to and note again that there isn't a single cortical area to which all the specialized visual areas report exclusively. It makes sense to suppose that the conscious awareness of the visual stimulus is made possible not only by the simultaneous and correlated activity of cells in two areas (say V1 and V5 in the motion example given above) but also by the re-entrant links between them. As another example, the conscious awareness of the colour of a surface is a feature of the neurophysiological machinery that links V1 and V2 re-entrantly to V4. And the clinical evidence makes such a suggestion plausible because the integrity of both areas is critical to see, and be consciously aware of having seen, both colour and motion.

It is important to emphasize here that the return pathways from V4 and V5 back to V1 and V2 are not the only pathways from these two areas, although they would appear, if the present analysis is correct, to be critical for the conscious awareness of these attributes of vision. The other pathways emanating from V4 and V5 to healthy and intact parts of the brain may be functioning quite normally. In other words, only some of the operational connections (see Chapter 21) from V4 and V5 may be compromised. This is nicely illustrated in a recent report[9] of a dissociation between perceiving objects and grasping them. A young woman who suffered irreversible brain damage following carbon monoxide poisoning was found to suffer from a profound 'visual form agnosia'. She showed 'poor perception of shape or orientation, whether this information was conveyed by colour, intensity, stereopsis, motion, proximity, continuity or similarity'. In spite of this, she was able to reach for the visual objects very precisely. Indeed, 'she oriented her hand appropriately very early in the reaching movement and grasped the object normally'. This leads the authors to conclude that a person 'with brain damage may retain the ability to calibrate normal aiming and prehension movements with respect to the orientation and dimensions of objects, despite a profound inability to report, either verbally or manually, these same visual properties. This dissociation suggests that at some level in normal brains the visual processing underlying "conscious" perceptual judgements must operate separately from that underlying the "automatic" visuomotor guidance of skilled actions of the hand and limb'.[9] It would seem therefore that there are several operational connections emanating from an area, that some can be compromised without the others, and that some are actively involved in conscious perception, whereas others are not. It would seem, in brief, that we are getting relatively close to dissecting out the nervous pathways involved in conscious perception.

The synchronous firing of different cells

If the integrity of both reciprocally linked areas, say V1 and V4, is critical for the conscious perception of colour, what kind of mechanism can we postulate to occur between them? We might expect that cells in both areas responding to the same stimulus might respond synchronously, and inform each other of this fact through reciprocal connections.[10] How can this be achieved? It has been evident for some time that there is an oscillatory component to the responses of cells in the retina,[11] lateral geniculate nucleus[12] and the cortex. In other words, when one examines the electrical discharge of a cell in response to a stimulus in greater detail, one finds that the response occurs in bursts which repeat themselves at certain frequencies, usually in the 40–60 Hz range. These bursts constitute the 'rhythmical oscillations'.[13] Although oscillations are not a prerequisite for the temporal synchrony of responses, it is nevertheless a matter of considerable interest that, in the visual cortex, the oscillatory responses of two cells responding to the same visual stimulus can be in synchrony.[14] If two cells in area V1 with similar orientational preferences are situated sufficiently close to one another to have overlapping receptive fields, they tend to synchronize their responses when shown a continuous line which invades the receptive field of both. Much more interesting are examples in which two cells with similar orientational preferences are located sufficiently apart in the cortex for their receptive fields not to overlap. Here again, it has been reported that cells synchronize their responses only when they are activated by a single stimulus which has the same orientation in both receptive fields. Even more interestingly, it has been reported that cells with similar orientational preferences in different visual areas, and even in different hemispheres[15] (see Figure 29.1), can synchronize their responses to the same stimulus falling in their receptive fields, provided that the stimulus is continuous.[16] 'Thus, synchrony in the oscillatory responses of spatially separate neuron clusters signals coherence inherent in the stimuli that gives rise to the responses. Particularly good synchronization is achieved among clusters of cells activated by colinear and continuous contours. But cell clusters also synchronize their respective responses if they are activated by spatially distributed pattern elements that share particular features such as the same orientation, or the same direction of motion'.[16] It is very likely that the reciprocal connections between cells of different visual areas or between neighbouring cells having the same specificities in the same visual area allow the responses of cells, whether oscillatory or not, to be in temporal synchrony.

There is a great deal more that we would like to learn about this phenomenon of synchronous oscillation. We should like to know, for example, whether there is a synchronous response when cells in two very different areas code for different attributes of the same object, let us say the colour and motion of a stimulus. This seems a possibility, particularly since there is at least one report (the patient of Gelb; see Chapter 30) of experiencing difficulty in integrating colour with objects, as if there was an absence of synchronous firing. Equally, we should like to learn whether in conditions of conflict there is a synchronous firing of cells in V1 and V5. Even without all this information, however, some see in this synchronous oscillation of cells the key to the problem of consciousness.[17] This may indeed be so, or it may be merely a partial clue to the problem or a partial solution of it. At present we do not have enough information to judge whether the phenomenon of synchronous oscillation is not supplemented by other strategies. In spite of this, we know a sufficient amount about this phenomenon to look again at the problem of plasticity and maps in the visual cortex and, beyond, to the synthetic visual image in the brain.

Synchronous responses and group formation

Cells in the visual cortex show a great deal of variability in their more intimate anatomy, suggesting that they could have a selective advantage in the competition for space on other cells[13] (see Chapter 22). Moreover, all the evidence indicates that connections can be established well into adult life, since the brain appears to maintain its plasticity to a remarkable extent. It has therefore been proposed that, where the activities of groups of cells are highly correlated, as in the examples given above, the cells could form groups or repertoires.[18] It is obvious that in the examples which I have given here, re-entry would be a critical feature. Take the example of a fence gate, given earlier. Cells in V1 specific for the horizontal orientation and on whose receptive fields different segments of the gate fall would fire in synchrony. But cells of area V3, which are also selective for the horizontal orientation and which receive their inputs from the stimulated V1 cells, would also have to fire in synchrony. To signal that both the cells in V1 and those in V3 are responding in synchrony to the same visual stimulus, and thus constitute a group, a re-entrant input from V3 to V1 is needed.

It is evident from this that group formation may be a temporary phenomenon or it may be longer lasting. The responses of some cells would always be very highly correlated while the responses of others may or may not be so highly correlated, depending upon the stimulus. Thus, two cells in V1 separated by short distances of less than 1 mm, with overlapping receptive fields and the same orientational selectivity, are much more likely to be activated by the same stimulus and to respond in synchrony. It is not surprising to find therefore that such cells 'always synchronize their oscillatory responses when they show the same orientation preference'.[16] By contrast, cells which are more distant in the cortex 'tend to synchronize their oscillatory responses'.[16] Thus we should not think of these groups as permanent ones, but as dynamic ones, the existence of some being even a temporary affair. Our earlier review of plasticity showed that the brain is able to form new connections even late in life, which implies that some degree of plasticity persists for a long time. There is therefore no reason to suppose that cells form only permanent and immutable repertoires. Depending upon the strength of the stimuli and the strength of the correlated responses that link them, the groups may be temporary and their allegiances may shift from one state to the next even over short periods.

References

1 Searle, J. (1987). Minds and brains without programs. In *Mindwaves*, edited by C. Blakemore & S. Greenfield, pp. 209–233. Basil Blackwell, Oxford.

2 Pöppel, E., Held, R. & Frost, D. (1973). Residual visual function after brain wounds involving the central visual pathways in man. *Nature* **243**, 295–296; Weiskrantz, L. (1986). *Blindsight*. Clarendon Press, Oxford; Perenin, M.T. (1978). Visual function within the hemianopic field following early cerebral hemidecortication in man. II. Pattern discrimination. *Neuropsychologia* **16**, 696–707; Perenin, M.T. & Jeannerod, M. (1978). Visual function within the hemianopic field following early hemidecortication in man. I. Spatial localization. *Neuropsychologia* **16**, 1–13; Weiskrantz, L. (1990). The Ferrier Lecture: Outlooks for blindsight: explicit methodologies for implicit processes. *Proc. R. Soc. Lond.* B **239**, 247–278; Heywood, C.A., Cowey, A. & Newcombe, F. (1991). Chromatic discrimination in a cortically colour blind observer. *Eur. J. Neurosci.* **3**, 802–812.

3 Celesia, G.G., Bushnell, D., Toleikis, S.C. & Brigell, M.G. (1991). Cortical blindness and residual vision: is the 'second' visual system in humans capable of more than rudimentary visual perception? *Neurology* **41**, 862–869.

4 Cowey, A. & Stoerig, P. (1991). Reflections on blindsight. In *The Neuropsychology of Consciousness*, edited by D. Milner & M. Rugg, pp. 11–37. Academic Press, London.

5 Henschen, S.E. (1910). Zentrale Sehstörungen. In *Handbuch der Neurologie*, Vol. 2, edited by M. Lewandowsky, pp. 891–918. Springer-Verlag, Berlin.

6 Yukie, M. & Iwai, E. (1981). Direct projection from the dorsal lateral geniculate nucleus to the prestriate cortex in macaque monkeys. *J. Comp. Neurol.* **201**, 81–97; Fries, W. (1981). The projection from the lateral geniculate nucleus to the prestriate cortex of the macaque monkey. *Proc. R. Soc. Lond.* B **213**, 73–80.

7 Horton, J.C. & Hoyt, W.F. (1991). Quadrantic visual field defects. *Brain* **114**, 1703–1718.

8 Edelman, G.M. (1989). *The Remembered Present*. Basic Books, New York.

9 Goodale, M.A., Milner, A.D., Jakobson, L.S. & Carey, D.P. (1991). A neurological dissociation between perceiving objects and grasping them. *Nature* **349**, 154–156.

10 Milner, P.M. (1974). A model for visual shape recognition. *Psychol. Rev.* **81**, 521–535.

11 Einthoven, W. & Jolly, W.A. (1908). The form and magnitude of the electrical response of the eye to stimulation by light at various intensities, *Quart. J. Exp. Physiol.* **1**, 373–416; Fröhlich, F.W. (1914). Beiträge zur allgemeinen Physiologie der Sinnesorgane. *Z. Psychol. Physiol. Sinnesorg. II. Abt. Sinnesphysiol.* **48**, 28–164;

Laufer, M. & Verzeano, M. (1967). Periodic activity in the visual system of the cat. *Vision Res.* **7**, 215–229.

12 Podvigin, N.F., Jokeit, H., Pöppel, E. *et al.* (1992). Stimulus-dependent oscillatory activity in the lateral geniculate body of the cat. *Naturwiss.* **79**, 428–431.

13 Einthoven, W. & Jolly, W.A. loc. cit [11].

14 Eckhorn, R., Bauer, R., Jordan, W. *et al.* (1988). Coherent oscillations: a mechanism of feature linking in the visual cortex? Multiple electrode and correlation analysis in the cat. *Biol. Cybern.* **60**, 121–130; Gray, C.M., König, P., Engel, A.K. & Singer, W. (1989). Oscillatory responses in cat visual cortex exhibit inter-columnar synchronization which reflects global stimulus properties. *Nature* **338**, B, 334–337.

15 Engel, A.K., König, P., Kreiter, A.K., & Singer, W. (1991). Interhemispheric synchronization of oscillatory neuronal responses in cat visual cortex. *Science* **252**, 1177–1179.

16 Singer, W. (1990). Search for coherence: a basic principle of cortical self-organization. *Concepts Neurosci.* **1**, 1–26.

17 Crick, F. & Koch, C. (1991). Some reflections on visual awareness. *Cold Spring Harb. Symp. Quant. Biol.* **55**, 953–962.

18 Edelman, G. (1987). *Neural Darwinism: The Theory of Neuronal Group Selection.* Basic Books, New York.

Epilogue

The scientific study of the brain is still in its infancy. Anyone who has managed to get to these last few pages will, perhaps, have been impressed by how little we know about the workings of even the most intensively studied part of the cerebral cortex, the visual cortex. I hope that they will have been equally impressed by how much we have learnt, especially in the last few years, and by the extraordinary beauty and subtlety of the machinery in our brains that allows us to gain our knowledge of the external world through the sense of vision. That beauty and that subtlety are best expressed, not in the experimental details laid out in these pages, but in the efficiency with which the visual cortex of the most humble man as well as that of the most sophisticated observer undertakes its daily tasks. This efficiency is so great that many have not realized the magnitude of the problems which the human brain, through evolution, has had to overcome to be able to obtain its knowledge of the external world so effortlessly and so reliably.

The acquisition of knowledge about the external world through the sense of vision has been the main theme of this book and its starting point. It is with this that we can equally end the book, by summarizing the major features of the visual system.

1 The brain strives to acquire a knowledge about the permanent, invariant and unchanging properties of objects and surfaces in our visual world. But the acquisition of that knowledge is no easy matter because the visual world is in a continual state of change. Thus, the brain can only acquire knowledge about the invariant properties of objects and surfaces if it is able to discard the continually changing information reaching it from the visual environment.

2 Functional specialization is the strategy developed by the brain to acquire a knowledge about the permanent properties of objects, since the machinery required to gain a knowledge about certain unchanging properties, such as reflectance and therefore colour, is different from the machinery required to gain a knowledge about other unchanging properties, such as form or motion.

3 While it solves one set of problems, functional specialization raises a host of new ones which have to be solved to generate the integrated visual image in the brain. Chief among these is the integration of the results of the operations undertaken by the different specialized areas in order to generate the unified visual image in the brain. The problem of integration is therefore a consequence of functional specialization. It demands that cells in different visual areas, registering different attributes of the visual scene, interact with one another.

4   This raises the problem of what anatomical and functional strategy the visual cortex uses for this interaction. All the anatomical evidence suggests that:

(a) there is no single area to which all the specialized visual areas project, and

(b) where two areas specialized for different attributes of the visual scene send outputs onto a third area, each maintains its own territory in the third, suggesting that any convergence must be brought about by local circuits.

Physiologically, the problem of integration demands that the cells respond with some kind of temporal synchrony, but this raises the question of who monitors the synchrony, a problem which also imposes itself when one asks who it is who monitors or 'sees' the integrated visual image.

5   One way of solving this problem is for the cells in the specialized visual areas to communicate directly and reciprocally, not only with each other but also with cells in areas V1 and V2 from which they receive their inputs. Such a postulated mechanism receives powerful support from the anatomical evidence which shows that the specialized visual areas are indeed reciprocally connected with one another and send diffuse return outputs back to areas V1 and V2. These reciprocal connections form the anatomical basis for re-entry.

6   Through re-entry, cells could establish groups or repertoires made up of cells in several different visual areas, all of which fire in temporal synchrony. Such groups will become stable if the chances of their responding in synchrony is high and unstable if the chances are low, with many gradations in between the two extremes. There is a sufficient degree of plasticity in the brain, even in the adult brain, to allow this to occur. It follows from this that some groups may be transient while others are more stable, and that one set of cells may take part in one group at one time and in another group at another time.

7   It follows from this, too, that the synthesis of the visual image in the brain depends not only on the simultaneous activity of cells in the different specialized visual areas, but also on the temporal synchrony of their responses. Moreover, this synchronous activity must also include areas such as V1 and V2 with which the specialized visual areas are reciprocally connected. From which it follows that the visual percept does not reside in any given visual area, even if that area is critical for certain features of that visual image. Rather it is the result of on-going activity in several re-entrantly connected visual areas.

8   A review of the experimental and clinical evidence suggests that, for the conscious perception of a visual stimulus and thus for the acquisition of knowledge about the visual world, the simultaneous activity of many visual areas is necessary and that a stimulus will not reach visual awareness unless this condition is satisfied, even if signals reach the specialized visual areas indirectly, by by-passing area V1. This is what is observed in blindsight, a condition in which subjects have no conscious awareness of the stimuli presented to their 'blind' fields and consequently have no knowledge of these stimuli, even if they can discriminate them. One can postulate therefore that blindsight is the consequence of a condition in which there is no synchronous firing of cells in the specialized visual areas with their counterparts in area V1, because the latter is damaged. More simply, the groups or repertoires necessary for the conscious perception of vision cannot be formed.

Naturally the above is a very general account and it will take many years of work to settle the many details that are involved. Naturally, too, there may be major flaws in the arguments presented, which future scientific results will uncover. There is nevertheless a certain coherence to the arguments and a strong link between them. Above all, there is the splendour of knowing that the problem of vision is a problem of knowledge and of consciousness, that one can dissect the cerebral pathways and functions which the brain uses to acquire its knowledge of the external world. More than that, there is the splendour of knowing that, in studying the complex pathways of the visual cortex and its normal and abnormal functioning, one is contributing not only to an understanding of the processes of vision but also to the much grander and more profound problems of knowledge and of consciousness, perennial problems that are at the heart of philosophical enquiry and at the heart of man's quest to know himself. Truly the study of the visual cortex gives one a vision of the brain.

Index